CONTENTS

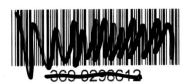

PRECIS

AN UPDATE IN OBSTETRICS AND GYNECOLOGY

Obstetrics

Fourth Edition

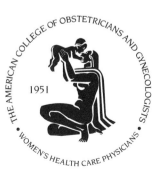

THE AMERICAN COLLEGE OF OBSTETRICIANS AND GYNECOLOGISTS · WOMEN'S HEALTH CARE PHYSICIANS · 1951

Library of Congress Cataloging-in-Publication Data

Precis : an update in obstetrics and gynecology. Obstetrics. -- 4th ed.
    p. ; cm.
Includes bibliographical references and index.
ISBN 978-1-934946-84-8 (alk. paper)
    1. Obstetrics--Outlines, syllabi, etc. I. American College of Obstetricians and Gynecologists. II. Title: Obstetrics.
    [DNLM: 1. Pregnancy. 2. Delivery, Obstetric. 3. Postpartum Period. 4. Pregnancy Complications. 5. Prenatal Care. 6. Prenatal Diagnosis. WQ 200 P917 2010]
RG533.P74 2010
618.2--dc22
    2009042547

The American College of Obstetricians and Gynecologists
409 12th Street, SW
PO Box 96920
Washington, DC 20090-6920
www.acog.org

12345/43210

CONTRIBUTORS

EDITORIAL TASK FORCE

Gary D. V. Hankins, MD, Chair

Nancy C. Chescheir, MD

Charles J. Lockwood, MD

Brian M. Mercer, MD

Thomas C. Peng, MD

Susan M. Ramin, MD

Andrew J. Satin, MD

ADVISORY COMMITTEE

Donald R. Coustan, MD, Chair

Jonathan Berek, MD

Roger P. Smith, MD

AUTHORS

William H. Barth Jr, MD

Michael A. Belfort, MD, PhD

Clarissa Bonnano, MD

Radek Bukowski, MD, PhD

Anne E. Burke, MD, MPH

Brian M. Casey, MD

Patrick M. Catalano, MD

Steven L. Clark, MD

Maged Costantine, MD

Donald R. Coustan, MD

Mary E. D'Alton, MD

Donna S. Dizon-Townson, MD

Christopher S. Ennen, MD

Harold E. Fox, MD

Larry C. Gilstrap III, MD

Jay P. Goldsmith, MD

William A. Grobman, MD, MBA

Wendy F. Hansen, MD

Cara C. Heuser, MD

David C. Jones, MD

Mark B. Landon, MD

George A. Little, MD

Charles J. Lockwood, MD

Judette M. Louis, MD, MPH

George A. Macones, MD

Gilbert I. Martin, MD

Brian M. Mercer, MD

Kenneth J. Moise Jr, MD

Manju Monga, MD

Tristi W. Muir, MD

Roger B. Newman, MD

Thomas E. Nolan, MD

Luis D. Pacheco, MD

Teri Pearlstein, MD

Thomas C. Peng, MD

J. Gerald Quirk, MD, PhD

Susan M. Ramin, MD

George Saade, MD

Andrew J. Satin, MD

Katherine M. Sharkey, MD, PhD

David E. Soper, MD

Catherine Y. Spong, MD

Zachary N. Stowe, MD

Rakesh B. Vadhera, MD

Katharine D. Wenstrom, MD

STAFF

Sterling B. Williams, MD, MS
Vice President for Education

Thomas Dineen
Director of Publications

Deirdre Allen, MPS
Editorial Director

Nikoleta Dineen, MA
Senior Editor

Mark D. Grazette
Senior Graphic Designer

PREFACE

Education is a lifelong process. In no field is this process more important than in medicine. As scientific advances unfold, new techniques and technologies emerge, knowledge expands, and the art and science of medicine undergo dynamic change. Progress in medicine is ongoing, and so too must be the continuing medical education of those who practice it.

Precis: An Update in Obstetrics and Gynecology is intended to meet the continuing education needs of obstetricians and gynecologists. It is a broad, yet concise, overview of information relevant to the specialty. As in earlier editions, the emphasis is on innovations in clinical practice, presented within the context of traditional approaches that retain their applicability to patient care.

Precis is an educational resource to be used in preparation for the cognitive assessment of clinical knowledge, regardless of the form of the assessment—formal or informal, structured or independent. It is one of the recognized vehicles useful in preparing for certification and accreditation processes, and it is designed to complement those evaluations while serving as a general review of the field.

Each year, one volume of this five-volume set is revised. This process provides continual updates that are critical to the practice of obstetrics and gynecology, and it echoes the dynamic nature of the field. The focus is on new and emerging techniques, presented from a balanced perspective of clinical value and cost-effectiveness in practice. Hence, discussion of traditional medical practice is limited. The information has been organized to unify coverage of topics into a single volume so that each volume can stand on its own merit.

This fourth edition of *Precis: Obstetrics* reflects current thinking on optimal practice. The information is intended to be a useful tool to assist practicing obstetrician–gynecologists in maintaining current knowledge in a rapidly changing field and to prepare them better for the role of women's health care physicians.

Some information from the previous edition continues to be of value and, thus, has been retained and woven into the new structure. The efforts of authors contributing to previous editions, as well as the work of those authors providing new material, must be recognized with gratitude. Collectively, they represent the expertise of the specialty. With such a breadth of representation, differences of opinion are inevitable and have been respected.

Other *Precis* volumes are *Primary and Preventive Care,* Fourth Edition; *Oncology,* Third Edition; *Gynecology,* Third Edition; and *Reproductive Endocrinology,* Third Edition. Each is an educational tool for review, reference, and evaluation. *Precis* establishes a broad scientific basis for the delivery of quality health care for women. Rather than being a statement of the American College of Obstetricians and Gynecologists (the College) policy, *Precis* serves as an intellectual approach to education. An effort has been made, however, to achieve consistency within *Precis* and with other College recommendations. Variations in patient care, based on individual needs and resources, are encouraged as an integral part of the practice of medicine.

—THE EDITORS

PRECIS

AN UPDATE IN OBSTETRICS AND GYNECOLOGY

Obstetrics

Fourth Edition

INTRODUCTION

Precis: Obstetrics strives to live up to its name by being concise and emphasizing areas of utmost importance to clinical practice. An area of particular importance is obesity. Because obesity is now pandemic, a completely new section, which includes the new Institute of Medicine guidelines and information on sleep apnea and bariatric surgery, has been added. Another new section is devoted to substance abuse, specifically, the latest information on maternal and fetal effects of illegal drugs, alcohol, and tobacco use. The topic of pain management in pregnancy was refocused from the use of obstetric analgesia and anesthesia to a new section on the management of chronic pain and headache. Other important advances, such as novel, but not yet standardized, screening and treatment modalities for intrauterine growth restriction and the new classification system for intrapartum fetal heart rate monitoring, and management are discussed within the contexts of their own sections. Also discussed is appropriate patient education, which is key to optimal patient care. Specific areas calling for patient counseling are identified throughout. Web sites that may be useful to patients and obstetrician–gynecologists seeking additional information are provided in Appendix A.

The members of the Editorial Task Force and Advisory Committee as well as other selected individuals have reviewed the content to ensure that the information is accurate, complete, and current. During this review, an effort was made to ensure consistency with the guidelines of the American College of Obstetricians and Gynecologists as well as to identify emerging areas. As advances unfold, physicians are urged to consult current recommendations.

—GARY D.V. HANKINS, MD
Chair, Editorial Task Force

PATIENT SAFETY

Andrew J. Satin, Christopher S. Ennen, and Harold E. Fox

The American College of Obstetricians and Gynecologists (the College) is committed to improving quality and safety in women's health care. The Institute of Medicine estimates that medical errors may account for up to 98,000 deaths each year in the United States (1). Although, there is a paucity of data specifically addressing medical errors in obstetrics, it stands to reason that with 4 million hospitalizations related to childbirth each year, strategies to reduce errors may benefit women and their children. Reasons for error may include human fallibility, medical complexity, system deficiencies, and defensive barriers. The College has codified a set of objectives to be adopted by clinicians to promote safety (Box 1). In an effort to promote safety initiatives the American Board of Obstetrics and Gynecology and the College have developed modules on patient safety as part of their maintenance of certification program.

Obstetricians should develop and adopt safe practices that reduce the likelihood of system failures that can cause adverse occurrences. Leadership is essential in facilitating an effective patient safety program. Optimizing communication and collaboration among members of the health care team are important in promoting safety. Most medical errors are associated with medications. Strategies to reduce medication errors include computerized order entry programs, the use of legible handwriting, and avoidance of nonstandard abbreviations. Patients should be encouraged to ask questions regarding their health care because those patients who are involved with their own health care have better outcomes than those who are not.

Box 1

Objectives to Promote Safety

- Develop a commitment to encourage a culture of patient safety
- Implement safe medication practices
- Reduce the likelihood of surgical errors
- Improve communication
- Identify and resolve system problems
- Establish a partnership with patients to improve safety
- Make safety a priority

Patient safety in obstetrics and gynecology. ACOG Committee Opinion No. 286. American College of Obstetricians and Gynecologists. Obstet Gynecol 2003;102:883–5.

Strategies to reduce errors and subsequently adverse outcomes have focused on teamwork and individual training; development of protocols, guidelines, and checklists; the use of information technology; and resident education. Information in this section provides an overview of the current trends and strategies in improving patient safety. It is not the authors' intention to highlight one system over another, draw conclusions, or issue recommendations for its use.

Teamwork Training

The Joint Commission, the College, and the Institute of Medicine all recognize teamwork as a critical element of patient safety (1–3). In a labor and delivery setting, the patient and her baby are cared for by obstetricians, nurses, anesthesia and pediatric providers, and support staff. Teamwork and communication failures account for 70% of sentinel events in obstetrics (1).

Investigators have evaluated the effect of teamwork training on maternal and fetal outcomes as well as the difference in team performance before and after teamwork training. Thus far, there is limited evidence that teamwork training may improve outcomes. The U.S. Department of Defense conducted a randomized study to evaluate the effect of teamwork training on adverse maternal and neonatal outcomes (4). The study was performed at 15 military and civilian hospitals with a combined annual delivery rate of more than 53,000. The institutions were randomly divided into two groups, balancing military and civilian institutions. The study group was randomly assigned to receive formal teamwork training while the other group served as a control. The MedTeams® teamwork training program was originally adapted from aviation crew resource management principles for emergency department personnel. The core concepts of crew resource management are leadership, mutual performance monitoring, backup behavior, adaptability, and team orientation (5). The curriculum was further adapted by the investigators for instruction of labor and delivery personnel. A total of 1,307 labor and delivery personnel were trained. Outcomes were recorded before and 5 months after teamwork training.

The researchers developed a composite maternal and neonatal outcome measure, called the Adverse Outcome Index, defined as the number of patients with one or more adverse outcomes, divided by the total number of deliveries (6). Adverse maternal outcomes recorded included maternal death, uterine rupture, unplanned admission to an intensive care unit, unplanned return to the operating room, blood transfusion, and third-degree or fourth-degree vaginal laceration. Neonatal outcomes recorded were intrapartum death of a fetus weighing at least 500 g at 24 or more weeks of gestation, death within 7 days of birth of an infant with birth weight of at least 2,500 g, neonatal birth trauma, unplanned admission of a term infant to the intensive care nursery, and 5-minute Apgar score of less than 7 in a term infant. In an attempt to evaluate teamwork, 11 process measures were used to evaluate length of stay and delays in action where multiple care providers were involved.

Approximately 14,000 deliveries occurred in each group during the study period. Outcomes of approximately 4,000 deliveries in each group were used for baseline comparisons and 10,000 for postintervention evaluation. There were no differences in baseline characteristics or outcomes between the groups. There was no statistically significant difference between the group that received formal teamwork training in the individual maternal and neonatal adverse outcomes or in the Adverse Outcome Index. Of the 11 process measures evaluated, the only significant difference between the groups was a reduction in the time from decision to proceed with immediate cesarean delivery and the time of incision from 33 minutes to 21 minutes. The authors attributed this finding to be related to the formation of contingency teams at the hospitals that received teamwork training. A contingency team on labor and delivery would typically consist of the obstetric and anesthesia attending physicians, obstetric chief resident, labor nurse, and surgical scrub nurse. The authors state that the formation of such teams is a relatively easy intervention and that the reduction in decision-to-incision time of 10 minutes may have clinical significance.

The lead civilian hospital in the described study worked with the U.S. Department of Defense in the creation of the teamwork-training curriculum, but its outcome data were not included in the analysis. Based on the study's findings, the hospital further modified the curriculum for their institution and implemented the training for all labor and delivery staff. The Adverse Outcome Index then was compared for the 3 years before the program implementation with the 4 years after implementation (7). A decrease in the Adverse Outcome Index from 5.9–4.6% was found, representing 300 fewer women experiencing an adverse event. Also reported was a decrease in high-severity malpractice claims from 13 cases to 5 cases. The authors theorize that the improvement in outcomes they found (versus the lack of difference in the original multicenter study results) may have been because of the length of follow up, the creation of other protocols not related to teamwork training, better integration of the teamwork training into practice, or a combination of these changes.

Critics of MedTeams® training cite its reliance on the concepts of crew resource management at the exclusion of other team training science. This led the U.S. Department of Defense to commission development of a more inclusive teamwork-training program. TeamSTEPPS™ (Team Strategies and Tools to Enhance Performance and Patient Safety) was thus created and has been implemented at many military hospitals (8). The Agency for Healthcare Research and Quality is now implementing TeamSTEPPS™ training nationwide. There are no trials on the impact of TeamSTEPPS™ training in reducing adverse obstetric outcomes.

Another large academic hospital instituted a comprehensive safety strategy including creation of standardized protocols, teamwork training, and training in the interpretation of fetal heart rate monitoring (9). The authors reported a significant decrease in the Adverse Outcome Index and a significant improvement in the safety climate as determined by provider survey. There were no significant improvements in the individual outcomes that comprise the Adverse Outcome Index other than a decrease in the rate of episiotomies performed. The rate of cesarean deliveries performed increased over the study period. A limitation of the study is that there was no means to determine which of the several safety interventions performed may have led to the modest improvement in outcomes.

To assess the benefit of teamwork training, a group in the United Kingdom evaluated team performance in a standardized eclampsia drill (10). All teams received training in eclampsia management, but one half of the teams was randomized to also receive formal training in teamwork theory. The groups also were randomized to receive training at their local hospital or at a regional simulation center. Teamwork was improved in all groups after the training, but there was no additional benefit found from the teamwork training. The authors suggested that the apparent lack of benefit of formal teamwork training may have been because the training used was inadequate. It also is possible that simply rehearsing the scenario was sufficient because of its relatively straightforward nature. In contrast, the introduction of annual team training for the management of umbilical cord prolapse resulted in a significant reduction in diagnosis-to-delivery interval from 25 minutes to 14 minutes (11). Critical to improving patient safety will be further study into the most effective combination of didactic, teamwork, and simulation training in reducing adverse events (12).

Simulation and Drills

Simulation in obstetrics has become a common method of training individuals and teams. Obstetricians can simulate procedures to improve technical skills. Emergency situations that arise infrequently can be recreated, allowing teams to practice required interventions in a safe environment. Simulation can identify opportunities for improvement. Another reason for the increasing interest in simulation is the desire to augment the reduction in clinical experience among obstetric–gynecologic residents.

One group investigated the benefit of a structured training course on neonatal outcomes (13). The course was a full day, with didactic training in electronic fetal monitoring in the morning, followed by an afternoon session of emergency drills to review the management of shoulder dystocia, postpartum hemorrhage, eclampsia, twins, breech presentation, and adult and neonatal resuscitation. The authors retrospectively reviewed neonatal outcomes before and after implementation of the training sessions and found a significant reduction in 5-minute Apgar scores of less than 7 and hypoxic–ischemic encephalopathy. They did not report on any maternal outcomes.

In a study performed in the United Kingdom, the authors compared team performance in an eclampsia drill before and after training (10). Groups were randomly assigned to training at their local hospital or in a regional simulation center. After training, teams completed more basic tasks and these tasks were completed more quickly. However, there was no difference between the teams trained locally or at a simulation center.

Shoulder dystocia is an obstetric emergency with the potential for serious neonatal and maternal adverse outcomes and usually is unpredictable and not preventable. Improper management of this emergency may worsen neonatal outcomes, highlighting the need for adequate training of delivery providers. The infrequent nature and special skills needed combine to make shoulder dystocia an obstetric emergency ideally suited for simulation.

Several studies have been able to identify deficiencies and demonstrate improvement in management and documentation of a simulated shoulder dystocia event after training for residents and attending physicians (14–16). Both low-fidelity and high-fidelity simulation of shoulder dystocia improve performance (17). Observations of many providers performing the same shoulder dystocia (or other emergency event) simulation can elucidate the most common mistakes, allowing for development of appropriate and efficient curriculum for future training (18, 19).

In a retrospective study, one group compared shoulder dystocia management and neonatal outcomes between 4-year periods before and after institution of a training program (20). Training consisted of didactic and practical training on risk factors, diagnosis, and proper management of shoulder dystocia. They found similar rates of shoulder dystocia (approximately 2%) during both periods, but a significant reduction in neonatal brachial plexus injury at birth from 9.3% to 2.3%.

They also reported a significant improvement in use of appropriate management techniques (McRoberts position, suprapubic pressure, internal rotation maneuvers, and the delivery of the posterior arm) and a significant decrease in inappropriate techniques (no recognized maneuvers performed, excessive traction, and fundal pressure). If training can help reduce adverse outcomes, it is important to know how frequently it must be performed. In a study of the management of shoulder dystocia using simulation, the authors sought to determine skill retention after training (21). Participants, including junior and senior physicians and midwives, performed a simulated delivery with a shoulder dystocia. The simulation ended when the participant delivered the posterior arm, elected to stop, or 5 minutes had elapsed. They were evaluated on whether delivery was successful, the head-to-body delivery interval, performance of appropriate actions, force applied, and communication. The participants did the simulation once before the training session and then 3 weeks, 6 months, and 12 months after training. The training session included a 40-minute practical workshop on shoulder dystocia management. The authors found that 49% of participants were able to deliver the fetus before training, and 82%, 84%, and 85% of participants were able to achieve delivery at the 3 weeks, 6 months, and 12 months of follow up, respectively. They offered additional training to the 18% of participants who were unable to deliver 3 weeks after the initial training and 79% of these individuals were able to achieve delivery at 12 months. The authors concluded that annual training is adequate for providers demonstrating competency after initial training. However, those that were unsuccessful 3 weeks after training should have remediation and be monitored more closely to ensure retention of skills. This study also highlights the fact that providers do not all learn in the same way or at the same rate and that, to achieve maximal benefit, some individualization of simulation training is required.

It is likely that lack of training in operative vaginal delivery contributes to an increase in cesarean deliveries. Teaching the proper use of obstetric forceps in the clinical setting is difficult because they are primarily used in urgent or emergency situations. The key maneuvers of blade placement by the learner are done in the vagina and, thus, the teacher is blind to whether placement is correct until it is complete. To overcome this obstacle, investigators created a forceps simulation system using blades that were implanted with position sensors, allowing real-time and postsimulation evaluation of blade trajectory during placement (22, 23). Based on objective assessment of blade trajectory and repeatability of insertion technique, they found that senior obstetricians performed forceps placements in an "excellent," "very good," or "good" manner 92% of the time, compared with only 38% of the time for junior obstetricians. Also they found that with more training, less experienced obstetricians' skills progressed, showing less hesitation and better following of a trajectory modeled by an expert operator (24). One study evaluated the effect of training in operative vaginal deliveries on maternal and neonatal outcomes (25). The training was an educational program that included training sessions with a senior staff member using lectures, videos, and a "doll and pelvis" model. The training emphasized techniques to minimize maternal and neonatal injury and to reduce the number of failed instrumental deliveries. The authors compared outcomes for all operative vaginal deliveries in the 4 months after initiation of the training program to a historical control group. They found no statistically significant difference in the incidence of failed forceps or vacuum delivery or maternal anal sphincter injury. There was a significant reduction in neonatal admissions to a special care nursery and in neonatal scalp and facial injuries. The authors theorized that the improvement in neonatal outcome may have been largely because of better understanding of the correct technique of vacuum delivery, given that this was the more commonly used method.

In 2007 the College convened the Task Force on Simulation for Obstetric and Gynecologic Residents that proposed a list of obstetric scenarios that may be amenable to simulation training, such as operative vaginal delivery, third-degree and fourth-degree laceration repair, breech vaginal delivery, shoulder dystocia, eclampsia, postpartum hemorrhage, amniocentesis, and cerclage. Eclampsia simulation has been performed and has offered insights into individual, team, and system errors that can be improved. Realism can be added to the simulation of eclampsia and hemorrhage with additions of actors and high fidelity trainers to commonly used models. The use of a high-fidelity simulator has been demonstrated to improve performance of trainees with amniocentesis (26). Vaginal breech delivery, like shoulder dystocia, is an event well suited for simulation in that it is a rare but critical occurrence. Simulation has been shown to improve the less experienced obstetrician's performance with vaginal breech deliveries (27). Although these simulations have been shown to improve performance in simulated scenarios, there is little but evolving evidence for improvement in maternal or neonatal outcomes.

Protocols, Guidelines, and Checklists

Based on experiences in military and commercial aviation it has been suggested that uniform medical practice could improve safety. A large hospital corporation published data on the effects of implementing a checklist-based system for oxytocin use (28). A "preoxytocin use" checklist required adequate documentation of a patient's eligibility for labor (estimated fetal weight, fetal presenta-

tion, clinical pelvimetry, and fetal assessment). An "oxytocin in-use" checklist was completed every 30 minutes while the patient received the medication. This checklist included fetal assessment by heart rate pattern and uterine assessment by pattern and strength of contractions (either by palpation or with an intrauterine pressure catheter). If each item on the checklist could not be completed, the administration of oxytocin was reduced or stopped. The infusion could be restarted if both the "preoxytocin use" and "oxytocin in-use" checklists were completed.

To evaluate the effect of these checklists, they were implemented at one hospital, and the authors reviewed the last 100 patients who received oxytocin before its implementation and the first 100 patients who received oxytocin using the checklist-based protocol. The groups were similar at baseline and the authors found no significant difference in total duration of oxytocin infusion, cesarean delivery rate, or specific neonatal outcomes (intensive care nursery admission, respiratory distress, and sepsis—suspected or confirmed). There was a clinically small, but statistically significant reduction in maximum oxytocin infusion rate from 13.8 mU/min to 11.4 mU/min and the number of neonates with any adverse outcome decreased from 31 to 18. In the subsequent year, they implemented the checklist across the entire hospital system and reported a decrease in cesarean rate from 23.6% to 21%. Weaknesses of the study include small numbers and lack of control for potentially confounding variables.

Based on the perceived success of the oxytocin checklists, the same hospital corporation instituted similar checklists for the use of misoprostol and magnesium sulfate as well as for the performance of operative vaginal delivery and the management of shoulder dystocia and abnormal fetal heart rate monitoring results (29). The investigators reported a decrease in litigation in addition to the 1-year reduction in cesarean delivery rate. No further data were provided about maternal or neonatal outcome.

In order to reduce the frequency of third-degree and fourth-degree lacerations associated with operative vaginal delivery, one institution instituted a training program and provided practice guidelines for this procedure (30). Recommendations included using a vacuum instead of forceps when possible, converting occiput posterior to occiput anterior before delivery, and performing a mediolateral episiotomy if an episiotomy was necessary. The guidelines were promulgated using methods such as departmental conferences and distribution of reading materials and instructional posters. The authors of the study reviewed outcomes in the 9 months before the intervention began and for the first 9 months afterwards. They found a significant reduction in the frequency of third-degree and fourth-degree lacerations after the training was initiated (from 41% to 26% of 115 and 100 operative vaginal deliveries, respectively). Of these patients, the incidence of fourth-degree lacerations decreased from 30% to 19%. There was a significant increase in the use of vacuum extraction over the use of forceps delivery.

After the deaths of two patients from hemorrhage, a hospital implemented a comprehensive program to improve patient safety (31). They created obstetric rapid response teams to respond to obstetric emergencies. Quarterly drills were performed for various emergencies. Clinical guidelines and pathways were created. The in-house obstetrician was relieved of caring for gynecologic emergencies and was expected to monitor all patients in labor and delivery, regardless of who their primary physician was. If there were disagreements about the care of patients, all members of the labor and delivery team were empowered to consult with a senior department member, who would immediately discuss the issue with the attending physician. Training sessions discussing the new guidelines as well as the recognition and management of severe obstetric hemorrhage were regularly performed. Finally, the hospital's trauma team was made available to consult on all cases of severe obstetric hemorrhage.

To compare the effect of this intervention, the team analyzed outcomes during the year before and the 4 years after its implementation. There was a significant increase in cesarean delivery rate, repeat cesarean delivery, and major obstetric hemorrhage. There was no difference in the rate of cesarean hysterectomy. Patient characteristics were similar between the two periods, as were the occurrence of placenta accreta and the severity of hemorrhage. Despite the increase in major obstetric hemorrhage cases, they found improved outcomes and fewer maternal deaths after implementing systemic approaches to improve patient safety.

Also in an effort to improve on the management of obstetric hemorrhage, one hospital evaluated all their cases of massive postpartum hemorrhage (defined as blood loss of greater than 1,000 mL) over a 6-month period (32). They evaluated each case to identify deviation from hospital guidelines. The guidelines were then revised and the staff was trained and practice drills were implemented. They then reviewed cases of hemorrhage during a subsequent 6-month period and compared outcomes to the original 6 months. They found deviation from guidelines of 37% in the first period versus none in the second period. They found a significant decrease in the incidence of massive postpartum hemorrhage from 1.7% to 0.45%. Also there were fewer blood transfusions and admissions to higher level care units.

Information Technology

A systematic review of 257 studies reviewed evidence on the effect of health information technology on quality, efficiency, and cost of care. Approximately 25% of studies emanated from four academic institutions. Three major benefits on quality were demonstrated: 1) adherence to guideline-based care, 2) enhanced surveillance and monitoring, and 3) decreased medication errors (33). Computer software may aid obstetricians by reminding them of milestones associated with antepartum care and tracking laboratory and imaging studies.

Resident Education and Work Hours

Arguably the biggest step to ensure patient safety occurred over a decade ago when obstetricians adopted 24-hour and 7-day in-house supervision of their residents. In 2003, the Accreditation Council for Graduate Medical Education established the 80-hour workweek for all residency programs. More recently, the Institute of Medicine released a report recommending adjustments to the Accreditation Council for Graduate Medical Education guidelines, including reductions in maximum shift length without time for sleep and number of consecutive night shifts (34).

These guidelines are based on research into sleep and human performance but were instituted without investigation into whether they would reduce adverse events. In addition, there was concern from medical educators about the impact on resident education. Two years after initiation of reduced work hours in New York, a survey of residents and attending physicians found significant improvement in resident lifestyle without a decrease in surgical case load (35). Importantly, there was no perceived improvement in quality of care.

In a survey of residents working before and after the initiation of the 80-hour work week responders reported increased satisfaction with personal lives but found no change in job satisfaction or the Council on Resident Education in Obstetrics and Gynecology scores (36). There was a statistically significant decrease in weekly work hours reported, from 89 hours to 83 hours. The residents, however, did not report an increased amount of sleep at home.

Educators surveyed regarding the impact of the reduction in resident work hours reported they felt that residents' interest in teaching, time available to teach, surgical volume and overall education were worse (37). However, resident morale was thought to be improved. The respondents did feel that reduced hours would have a positive effect on medical student recruitment into obstetrics and gynecology. Residents and interns found that residents spent less time teaching with reduced work hours.

The mandated reduction in obstetric resident work hours has not been found to reduce adverse obstetric outcomes. In one study in a metropolitan hospital, the authors compared outcomes during the year before and after the initiation of the 80-hour workweek (36). They found a slight decrease in maternal hemorrhage (from

2% to 1.2%) and slight increase in primary cesarean delivery rate (from 14.5% to 16.1%). Other obstetric outcomes were the same. In the survey of educators there was no perceived difference in patient safety after the enactment of reduced work hours (37).

Thus, despite limited evidence of improvement in patient safety, teamwork training is well accepted by trainees, and likely to remain a part of obstetric training. Simulation training improves resident performance and is becoming more widely embraced by experienced obstetricians and perinatal teams. Obstetricians are encouraged to promulgate safety principles in the hospitals and other settings where they practice. Committee Opinions from the College's Committee on Patient Safety and the Patient Safety Toolkit CD-ROM are good resources for understanding and initiating safety principles.

References

1. Institute of Medicine. To err is human: building a safer health system. Washington, DC: National Academy Press; 2000.

2. Patient safety in obstetrics and gynecology. ACOG Committee Opinion No. 286. American College of Obstetricians and Gynecologists. Obstet Gynecol 2003;102:883-5.

3. The Joint Commission. Preventing infant death and injury during delivery. Sentinel Event Alert 2004;(30):1-3.

4. Nielsen PE, Goldman MB, Mann S, Shapiro DE, Marcus RG, Pratt SD, et al. Effects of teamwork training on adverse outcomes and process of care in labor and delivery: a randomized controlled trial. Obstet Gynecol 2007;109:48-55.

5. Mann S, Pratt SD. Team approach to care in labor and delivery. Clin Obstet Gynecol 2008;51:666-79.

6. Mann S, Pratt S, Gluck P, Nielsen P, Risser D, Greenberg P, et al. Assessing quality obstetrical care: development of standardized measures. Jt Comm J Qual Patient Saf 2006;32:497-505.

7. Pratt SD, Mann S, Salisbury M, Greenberg P, Marcus R, Stabile B, et al. John M. Eisenberg Patient Safety and Quality Awards. Impact of CRM-based training on obstetric outcomes and clinicians' patient safety attitudes. Jt Comm J Qual Patient Saf 2007;33:720-5.

8. Alonso A, Baker DP, Holtzman A, Day R, King H, Toomey L, et al. Reducing medical error in the Military Health System: how can team training help? Hum Resour Manage Rev 2006;16:396-415.

9. Pettker CM, Thung SF, Norwitz ER, Buhimschi CS, Raab CA, Copel JA, et al. Impact of a comprehensive patient safety strategy on obstetric adverse events. Am J Obstet Gynecol 2009;200:492.e1-492.e8.

10. Ellis D, Crofts JF, Hunt LP, Read M, Fox R, James M. Hospital, simulation center, and teamwork training for eclampsia management: a randomized controlled trial. Obstet Gynecol 2008;111:723-31.

11. Siassakos D, Hasafa Z, Sibanda T, Fox R, Donald F, Winter C, et al. Retrospective cohort study of diagnosis-delivery interval with umbilical cord prolapse: the effect of team training. BJOG 2009;116:1089-96.

12. Ennen CS, Satin AJ. Reducing adverse obstetrical outcomes through safety sciences. In: Lockwood CJ, editor. Wellesley (MA): UpToDate; 2009.

13. Draycott T, Sibanda T, Owen L, Akande V, Winter C, Reading S, et al. Does training in obstetric emergencies improve neonatal outcome? BJOG 2006;113:177-82.

14. Gurewitsch ED. Optimizing shoulder dystocia management to prevent birth injury. Clin Obstet Gynecol 2007; 50:592-606.

15. Deering S, Poggi S, Macedonia C, Gherman R, Satin AJ. Improving resident competency in the management of shoulder dystocia with simulation training. Obstet Gynecol 2004;103:1224-8.

16. Goffman D, Heo H, Pardanani S, Merkatz IR, Bernstein PS. Improving shoulder dystocia management among resident and attending physicians using simulations. Am J Obstet Gynecol 2008;199:294.e1-294.e5.

17. Crofts JF, Bartlett C, Ellis D, Hunt LP, Fox R, Draycott TJ. Training for shoulder dystocia: a trial of simulation using low-fidelity and high-fidelity mannequins. Obstet Gynecol 2006;108:1477-85.

18. Crofts JF, Fox R, Ellis D, Winter C, Hinshaw K, Draycott TJ. Observations from 450 shoulder dystocia simulations: lessons for skills training. Obstet Gynecol 2008;112:906-12.

19. Maslovitz S, Barkai G, Lessing JB, Ziv A, Many A. Recurrent obstetric management mistakes identified by simulation. Obstet Gynecol 2007;109:1295-300.

20. Draycott TJ, Crofts JF, Ash JP, Wilson LV, Yard E, Sibanda T, et al. Improving neonatal outcome through practical shoulder dystocia training. Obstet Gynecol 2008;112:14-20.

21. Crofts JF, Bartlett C, Ellis D, Hunt LP, Fox R, Draycott TJ. Management of shoulder dystocia: skill retention 6 and 12 months after training. Obstet Gynecol 2007;110:1069-74.

22. Dupuis O, Moreau R, Silveira R, Pham MT, Zentner A, Cucherat M, et al. A new obstetric forceps for the training of junior doctors: a comparison of the spatial dispersion of forceps blade trajectories between junior and senior obstetricians. Am J Obstet Gynecol 2006;194:1524-31.

23. Dupuis O, Moreau R, Pham MT, Redarce T. Assessment of forceps blade orientations during their placement using an instrumented childbirth simulator. BJOG 2009;116:327-32; discussion 332-3.

24. Moreau R, Jardin A, Pham MT, Redarce T, Olaby O, Dupuis O. A new kind of training for obstetric residents: simulator training. Conf Proc IEEE Eng Med Biol Soc 2006;1:4416-9.

25. Cheong YC, Abdullahi H, Lashen H, Fairlie FM. Can formal education and training improve the outcome of instrumental delivery? Eur J Obstet Gynecol Reprod Biol 2004;113:139-44.

26. Pittini R, Oepkes D, Macrury K, Reznick R, Beyene J, Windrim R. Teaching invasive perinatal procedures: assessment of a high fidelity simulator-based curriculum. Ultrasound Obstet Gynecol 2002;19:478-83.

27. Deering S, Brown J, Hodor J, Satin AJ. Simulation training and resident performance of singleton vaginal breech delivery. Obstet Gynecol 2006;107:86–9.

28. Clark S, Belfort M, Saade G, Hankins G, Miller D, Frye D, et al. Implementation of a conservative checklist-based protocol for oxytocin administration: maternal and newborn outcomes. Am J Obstet Gynecol 2007;197:480. e1–480.e5.

29. Clark SL, Belfort MA, Byrum SL, Meyers JA, Perlin JB. Improved outcomes, fewer cesarean deliveries, and reduced litigation: results of a new paradigm in patient safety. Am J Obstet Gynecol 2008;199:105.e1–105.e7.

30. Hirsch E, Haney EI, Gordon TE, Silver RK. Reducing high-order perineal laceration during operative vaginal delivery. Am J Obstet Gynecol 2008;198:668.e1–668.e5.

31. Skupski DW, Lowenwirt IP, Weinbaum FI, Brodsky D, Danek M, Eglinton GS. Improving hospital systems for the care of women with major obstetric hemorrhage. Obstet Gynecol 2006;107:977–83.

32. Rizvi F, Mackey R, Barrett T, McKenna P, Geary M. Successful reduction of massive postpartum haemorrhage by use of guidelines and staff education [published erratum appears in BJOG 2007;114:660]. BJOG 2004;111: 495–8.

33. Chaudhry B, Wang J, Wu S, Maglione M, Mojica W, Roth E, et al. Systematic review: impact of health information technology on quality, efficiency, and costs of medical care. Ann Intern Med 2006;144:742–52.

34. Institute of Medicine. Resident duty hours: enhancing sleep, supervision, and safety. Washington, DC: National Academies Press; 2009.

35. Kelly A, Marks F, Westhoff C, Rosen M. The effect of the New York State restrictions on resident work hours. Obstet Gynecol 1991;78:468–73.

36. Bailit JL, Blanchard MH. The effect of house staff working hours on the quality of obstetric and gynecologic care. Obstet Gynecol 2004;103:613–6.

37. Espey E, Ogburn T, Puscheck E. Impact of duty hour limitations on resident and student education in obstetrics and gynecology. J Repro Med 2007;52:345–8.

ANTEPARTUM MANAGEMENT

Preconception Care

Katharine D. Wenstrom and Charles J. Lockwood

The three main components of preconception care are screening for risks, providing health education, and instituting effective interventions. Some aspect of preconception care can be provided at every office visit; the ideal time to assess the health and childbearing plans of reproductive age patients is during the annual examination. The ultimate goal of preconception care is to help each woman to be optimally prepared for pregnancy. Although some patients plan their pregnancies and seek medical advice before conception, approximately 50% of pregnancies in the United States are unintended and many women and teenagers seek medical care only after they become pregnant. The critical period of organogenesis—17–56 days after fertilization—occurs before most women become aware that they are pregnant. Women in whom preconception screening reveals risk factors should receive information and advice on how to minimize identified risks and referral services as appropriate. Patients with unresolved issues (potentially harmful lifestyle habits, medical conditions, and other risk factors) should be provided with contraception counseling to reduce the likelihood of an unplanned pregnancy followed by targeted interventions. Screening, health maintenance, and continued education in the primary care setting, combined with preconception care in obstetric practice, can promote healthy pregnancies.

Preconception care should begin with an assessment of a woman's current health, including immunity to certain infections and the need for immunization, the presence and status of medical conditions, current use of specific drugs and medications, use of alternative or complementary medicine, and nutrition. Factors influencing health and reproduction that also should be assessed include the patient's reproductive history, family medical history and risk of genetic disease, substance abuse, exposure to domestic violence, and occupational exposures (Box 2). Women contemplating infertility treatments should be encouraged to consider the possibility of multiple gestation and their options to minimize this risk. Women also should be informed of the increased risks of fertility problems and of aneuploidy associated with advancing age.

Infection

All women should be tested for immunity to rubella, and those who are not immune should be vaccinated (Box 3). Ideally, it should be recommended to these women to delay pregnancy by at least one month. Women who do not report having chickenpox as a child should be tested and offered vaccination if they are not immune. Women at risk of hepatitis B infection should be offered vaccination. Diphtheria and reduced tetanus toxoids and acellular pertussis vaccine (Tdap) should be given every 10 years to all adults. If a woman has not received the Tdap, has not received it after the age of 18 years, or cannot remember receiving it, she should receive the full vaccine, which is a series of three shots (one dose of Tdap and two doses of tetanus and diphtheria [Td] vaccine). Women who have been vaccinated

---

Box 2

Components of Preconception Care

- Systematic identification of preconception risks through assessment of medical, social, reproductive, and family histories, including genetic risk, drugs, and medication history

- Discussion of possible effects of pregnancy on medical conditions for both the prospective mother and the fetus and introduction of interventions, if appropriate and desired

- Determination of risk of infection and, if indicated, testing and vaccination (if available)

- Nutritional counseling regarding appropriate weight for height, nutrient sources, and importance of folic acid, and avoidance of vitamin oversupplementation (especially vitamin A) and referral for in-depth nutrition counseling, if appropriate and desired

- Discussion of social, financial, and psychologic issues in preparation for pregnancy, including lifestyle habits, alcohol and recreational drug use, and domestic violence screening

- Review of alternative and complementary medicine practices

- Provision of education based on risks

- Discussion of birth spacing and real and perceived barriers to achieving desires, including problems with contraceptive use

- Recommendation to keep menstrual calendar

- Emphasis on importance of early and continuous prenatal care and discussion of how care will be structured based on the woman's risks and concerns

against tetanus and diphtheria should receive one dose of the Tdap vaccine to prevent pertussis (1).

All women should be offered testing for human immunodeficiency virus (HIV) infection, with appropriate counseling and consent. For women who already are pregnant, the Institute of Medicine and the American College of Obstetricians and Gynecologists recommend universal screening after patient notification. Patients can be told that HIV testing is part of a recommended battery of tests performed to help increase the likelihood of a healthy pregnancy outcome and that they can choose not to be tested. Although testing can be done without an obligation to provide extensive pretest counseling, counseling should be offered if possible. Screening for sexually transmitted diseases (STDs) may be performed as part of the risk assessment.

The preconception period may be an important time to screen and counsel at-risk patients for other infectious disorders, such as toxoplasmosis and cytomegalovirus (CMV). At-risk patients who test negative for antitoxoplasmosis immunoglobulin M (IgM) and immunoglobulin G (IgG) should be advised to wear gloves during and wash hands after gardening, avoid contact with cat litter, wash fruits and vegetables, and thoroughly cook meat. Patients with exposures to CMV (child care and health care workers) who have negative CMV IgG and IgM should be encouraged to use precautions, particularly frequent hand washing. Conversely, they should be counseled that the presence of CMV IgG and CMV IgM in an individual does not absolutely protect against recurrent infection.

Medical Conditions

Cardiac Disease

Certain medical conditions may entail risks for both mother and fetus. For example, a woman with congenital heart disease may be at increased risk of having a cardiovascular complication during pregnancy, whereas her fetus has a 2–10% risk of having a congenital heart defect. Certain cardiac anomalies, such as uncorrected coarctation of the aorta, pulmonary hypertension, Eisenmenger syndrome, or Marfan syndrome with aortic root dilatation greater than 4 cm, pose a serious risk to the mother's life, and this risk should be fully explained to the affected woman before conception. Patients with chronic hypertension and cardiac arrhythmias may continue taking certain medications, such as β-adrenergic blocking agents, long-acting calcium channel blockers, and digoxin, but angiotensin-converting enzyme inhibitors and angiotensin-receptor antagonists have adverse fetal effects in all three trimesters and, thus, use of these medications should be discontinued before conception. Women who have a positive result on a pregnancy test and who are taking warfarin for anticoagulation should be informed of this medication's teratogenic potential and, if possible, be switched to therapy with unfractionated or low molecular weight heparins, which do not cross the placenta or reach the fetus. Women with a mechanical heart valve have a difficult decision to make and should receive detailed counseling; warfarin therapy is optimal for preventing maternal thromboembolism but is teratogenic, whereas heparin, although safe for the fetus, may not adequately prevent maternal thrombosis (see the section "Deep Vein Thrombosis and Pulmonary Embolism").

Diabetes Mellitus

Women with pregestational diabetes mellitus should be counseled about the many benefits of preparing for pregnancy. A large body of evidence confirms that strict preconceptional glucose control significantly reduces the incidence of serious congenital malformations in offspring with a preconceptional hemoglobin A_{1C} level of less than 6% being an optimum target. Women with diabetes mellitus may benefit from a prepregnancy evaluation for retinopathy and cardiovascular or renal disease, with treatment as necessary. The importance of an appropriate diet and sufficient exercise should be emphasized, and women with diabetes mellitus who are overweight should be urged to reduce their weight before conception. Normalization of weight has been shown to improve glucose control while decreasing the

---

Box 3

Contents of Preconception History

The following information should be obtained during the preconception period:

I. Immunization—if serology indicates lack of immunity
   A. Rubella
   B. Varicella
   C. Hepatitis B
   D. Tetanus–diphtheria–pertussis

II. Occupational and household risks
   A. Workplace exposure
   B. Cytomegalovirus
   C. Human immunodeficiency virus (HIV)
   D. Toxoplasmosis

III. Genetic history risks—carrier status
   A. Autosomal recessive genes (eg, Tay–Sachs disease, cystic fibrosis, Canavan disease, and sickle cell anemia)
   B. X-linked mental retardation (eg, fragile X syndrome)
   C. Population-specific risk

amount of insulin required and to reduce the risk of adverse pregnancy outcomes, such as pregnancy-associated hypertension, cesarean delivery, and postoperative infection (see the section "Diabetes Mellitus").

Thyroid Disorders

It recently has been shown that untreated maternal hypothyroidism has adverse effects on fetal neurodevelopment. Euthyroid women who have known autoimmune thyroiditis, a history of treated hyperthyroidism, or other risk factors for hypothyroidism (eg, family history of thyroid disorders or related autoimmune conditions) should have their thyroid function tested before conception and treated medically if necessary. They should then be reassessed for the emergence of hypothyroidism in their first trimester of pregnancy.

Neurologic Disorders

The offspring of women with epilepsy have a higher rate of malformations than the general population, primarily related to treatment with teratogenic medications (2). Newer medications that appear to have less teratogenic potential are only gradually being used in the pregnant population. However, maternal seizures also can have adverse effects on the developing fetus. If a woman has been seizure free for 2 years, a trial of discontinuation of antiepileptic medication should be discussed during the prepregnancy period in consultation with her neurologist. If possible, women who must continue to take medication should be switched to one of the newer and potentially lower-risk antiepileptic drugs or be switched to monotherapy and take the lowest dose associated with seizure control. Preconception folate supplementation (4 mg/d) should be recommended. Predelivery vitamin K supplementation is controversial; it is not clear if maternally ingested vitamin K crosses the placenta, and most infants are given vitamin K immediately after birth.

Deep Vein Thrombosis and Pulmonary Embolism

Women with a history of thromboembolism while not pregnant should undergo a thorough review of their medical history and be screened for thrombophilias and antiphospholipid antibody syndrome (3). Detailed recommendations for prophylaxis can be found in the section "Deep Vein Thrombosis and Pulmonary Embolism."

Depression and Other Mood Disorders

Many reproductive-aged women take medication for mood disorders or other psychiatric illnesses, and some may be able to safely stop using their medication before pregnancy. However, more severely affected women may need to continue taking their medication to prevent morbidity. For example, data indicate that two thirds of women with severe depressive illness who stop taking their antidepressant medication during pregnancy will experience a relapse of severe depression during pregnancy, severe postpartum depression, or postpartum psychosis (4). Untreated maternal depression leads not only to poor nutrition, abnormal sleep patterns, and a general inability to attend to activities of daily living, but has been associated with poor mother–infant bonding and developmental delay in the child (5). Each case must be assessed individually.

Recent reports suggest that malformations occur more frequently in pregnant women who have used selective serotonin reuptake inhibitors in the first trimester of pregnancy, but there is no consistent pattern of defects associated with the use of individual agents or classes of agents. A single study found that selective serotonin reuptake inhibitor use after 20 weeks of gestation was associated with persistent pulmonary hypertension in 6–12 neonates per 1,000 compared with a baseline rate of 1–2 neonates per 1,000 (6).

Women with mild symptoms who may be able to discontinue the use of antidepressants or mood stabilizers before attempting to conceive should be instructed to taper their dose slowly over at least 2 weeks to avoid the kind of symptomatic recurrence that often follows abrupt discontinuation. Women with severe depression, bipolar disorder, or schizophrenia who may not be able to safely discontinue medication without increasing morbidity to themselves and their fetuses should be taking the fewest number of drugs at the lowest effective doses whenever possible (7). Illness should be deemed severe if a patient's history includes self-harm, protracted recovery time, impaired insight, or inability to manage activities of daily living when unmedicated (see the section "Depression").

Medications

A patient's use of alternative or complementary medicine should be noted when current medications are reviewed, and patients should be counseled about the safe use and potential interaction of these therapies with conventional medicine. Conventional medication use should be reviewed with the goal of discontinuing unnecessary medications and substituting safe medications for potential teratogens (see the section "Teratogenic Exposures").

Diet and Nutrition

Nutrition and its importance in reproductive outcome should be emphasized during all preconception counseling visits. Appropriateness of the patient's weight for height; adherence to special diets, such as those required for patients with diabetes mellitus, celiac disease, or phenylketonuria; and nutrition patterns, such as vegetarianism or high-protein diets should be thoroughly reviewed. Information about abnormal eating patterns, including anorexia nervosa, bulimia nervosa, and pica, may be elicited by asking specific questions about diet and weight gain. Women with poorly controlled eating disorders should be discouraged from beginning a pregnancy until their eating patterns and weight have stabilized.

The importance of vitamin supplementation should be emphasized as well as the potential teratogenic risks of oversupplementation with vitamin A and other fat-soluble vitamins. For example, although vitamin A promotes bone growth, healthy skin and eye sight, excessive supplementation (per some studies, more than 10,000 international units per day) may be associated with fetal malformations. The U.S. Public Health Service recommends that all women of reproductive age take 0.4 mg (400 micrograms) of supplemental folic acid per day. Women who have had a child with a neural tube defect (NTD) and women with seizure disorders who are being treated with valproic acid or carbamazepine should use a higher dose of folic acid supplements (4 mg/d) for 3 months before a planned pregnancy and throughout the first trimester. Although type 2 diabetes mellitus is associated with a 1% risk of NTDs, it does not appear that these defects are associated with folic acid metabolism. Strict blood sugar control during the first trimester of pregnancy is the most effective method for prevention of NTDs and other fetal anomalies. Folic acid supplementation also prevents megaloblastic anemia, an uncommon condition that can cause nausea, vomiting, and anorexia nervosa during pregnancy. Megaloblastic anemia almost always results from folic acid deficiency, and usually is found in women who do not consume fresh, leafy green vegetables or foods with a high content of animal protein.

Reproductive History

Reviewing the reproductive history helps to identify conditions that may have contributed to a previous adverse pregnancy outcome and that can be treated before a subsequent pregnancy. Adverse pregnancy outcomes should be categorized according to the trimester of their occurrence to provide clues to their etiology and areas for evaluation. First trimester pregnancy losses typically result from fetal genetic abnormalities, such as aneuploidy, or acute maternal infection. Second trimester pregnancy losses may be related to anatomic abnormalities, such as rare primary cervical insufficiency, a uterine septum or submucous leiomyomas, or antiphospholipid antibodies and possibly inherited thrombophilias. Third trimester pregnancy losses often involve chronic maternal medical conditions, antiphospholipid antibodies, and possibly inherited thrombophilias, or pregnancy complications, such as placental abruption, severe preeclampsia,

or preterm birth. Interventions, such as anticoagulation, cervical cerclage, surgical removal of a uterine septum or myoma, progesterone supplementation, or optimal control of maternal chronic disease may significantly improve outcome in a subsequent pregnancy. A consultation with a maternal–fetal medicine specialist may be helpful in identifying potentially treatable problems and the most appropriate intervention.

Family Medical History and Risk of Genetic Disease

A patient's personal and family medical histories and her ethnic or racial background may reveal an increased risk of birth defects or genetic diseases. Construction of a genetic pedigree is especially useful for assessing the risk of heritable disease. Women of African descent are at an increased risk of having offspring with hemoglobinopathies, such as sickle cell anemia or hemoglobin C disease. Women of Middle Eastern or Far Eastern origin are at increased risk of α-thalassemia or β-thalassemia. Caucasian women of Northern European origin are at increased risk of cystic fibrosis, and those of Jewish ancestry are at increased risk of Tay–Sachs disease and a variety of other enzyme deficiency diseases. Molecular genetic testing to determine carrier status is available for many single gene disorders and should be offered to high-risk women and their partners (see the section "Prenatal Diagnosis of Genetic Disorders").

Some women have a genetic disease that could affect their pregnancy and fetus. For example, women with phenylketonuria or atypical hyperphenylalanemia with blood phenylalanine levels greater than 10 mg/dL are at increased risk of having a child with microcephaly, mental retardation, congenital heart disease, and intrauterine growth restriction. These adverse outcomes can be avoided by adopting a strict phenylalanine-free diet and maintaining a maternal blood phenylalanine level in the range of 6 mg/dL, starting before conception and continuing throughout pregnancy. Women with myasthenia gravis should avoid certain drugs that are commonly used during pregnancy, such as magnesium sulfate and certain anesthetic agents, because of their effects on neuromuscular function, whereas women with Marfan syndrome should undergo echocardiography to evaluate for possible aortic valve root dilation. Consideration should be given to the referral of women with genetic syndromes or diseases for preconception counseling by a genetics professional (see the section "Prenatal Diagnosis of Genetic Disorders").

Substance Abuse

An accurate history of alcohol use, taken in a nonthreatening manner, is a critical component of the preconception visit. A number of techniques have been successful for identifying problem drinkers, such as the TWEAK test, the CAGE test, the T-ACE questionnaire, or the National Institute on Alcohol Abuse and Alcohol questionnaire (see the sections "Substance Abuse" in this book and in *Precis: Primary and Preventive Care*, Fourth Edition.)

References

1. Update on immunization and pregnancy: tetanus, diphtheria, and pertussis vaccination. ACOG Committee Opinion No. 438. American College of Obstetricians and Gynecologists. Obstet Gynecol 2009;114:398–400.

2. Holmes LB, Harvey EA, Coull BA, Huntington KB, Khoshbin S, Hayes AM, et al. The teratogenicity of anticonvulsant drugs. N Engl J Med 2001;344:1132–8.

3. Smoking cessation during pregnancy. ACOG Committee Opinion No. 316. American College of Obstetricians and Gynecol-ogists. Obstet Gynecol 2005;106:883–8.

4. Cohen LS, Altshuler LL, Harlow BL, Nonacs R, Newport DJ, Viguera AC, et al. Relapse of major depression during pregnancy in women who maintain or discontinue antidepressant treatment [published erratum appears in JAMA 2006;296:170]. JAMA 2006;295:499–507.

5. Deave T, Heron J, Evans J, Emond A. The impact of maternal depression in pregnancy on early child development. BJOG 2008;115:1043–51.

6. Chambers CD, Hernandez-Diaz S, Van Marter LJ, Werler MM, Louik C, Jones KL, et al. Selective serotonin-reuptake inhibitors and risk of persistent pulmonary hypertension of the newborn. N Engl J Med 2006;354:579–87.

7. The management of depression during pregnancy: a report from the American Psychiatric Association and the American College of Obstetricians and Gynecologists. Obstet Gynecol 2009;114:703–13.

Routine Care

Charles J. Lockwood

The major goal of prenatal care is to increase the probability of a healthy infant and mother. The *Antepartum Record* (see Appendix B) or equivalent electronic medical record provides useful checklists to improve the likelihood that key medical, genetic, and obstetric data will be gathered and acted on so that potential problems can be anticipated, prevented, or ameliorated. Also they provide reminders to enhance patient education and communication.

Diagnosis of Pregnancy

All commercial pregnancy tests depend on the detection of human chorionic gonadotropin (hCG) by an antibody. The various techniques used to detect hCG include agglutination inhibition, radioimmunoassay, enzyme-linked immunosorbent assay, and immunochromatography. Some tests can detect hCG levels as low as 25 mIU/mL or as early as 1 week after implantation.

History and Physical Examination

The American College of Obstetricians and Gynecologists (the College) currently recommends that screening for cystic fibrosis with a minimal panel of 25 common mutations be offered to all white patients and patients of European or Ashkenazi Jewish ethnicity or when there is a family history of the disease. It is reasonable to offer cystic fibrosis carrier screening to all couples, regardless of race or ethnicity, as an alternative to selective screening (1).

An important part of the initial physical assessment is the pelvic examination to ascertain uterine size and gestational age and to estimate the expected date of delivery. If there is a discrepancy between uterine size and the last menstrual period or if the latter is unknown, first-trimester or early second-trimester ultrasonography will help establish an expected date of delivery. Ultrasound measurement of the crown–rump length at 6–12 weeks of gestation is the most accurate technique for estimation of gestational age.

Laboratory Tests

All pregnant women in the United States should undergo human immunodeficiency virus (HIV) infection testing as early in pregnancy as possible. Testing should be conducted after the woman is notified that she will be tested for HIV as part of the routine panel of prenatal tests, unless she declines the test. The College and the Centers for Disease Control and Prevention (CDC) also recommend that obstetrician–gynecologists should follow opt-out prenatal HIV screening where legally possible. Repeat testing in the third trimester is an additional strategy to further reduce the rate of perinatal HIV transmission. The health care providers should be aware of state laws and hospital practices and comply with them (2).

All pregnant women at high risk for hepatitis C infection should be tested for hepatitis C antibodies at the first prenatal visit. Women at high risk include those with a history of injection-drug use and those with a history of blood transfusion or organ transplantation before 1992.

Nutrition and Weight Gain

All pregnant women should be encouraged to eat a well-balanced diet. Of particular note, the CDC has recommended supplemental folic acid in the preconceptional and early prenatal period to prevent neural tube defects (see the section "Preconception Care").

Recommendations for weight gain during pregnancy are based on a prepregnancy body mass index (BMI), defined as weight in kilograms divided by height in meters squared (the BMI calculator is available at www.nhlbisupport.com/bmi). Current information is based on the Institute of Medicine's May 2009 recommendations for total weight gain during pregnancy (3). Underweight women (those with a BMI of less than 18.5) should have a weight gain of 12.5–18 kg (28–40 lb), whereas overweight women (those with a BMI of 25–29.9) should have a weight gain of 7–11.5 kg (15–25 lb) and obese women (those with a BMI of 30 or greater) should have a weight gain of 5–9 kg (11–20 lb). The recommended weight gain for women of average weight (those with a BMI of 18.5–24.9) is 11.5–16 kg (25–35 lb).

Domestic or Intimate Partner Violence

Domestic violence is defined as violent, abusive, or controlling behavior and language perpetrated by a current or past intimate partner. Approximately 7–17% of all women screened report abuse during pregnancy. Domestic violence has many adverse effects on the woman and her fetus and is associated with late entry to prenatal care, substance abuse during pregnancy, inadequate maternal weight gain, fetal growth restriction, preterm birth, and other poor pregnancy outcomes. Although women at increased risk tend to be young and single, live alone, have a low socioeconomic status, and have a partner or ex-partner who abuses alcohol and other recreational drugs, intimate partner violence can happen to anyone, and pregnancy increases the risk (4). Thus, screening for domestic violence should be part of the preconception assessment or the first prenatal visit. A history of intimate partner violence or abuse is more likely to be elicited by a structured screening tool than by general questioning. One tool of documented efficacy during pregnancy is the Abuse Assessment Screen, developed by the Nursing Research Consortium on Violence and Abuse, which uses five questions to elicit a history of remote or current physical or sexual violence.

When a history of domestic violence is elicited, the woman should be referred to a health care professional or social worker for counseling and assessment of the need for alternative shelter and legal aid as appropriate. If violence is associated with substance abuse, counseling and intervention for that problem also should be provided.

Work During Pregnancy

The Pregnancy Discrimination Act requires that employers offering medical disability benefits must treat pregnancy-related disabilities as they do all other disabilities. Pregnant workers must be provided the same insurance benefits, sick leave, seniority credits, and reinstatement privileges that are awarded to workers who are disabled by other causes.

Work may be limited or contraindicated during pregnancy in patients with vaginal bleeding, cervical insufficiency, uterine malformation associated with perinatal loss, gestational hypertension, intrauterine growth restriction, multiple gestations, a history of preterm birth, or hydramnios.

Air Travel During Pregnancy

In the absence of obstetric or medical complications, pregnant women can observe the same precautions for air travel as the general population and can fly safely. Pregnant women should be instructed to continuously use their seat belts while seated, as should all air travelers. Pregnant air travelers may take precautions to ease in-flight discomfort and preventive measures to minimize risks of venous thrombosis, although no hard evidence exists regarding increased risks of this condition for pregnant air travelers. For most air travelers the risks to the fetus from exposure to cosmic radiation are negligible. For pregnant aircrew members and other frequent flyers, this exposure may be higher (5). Information is available from the Federal Aviation Administration to estimate this exposure (http://jag.cami.jccbi.gov/cariprofile.asp).

Exercise During Pregnancy

A pregnant woman may engage in a moderate level of physical activity if she has no obstetric or medical complications (Box 4 and Box 5). According to the CDC and the American College of Sports Medicine, this amounts to 30 minutes or more of moderate exercise on most, if not all, days of the week. Exercise helps a woman to maintain cardiorespiratory and muscular fitness throughout her pregnancy and may be particularly helpful in obese women and other women at high risk for gestational diabetes mellitus. Preliminary data suggests that exercise during pregnancy also may help long-term health. Compared with women who stop

---

Box 4

Absolute Contraindications to Aerobic Exercise During Pregnancy

- Gestational hypertension
- Hemodynamically significant heart disease
- Restrictive lung disease
- Preterm premature rupture of membranes
- Preterm labor during the current pregnancy
- Multiple gestations at risk for preterm labor
- Cervical insufficiency
- Second-trimester or third-trimester bleeding

Exercise during pregnancy and the postpartum period. ACOG Committee Opinion No. 267. American College of Obstetricians and Gynecologists. Obstet Gynecol 2002;99: 171–3.

Box 5

Relative Contraindications to Aerobic Exercise During Pregnancy

- Severe Anemia
- Unevaluated maternal cardiac arrhythmia
- Chronic bronchitis
- Poorly controlled type 1 diabetes mellitus
- Extreme underweight (body mass index [expressed as weight in kilograms divided by height in meters squared] less than 12)
- History of extremely sedentary lifestyle
- Intrauterine growth restriction in current pregnancy
- Poorly controlled hypertension or preeclampsia
- Orthopedic limitations
- Poorly controlled seizure disorder
- Poorly controlled thyroid disease
- Heavy smoker

Exercise during pregnancy and the postpartum period. ACOG Committee Opinion No. 267. American College of Obstetricians and Gynecologists. Obstet Gynecol 2002; 99:171–3.

---

exercising with pregnancy, women who continue their exercise regimens gain less weight and have a lower cardiovascular risk profile over time (6).

For women who do not have any additional risk factors for adverse maternal or perinatal outcomes, exercise should be considered in consultation with the obstetric provider. The College recommends the following guidelines for exercise during pregnancy:

- Women can continue to exercise and derive health benefits even from mildly to moderately strenuous exercise routines. Regular exercise on most days of the week is preferable to intermittent activity.

- Women should avoid exercise in the supine position after the first trimester of pregnancy. Such a position is associated with decreased cardiac output in most pregnant women. Because the remaining cardiac output will be preferentially distributed away from the splanchnic beds (including the uterus) during vigorous exercise, such regimens are best avoided during pregnancy. Prolonged periods of motionless standing also should be avoided.

- Pregnant women should be aware of the decreased oxygen available for aerobic exercise. They should be encouraged to modify the intensity of their exercise according to their symptoms. Pregnant women should stop exercising when fatigued and not exercise to exhaustion. Weight-bearing exercises may, under most circumstances, be continued throughout pregnancy at intensities similar to those before pregnancy. Nonweight-bearing exercises, such as stationary cycling, swimming and water aerobics, will minimize the risk of injury and facilitate the continuation of exercise during pregnancy.

- Morphologic changes in pregnancy should serve as a relative contraindication to types of exercise in which loss of balance could be detrimental to maternal or fetal well-being, especially in the third trimester. Furthermore, any type of exercise involving the potential for even mild abdominal trauma should be avoided. Scuba diving should be avoided throughout pregnancy.

- Pregnancy requires an additional 300 kcal/d in order to maintain energy balance. Thus, women who exercise during pregnancy should be particularly careful to ensure an adequate diet.

- Pregnant women who exercise in the first trimester should augment heat dissipation by ensuring adequate hydration, appropriate clothing, and optimal environmental surroundings during exercise. There are no reports linking hyperthermia associated with exercise and congenital malformations.

Many of the physiologic and morphologic changes of pregnancy persist for 4–6 weeks postpartum. Thus, prepregnancy exercise routines should be resumed gradually based on a woman's physical capability (7).

Follow-up Visits

The interval for prenatal visits should be individualized according to the patient's needs. More frequent visits are of benefit in monitoring women with diabetes mellitus, hypertension, threatened preterm birth, and postterm pregnancies.

References

1. American Academy of Pediatrics, American College of Obstetricians and Gynecologists. Guidelines for perinatal care. 6th ed. Elk Grove Village (IL): AAP; Washington, DC: American College of Obstetricians and Gynecologists; 2007.

2. Prenatal and perinatal human immunodeficiency virus testing: expanded recommendations. ACOG Committee Opinion No. 418. American College of Obstetricians and Gynecologists. Obstet Gynecol 2008;112:739–42.

3. Rasmussen KM, Yaktine AL. Weight gain during pregnancy: reexamining the guidelines. Institute of Medicine. Washington, DC: National Academies Press; 2009.

4. Norton LB, Peipert JF, Zierler S, Lima B, Hume L. Battering in pregnancy: an assessment of two screening methods. Obstet Gynecol 1995;85:321–5.

5. Air travel during pregnancy. ACOG Committee Opinion No. 264. American College of Obstetricians and Gynecologists. Obstet Gynecol 2001;98:1187–8.

6. Clapp JF 3rd. Long-term outcome after exercising throughout pregnancy: fitness and cardiovascular risk. Am J Obstet Gynecol 2008;199:489.e1–489.e6.

7. Exercise during pregnancy and the postpartum period. ACOG Committee Opinion No. 267. American College of Obstet-ricians and Gynecologists. Obstet Gynecol 2002; 99:171–3.

Substance Abuse

Katharine D. Wenstrom

The 2007 National Survey on Drug Use and Health by the Department of Health and Human Services Substance Abuse and Mental Health Services Administration surveyed the use of illicit substances, including cocaine, crack, heroin, hallucinogens, inhalants, methamphetamines, and marijuana as well as the nonmedical use of prescription psychotherapeutic drugs and prescription pain relievers, and found that 22.6% of women aged 15–17 years, 7.2% of women aged 18–25 years, and 3% of women aged 26–44 years engaged in illicit drug use during pregnancy (1). Approximately 12% of pregnant women aged 15–44 years drank alcohol, and 6.6% of these women reported binge drinking during the first trimester of pregnancy. More than one quarter of all women smoke, and 16.4% continue to smoke during pregnancy.

Screening for Drug Use

Substance abuse is defined as a maladaptive pattern of use leading to clinically significant impairment, occurring within a 12-month period. Substance abuse is likely when drug use results in any of the following situations:

- Failure to fulfill major role obligations at work (absences or poor performance), at school (absences, suspensions, or expulsions), or at home (neglect of children or household)

- Use of a drug in physically hazardous situations (eg, driving while intoxicated)

- Recurrent substance use-related legal problems

- Continued drug use despite the fact that it causes or exacerbates persistent or recurrent problems, including social and interpersonal problems.

Substance dependence is substance abuse characterized by three or more of the following factors:

- Tolerance (a decreasing response to repeated constant doses of a substance or the need for increasing doses to maintain a constant response)

- Withdrawal (characteristic symptoms of withdrawal or the need to take the substance to prevent withdrawal)

- Consuming larger amounts of substance over a longer period than intended

- The desire to cut down or control use

- A lot of time spent in substance-related activities, such as obtaining the substance, using it, and recovering from its use

- Giving up important social, occupational, or recreational activities because of substance use

- Continued use of the substance despite recurrent psychologic or physical problems caused or exacerbated by its use

Asking detailed questions about the frequency and magnitude of alcohol, drug, or cigarette use has been shown to be more effective for obtaining accurate information than using a standard pregnancy screening form that requests affirmative or negative answers to smoking and alcohol and drug use (2). During the patient interview, asking specific questions in a nonthreatening manner (Do you drink a fifth a day? A quart?) is likely to yield more accurate responses than asking accusatory (You don't drink, do you?) or open-ended (How much do you drink?) questions. There also are several simple screening tests that have been validated for use with pregnant women (see Box 6 and Box 7).

Box 6

The TWEAK Screening Test

The TWEAK test, which screens for alcohol abuse, is a self-administered test that includes five questions:

T　　　**T**olerance—How many drinks can you hold?

　　　　(If 5 or more drinks, score 2 points.)

W　　　Have close friends or relatives **W**orried or complained about your drinking in the past year?

　　　　(If "Yes," score 2 points.)

E　　　**E**ye Opener—Do you sometimes take a drink in the morning when you get up?

　　　　(If "Yes," score 1 point.)

A　　　**A**mnesia—Has a friend or family member ever told you about things you said or did while you were drinking that you could not remember?

　　　　(If "Yes," score 1 point.)

K(C)　　Do you sometimes feel the need to **C**ut down on your drinking?

　　　　(If "Yes," score 1 point.)

The TWEAK test is used to screen for pregnant at-risk drinking, defined here as the consumption of 1 oz or more of alcohol per day while pregnant. A total score of 2 points or more indicates a positive result for pregnancy risk drinking.

Modified from Chan AW, Pristach EA, Welte JW, Russell M. Use of the TWEAK test in screening for alcoholism/heavy drinking in three populations. Alcohol Clin Exp Res 1993; 17:1188–92.

Box 7

The CAGE Screening Test

The CAGE test, another simple test that can be used for either alcohol or illicit drug screening, is based on four questions:

1. Do you feel that you should **C**ut down on your narcotic or alcohol use?

2. Have you been **A**nnoyed by people criticizing your narcotic or alcohol use?

3. Do you ever feel **G**uilty about narcotic or alcohol use?

4. Do you feel **E**dgy if you do not use narcotics or alcohol? or Do you ever need an **E**ye opener to get going in the morning?

Two affirmative answers to the CAGE test indicate problems with narcotics or alcohol.

Women with substance abuse problems frequently experience concurrent psychiatric or social problems, which both identify the patient as a possible substance abuser and complicate diagnosis and therapy. Depression is especially common among addicts—78% of female drug abusers met criteria for clinical depression in one study—as are borderline depression, antisocial disorder, or narcissistic personality disorder (3). A narcissistic patient may not be identified by their responses to the TWEAK or CAGE questions because those questions rely on an understanding of other people's feelings that narcissists usually do not have. The substance abuser also may be a victim of domestic or intimate partner violence or sexual assault. The physician should be aware of the possibility of concurrent psychiatric or social problems when substance abuse is identified, and conversely should query women with depressive symptoms or poor social situations about substance abuse. Consultation with a mental health professional or social worker may be an important adjunct to substance abuse intervention.

Health Consequences of Substance Abuse

Women who use recreational drugs, and their fetuses, are at increased risk of having a variety of health problems resulting from the effects of the drug itself, the interaction of several drugs, the method of drug delivery, and associated adverse health behaviors or socioeconomic factors, such as poor nutrition, smoking, violence, and increased stress. An understanding of the maternal, fetal, and obstetric effects of currently popular recreational drugs is essential for obstetricians. Such knowledge can be used to guide medical care during pregnancy and should be provided to women at risk of drug abuse during preconception counseling. The reproductive age woman who uses recreational drugs should be made aware of the clinical and psychologic effects of drug use on both her own health and on the health of a fetus. She also should be educated about the obstetric complications associated with substance abuse, many of which result in early preterm birth, with all its adverse health consequences for the infant, or pregnancy loss. Understanding what recreational drug use can do to a fetus is a powerful motivator for many women and likely explains the observed decrease in drug and alcohol use during pregnancy.

Opiods

Opioid use is widespread in the United States. Currently popular opioid narcotics include heroin, morphine, codeine, oxycodone, narcotic analgesics, buprenorphine, and methadone. Opioid use results in a host of morbidities that can be roughly categorized as problems caused by vasospasm and vascular disease (thrombophlebitis, pulmonary embolism, acute myocardial infarction, rupture of the ascending aorta, cardiac arrhythmias, cerebrovascular accidents, seizures, and bowel ischemia), many different kinds of infections (pneumonia; endocarditis; hepatitis; sexually transmitted diseases [STDs], including human immunodeficiency virus [HIV] infection; urinary tract infections; or cellulitis), and problems related to adverse lifestyle, such as hypothermia or anemia. These problems may be exacerbated by coexistent psychologic problems, most notably depression, and by the concurrent use of other illicit substances.

Physical findings suggestive of opioid abuse include signs of intoxication and signs of withdrawal. The signs of intoxication are euphoria, constriction of the pupils, flushing of the face and neck, drowsiness, analgesia, nausea or vomiting, constipation and difficulty urinating, and decreased respiratory drive. Drug seeking behavior decreases during intoxication, and there also is decreased libido. The signs of narcotic withdrawal in the pregnant adult include anorexia; vomiting; diarrhea; abdominal cramps; flushing; chills, sweating, or both; tachycardia; hypotension or hypertension; and tremors, along with increased fetal activity and uterine irritability. The physical examination may reveal needle tracks, skin ulcers, or cellulitis. Intravenous drug users may have evidence of venous thrombosis, including foreign body embolism in the eye grounds, and nasal hyperemia. The cardiac examination may reveal abnormal rubs or murmurs consistent with previous episodes of endocarditis.

If withdrawal is suspected, a thorough examination to assess neurologic function and an examination for infection should be performed. Symptoms of withdrawal may be treated with methadone; after an initial dose of 1–20 mg is given orally, the patient should be reevaluated every 6 hours and given more methadone as needed. Blood pressure and fetal heart rate should be monitored closely. Methadone use, in high doses, occasionally has been associated with long QT syndrome. Some authors recommend obtaining electrocardiography results before initiation of the methadone treatment and during the treatment (4). Diarrhea can be treated with loperamide, decongestants may be given, and pain can be treated with nonopioid analgesics, such as ibuprofen. Sympathetic activity and jitteriness may be decreased with clonidine, low-dose benzodiazepine, or both.

Narcotic overdose is characterized by hypoxia caused by severe respiratory depression; somnolence, unconsciousness, or coma; pinpoint pupils (except with overdose of meperidine); inability to protect the airway; and seizures. Narcotic overdose is life threatening to both mother and fetus and should be treated aggressively. An airway must be established and protected, and naloxone, a short-acting narcotic antagonist, should be given intravenously at a dose of 0.01 mg per kilogram of body weight. The fetal heart rate should be monitored and may indicate fetal stress related to either the maternal overdose or acute withdrawal precipitated by the treatment. If possible, and especially if the fetus is very premature, in utero resuscitation should be allowed to occur. As the mother's condition stabilizes the fetal heart rate should stabilize as well. A toxicology screen should be performed on admission to determine what drugs the patient used and to assist the pediatricians caring for the infant if delivery occurs. Although withdrawal generally is not life threatening to the mother, it can result in fetal stress and eventual fetal demise. Both withdrawal and repeated intoxication–withdrawal cycles can be prevented, and other narcotics-associated morbidities avoided, by methadone maintenance.

Infants born to women who used heroin, methadone, or other opiates during pregnancy may be either depressed as the result of recent maternal use or will experience withdrawal, characterized by hyperirritability, increased muscle tone, tremors, tachypnea, vomiting, diarrhea, abdominal cramps, flushing, and a high-pitched cry. Studies of the relationship between maternal methadone dose and the risk of neonatal withdrawal are controversial (5, 6). Withdrawal is most severe in infants born preterm and in those chronically exposed to high narcotic doses. Prenatally, opiates increase the length of rapid-eye-movement sleep, leading to a hyperactive state and increased oxygen consumption. Maternal withdrawal has similar effects, increasing fetal oxygen consumption by triggering fetal hyperactivity and catecholamine release. Both situations can lead to fetal hypoxemia or asphyxia. Maternal methadone use has been associated with neonatal thrombocytosis, with resultant focal cerebral infarctions and subarachnoid hemorrhage.

Cocaine

Cocaine use causes intense sympathomimetic effects, including vasoconstriction, acute arterial hypertension, and tachycardia. Maternal cocaine use is a recognized cause of myocardial infarction, aortic rupture, cardiac arrhythmia, hemorrhagic stroke, seizures, bowel ischemia, and sudden death. Cocaine use during pregnancy significantly increases the risk of placental abruption and may provoke preterm labor and preterm birth.

There are many reports of an association between prenatal exposure to cocaine and birth defects caused by vascular disruption and hypoxemia, such as skull defects, cutis aplasia, porencephaly, subependymal and periventricular cysts, microcephaly, ileal atresia, visceral infarcts, urinary tract anomalies, and cardiac anomalies (see Reprotox in Resources). Exposed infants also are at increased risk of having behavioral problems, cognitive deficits, and developmental delay. The effects of maternal cocaine use frequently are compounded by concurrent adverse health habits, including late entry to prenatal care, poor nutrition, and the abuse of other drugs, including tobacco and alcohol.

Methamphetamine

Methamphetamine is a sympathomimetic drug that causes dopamine release, leading to intense feelings of well-being, alertness, and euphoria. Use of methamphetamine has been associated with serious neurologic morbidity, including hemorrhagic or ischemic brain infarction, subarachnoid hemorrhage, memory loss, and psychosis. Use during pregnancy has been associated with cardiovascular collapse and seizures. Methamphetamine use is associated with the same obstetric complications as cocaine, including placental abruption, preterm birth, growth restriction, and fetal stress or intolerance of labor. The effects of methamphetamine use often are confounded by concurrent use of cigarettes and alcohol.

Neonates exposed prenatally to methamphetamines are at increased risk of growth restriction, which may be exacerbated by maternal smoking and alcohol abuse. There have been sporadic reports of specific anomalies in fetuses exposed prenatally to methamphetamines, including cleft lip, cardiac defects, and biliary atresia, but no syndrome or recurring defect has been identified. One half of all neonates exposed to methamphetamines experience withdrawal, with symptoms including continuous high-pitched cry, sweating, hyperthermia, insomnia, tremors, hypertonicity, seizures, tachypnea, poor feeding, vomiting, and diarrhea (7).

Nonnarcotic Hypnotics or Sedatives

Nonnarcotic hypnotics are used illicitly to reduce anxiety, remove inhibitions, and to treat the effects of stimulant drugs. Generally only short-acting barbiturates, such as secobarbital, are abused because they rapidly cross the blood brain barrier and produce the desired effects within 30 minutes. The effect of the drug is determined by the dose and the circumstances in which it is taken. For example, taking secobarbital at bedtime with the intention of going to sleep produces somnolence, while taking it to "get high" produces intoxication, disinhibition, and excitement. Chronic use of barbiturates produces tolerance, and taking 600–800 mg per day for a month or longer produces dependence. Once dependence develops, abrupt discontinuation of the drug results in withdrawal symptoms similar to delirium tremens, with insomnia, sweating, tremors, hyperreflexia, agitation, disorientation, visual hallucinations, seizures, and hyperthermia.

Barbiturate overdose results in severe lethargy or coma. The pupils are constricted, and there is hypotension, respiratory depression, and hypothermia. Because opiate overdose produces a similar clinical picture, some authorities advise giving intravenous naloxone once the airway has been established and the patient is stabilized; if the patient does not respond to this therapy, opioid use is ruled out and barbiturate use is more likely. Patients who are conscious and have an intact gag reflex should be given activated charcoal and a cathartic. Comatose patients should have an endotracheal tube placed and then receive gastric lavage and charcoal.

Barbiturates cross the placenta freely, and chronic use during pregnancy can cause neonatal abstinence syndrome (withdrawal), beginning approximately 4–7 days after birth and lasting for up to 4 months. Symptoms include insomnia, tremors, overactivity, vasomotor instability, hypertonicity, and restlessness (8). Decreased verbal IQ scores have been reported in adults who were exposed to barbiturates in utero, particularly in the third trimester of pregnancy (9).

Phencyclidine

Phencyclidine (PCP), also called angel dust, is a synthetic hallucinogen originally developed for surgical anesthesia and analgesia. However, it rapidly lost favor because patients given PCP often became agitated, confused, and even psychotic, with psychotic episodes lasting up to 10 days. Phencyclidine appears to have stimulant, depressant, hallucinogenic, anesthetic, and analgesic properties. Depending on the dose, it can cause altered perception and euphoria, acute confusional states, loss of response to pinprick and other anesthetic effects, as well as seizures and cardiovascular abnormalities. Its propensity for causing paranoid delusion, auditory hallucinations, and psychotic reactions has resulted in its being considered a model for schizophrenia; in one report from a community mental health center in Washington, DC, all of the patients who reported symptoms of schizophrenia were found to have used PCP (10). Phencyclidine usually is sold as a powder that can be swallowed or smoked, often mixed with tobacco.

Prenatal exposure to PCP can lead to growth restriction and abnormal neurodevelopment. Neonates who were exposed prenatally often have tremors, hypertonicity, diarrhea, and bizarre eye movements and facial twitches, and may rapidly change their level of consciousness from irritability to lethargy. These effects have been observed in children up to 18 months old, suggesting that they are not caused solely by either PCP intoxication or withdrawal (11).

Alcohol

Chronic alcohol abuse results in fluctuating hypertension, cardiac arrhythmias, and frequent bouts of pneumonia and other infections. Long-standing use leads to cirrhosis, hepatitis, or both; pancreatitis; cardiomyopathy; decreased bone density with increased risk of fractures; and peripheral neuropathy. Female alcohol abusers frequently have menstrual irregularity and reduced fertility. Alcoholics also are at an increased risk of developing cancer of the head, neck, esophagus, or stomach.

Acute alcohol withdrawal can lead to a constellation of symptoms, ranging from mild to severe. The most serious is a severe dysautonomic encephalopathic state called delirium tremens. Withdrawal typically occurs 24–48 hours after the last drink in a patient with a history of chronic heavy alcohol use. The symptoms of alcohol withdrawal syndrome include anxiety, tremor, headache, anorexia, nausea and vomiting, diaphoresis, hyperflexia, tachycardia, hypertension, hyperventilation, and seizures. Delirium tremens is characterized by the usual withdrawal symptoms plus a severe hyperadrenergic state, disorientation, impaired attention and consciousness, and visual and auditory hallucinations. Although older studies suggested that up to one third of patients with delirium tremens died, more recent studies indicate that death is unlikely if there are no concurrent medical problems. In one series of 35 patients with delirium tremens, hyperthermia, and persistent tachycardia were significantly associated with mortality (12).

The patient presenting with symptoms of alcohol withdrawal may or may not give a history consistent with alcohol abuse. If the patient is unwilling or unable to provide a history, blood tests that may be helpful in identifying alcohol abuse include elevated levels of gamma glutamyl transferase (greater than 30 units) and carbohydrate deficient transferrin (greater than 20 units/L), which together have up to 80% sensitivity and specificity for identifying individuals who regularly imbibe at least 6–8 drinks per day. In addition, alcoholics often will have a high normal mean corpuscular volume (ie, greater than 91) and an elevated uric acid level (greater than 416 mol/L or 7 mg/dL) (13).

Severe withdrawal symptoms require pharmacologic treatment, usually in the form of a benzodiazepine. One method for assessing severity is the Clinical Institute Withdrawal Assessment Scale, which assesses the presence and severity of nausea, sweating, agitation, headache, anxiety, tremor, sensory disturbances and disorientation. For each symptom, a score of 0 (normal) to 7 (severe) is given. A score of 10 or more indicates the need for pharmacologic therapy. A benzodiazepine is given and assessment is repeated hourly. Additional dosing is given until the score is less than 9. Assessment is then repeated every 8 hours and discontinued when there has been a score of less than 6 on four consecutive assessments. There is no consensus on which type of benzodiazepine to use. Long acting agents, such as diazepam, seem to make withdrawal smoother and prevent delirium tremens but can have unpredictable effects in patients with liver disease. Although intermediate acting agents, such as lorazepam, may be safer if there is hepatic dysfunction, more frequent dosing is required because it has a shorter half-life.

Portal hypertension is a complication of alcoholism that can be life threatening during pregnancy (14). Up to 60% of patients with hepatic cirrhosis have portal hypertension, which can lead to esophageal varices, splenomegaly, and increased retrograde flow to the systemic venous circulation, resulting in hemorrhoids and enlargement of the periumbilical or abdominal wall collateral circulation (caput medusae). The increased intravascular volume of pregnancy can exacerbate portal hypertension, resulting in increased blood volume draining into the esophageal circulation and increased risk of variceal bleeding. Up to 50% of women with esophageal varices experience hemorrhage during pregnancy, which results in maternal death in 18% of patients.

Alcohol is the most widely used human teratogen, and prenatal exposure to alcohol is both the leading known cause of mental retardation and the leading preventable cause of birth defects in the western world. Fetuses exposed to alcohol are at risk of developing some or all features of the fetal alcohol syndrome, which includes varying degrees of mental retardation, developmental delay, hyperactivity and other behavioral abnormalities, along with prenatal and postnatal growth restriction, dysmorphic facies, microcephaly, joint contractures, and cardiac defects. The incidence of fetal alcohol syndrome among the offspring of pregnant women who consume four drinks per day during pregnancy is approximately 20%; this risk increases to 40% with six drinks per day, and up to 50% with eight drinks per day. Although it appears that binge drinking entails the highest risk of fetal alcohol syndrome, most studies of alcohol use during pregnancy have not monitored exposed children to adulthood. Thus, many subtle or age-specific alcohol related problems would not have been detected. Thus, a woman planning pregnancy should be advised not to drink any alcohol during gestation.

Marijuana

Cannabis use results in euphoria, relaxation, altered perception, and intensification of sensations. Occasionally, it may provoke anxiety or a full-blown panic attack. Short-term memory, motor skills, and reaction time are impaired while intoxicated, and there may be increased heart rate and blood pressure (15). Marijuana use rarely results in acute toxicity or dependence. However, chronic use can cause bronchitis and most likely increases the risk of lung cancer, similar to cigarette smoking.

Chronic marijuana use during pregnancy can result in low birth weight, although the effects of marijuana may be confounded by concurrent tobacco and alcohol use and poor nutrition. Neonates exposed prenatally to heavy maternal marijuana use have an exaggerated startle response, tremors, a high-pitched cry, and poor habituation to visual stimuli (16). In early childhood, exposed children score lower on tests of verbal ability than the children of nonusers, although by age 5–6 years this difference is no longer demonstrable.

Smoking

The many adverse clinical consequences of cigarette smoking have been well documented and include bronchitis, emphysema, cardiovascular disease, peripheral vascular disease, stroke, and a variety of malignancies, including lung cancer, colorectal cancer, bladder cancer, and pancreatic cancer. Smoking during pregnancy increases the risk of spontaneous abortion, placental abruption resulting in fetal death, preterm delivery, and premature preterm rupture of membranes.

The infants of smoking women are more likely to have low birth weight and have higher rates of respiratory distress syndrome than infants of nonsmoking women. Smokeless tobacco, which increases blood nicotine levels to those associated with cigarette smoking, appears to result in similarly decreased birth weight, and passive smoking also may have adverse clinical effects. The infants born prematurely as a consequence of preterm rupture of the membranes or uteroplacental insufficiency face all the morbidities of prematurity, and those whose births were complicated by placental abruption may be damaged by acute hypoxemia. Infants exposed to maternal smoking also have higher rates of sudden infant death syndrome and developmental delay (17).

Obstetric Care for Women With Substance Abuse

The pregnancies of substance abusers usually are considered high risk because of ongoing drug abuse; concurrent use of other substances, such as cigarettes; a history of adverse pregnancy outcomes; low socioeconomic status and poor social situation; and adverse health behaviors. Because the timing of antepartum surveillance and all interventions requires accurate pregnancy dating, an ultrasound examination should be performed at the first prenatal visit. The patient also should be screened for STDs and her HIV and hepatitis status determined (18). Depending on the patient's history, a tuberculosis skin test or chest X-ray may be appropriate. Intravenous drug users should be carefully examined for evidence of current drug use as well as cellulitis or thrombophlebitis. A targeted ultrasound examination to evaluate fetal anatomy should be done in the second trimester. In addition, depending on the patient's history, weight gain and other factors, serial ultrasound examinations to monitor fetal growth may be necessary. Screening for STDs should be repeated in the third trimester.

Late entry to prenatal care, multiple missed appointments, noncompliance with prenatal care, trouble with the law, and recurrent marital or family disputes are all warning signs of continued substance abuse. If substance abuse or withdrawal is suspected or the patient has an obstetric complication that could be related to substance abuse, such as placental abruption, spontane-

ous preterm labor, fetal demise, or severe growth restriction, a urine toxicology screen should be performed. Most illicit drugs also can be detected in blood and saliva, but for a much shorter interval after the last use.

If acute substance abuse is suspected at the time of delivery, urine toxicology screening is important. Ideally, the maternal urine specimen should be obtained immediately upon admission and before the patient has received any medication. If the maternal screening result is positive or if it was inadvertently omitted, a neonatal urine specimen should be sent for screening as soon as possible (19). Depending on the identity of the drug and the timing of its use, the urine screen may not accurately reflect maternal substance abuse. Although false-positive results are unlikely with current assays, an unexpected result should be confirmed by the laboratory. It takes at least 6 hours for most drugs to be metabolized and excreted in urine, after which they are detectable for only a few hours to a few days. Thus, a negative initial blood or urine toxicology screening result does not rule out drug use if clinical suspicion is high. Testing of a hair sample can detect use of illicit substances at any time in the past 90 days, but results usually take several days to return. Table 1 lists current drugs of abuse and the length of time they can be detected in urine and blood.

Women on methadone maintenance should continue to receive it at the usual daily oral dose during labor; if it must be given parenterally, the dose should be halved. Methadone users may need additional narcotics for pain relief, at higher doses than usual because of drug tolerance. There are no data to support the belief that giving a methadone user narcotics for pain relief will result in a relapse. All substance abusers should be kept comfortable during labor. Addicts who receive adequate analgesia have infants with better Apgar scores, whereas addicts who go into withdrawal during labor are more likely to have a compromised fetus because of increased oxygen consumption by both mother and fetus and other factors (20). Regional anesthesia is preferred because it does not increase the risk of neonatal depression. If general anesthesia is needed, the narcotized patient generally requires less barbiturate during induction. Unexplained hypotension during general anesthesia may be a sign of opioid withdrawal, and the patient should respond positively to opioid administration.

Intervention

The following section discusses the intervention techniques used in the management of substance abuse. Many of these modalities can be modified and used interchangeably for all substances of abuse.

Alcohol

No discrete cause for alcoholism has ever been identified. Current data indicate that alcohol addiction devel-

Table 1. Limits of Drug Detection in Urine and Blood Samples According to Length of Time From Last Use

Substance	Urine	Blood
Alcohol	12 hours	12 hours
Amphetamine (except methamphetamine)	1–2 days	12 hours
Methamphetamine	1–2 days	1–3 days
MDMA (Ecstasy)	1–2 days	25 hours
Barbiturates (except phenobarbital)	Short acting: 2 days Long acting: 1–3 weeks	1–2 days 2–3 weeks
Phenobarbital		4–7 days
Benzodiazepines	Therapeutic use: 3 days Chronic use: 4–6 weeks	6–48 hours
Cannabis	Single use: 2–7 days Prolonged use: 1–2 months	Infrequent use: 2–3 days Frequent use: up to 2 weeks
Cocaine	2–4 days	24 hours
Codeine	2 days	12 hours
Cotinine (metabolite of cigarettes)	2–4 days	2–4 days
Morphine	2 days	6 hours
Heroin	2 days	6 hours
LSD	1–3 days	0–3 hours
Methadone	3 days	24 hours
PCP	Single use: 14 days Chronic use: up to 30 days	1–3 days

Abbreviations: LSD indicates lysergic acid diethylamide; MDMA, 3,4-methylenedioxymethamphetamine; PCP, phencyclidine.

ops as the result of a combination of genetic factors; psychologic problems, such as depression, anxiety, low self esteem, and unresolved conflicts; social acceptance and promotion of alcohol use; peer pressure; and a stressful environment or lifestyle. Successful abstinence and ongoing sobriety are most likely if these factors are addressed through major lifestyle changes, psychiatric therapy, and ongoing social support. Alcoholics Anonymous and the 12 Steps programs are self help groups that model abstinence and provide emotional support for addicts who wish to stay sober and are examples of the kind of support programs that are essential to ongoing recovery (21). Although one study suggested that Alcoholics Anonymous may be more successful in helping patients to accept and stay in treatment than other programs, a meta-analysis of eight trials involving Alcoholics Anonymous and other support groups showed that most programs have similar success rates (22).

Pharmacologic therapies for alcohol abuse include the use of disulfiram, naltrexone, and acamprosate. Disulfiram prevents the liver from fully metabolizing alcohol, causing acetaldehyde to accumulate. If disulfiram is taken and alcohol use continues, the increasing acetaldehyde will result in nausea, flushing, headache, hypertension, and chest pain. During pregnancy, if disulfiram is taken and alcohol use continues, the risk of fetal alcohol syndrome is increased, most likely because acetaldehyde is embryotoxic or potentiates the embryotoxic effects of ethanol. Naltrexone and acamprosate work by different mechanisms to decrease the pleasurable reinforcing effects of alcohol. There is not sufficient data about either naltrexone or acamprosate to assure their safety for use during pregnancy.

Opioids

Intervention for opioid addiction is most successful when psychosocial support is combined with pharmacologic therapy (23). In fact, a meta-analysis of five randomized trials of various psychosocial interventions for opioid addiction found no evidence that psychosocial support alone is effective (24). Methadone has been used safely in pregnancy for many years, and although it readily crosses the placenta and binds to fetal tissues, it does not appear to have any long-lasting adverse effects on the fetus and in fact is associated with improved compliance. Although maternal methadone treatment is associated with higher birth weights and better neonatal outcome (20), it also may result in a more prolonged neonatal withdrawal syndrome than occurs after prenatal exposure to heroin (25). However, there does not appear to be a correlation between the incidence and severity of neonatal withdrawal symptoms and the maternal methadone dose (5). Thus, limiting the maternal dose out of concern for neonatal well-being is not necessary, and the dose should be titrated to reduce maternal symptoms. Hospitalization may be required for initiation of methadone maintenance, although outpatient treatment of pregnant addicts has been described (26). Buprenorphine is an opioid analgesic similar to morphine but with greater potency, and naltrexone is an opioid antagonist. Because buprenorphine does not cross the placenta as readily as methadone, it may result in less fetal exposure. All three drugs can cause neonatal abstinence syndrome.

Smoking

Interventions for smoking include counseling on how to stop smoking, behavioral or cognitive therapy, peer group support, hypnosis, and acupuncture. In a review of 64 trials of interventions to reduce smoking during pregnancy it was concluded that most interventions do reduce the number of women who continue to smoke or reduce the number of cigarettes smoked per day (27). If prior attempts to quit smoking without medications have failed, prescription of smoking cessation medications may be necessary. There are a wide variety of nicotine replacement systems available as well as drugs that have been shown to reduce the symptoms of nicotine withdrawal.

Because cigarette smoke contains hundreds of harmful chemicals, including reproductive toxins, the use of a nicotine replacement system, although not ideal, probably poses fewer risks than continued smoking during pregnancy (28). Results from a recent trial in which pregnant smokers received individualized behavioral counseling along with either nicotine gum or placebo showed that, although the nicotine gum did not significantly reduce the number of women who continued to smoke, it did significantly reduce the number of cigarettes smoked per day (29). Importantly, infants of women who received nicotine instead of placebo had a ninefold lower incidence of low birth weight and one half the rate of preterm birth. In addition, the number of serious adverse pregnancy outcomes was one third lower in the nicotine group. Nicotine gum or lozenges, which provide episodic nicotine, should be tried before the nicotine patch, which provides continuous nicotine. Most nicotine gum products contain 2–4 mg of nicotine per piece, whereas one cigarette delivers approximately 11 mg of nicotine. Heavy smokers will need gum with 4 mg of nicotine, whereas lighter smokers can use the 2-mg dose. One piece of gum should last 1–2 hours. Users should be advised to chew the gum slowly until they note a peppery taste, then position it between the cheek and the gum until it no longer produces a tingle. The recommended daily dose is 9–12 pieces of gum per day, with a maximum of 20–30 pieces per day (30).

Patients should be warned that if they use nicotine replacement therapy, especially the nicotine patch, and continue to smoke they are at risk of developing nicotine toxicity. Nicotine toxicity is heralded by nausea, abdominal pain, vomiting, diarrhea, diaphoresis, flushing, dizziness, hearing and vision disturbances, weakness, palpitations, hypotension, and altered perception (30).

Other drugs used for smoking cessation include bupropion, clonidine, nortriptyline, and selective serotonin reuptake inhibitors (30). Bupropion is an aminoketone antidepressant medication with a low incidence of side effects, which is believed to antagonize nicotine receptors in the brain and block nicotine's reinforcing effects. It can be used as a first-line drug, as an alternative for patients who dislike or have not had success using nicotine replacement, or in combination with nicotine replacement. Clonidine also has been used successfully for smoking cessation, and appears to suppress the anxiety, irritability, and restlessness that accompany smoking cessation and to decrease both craving and withdrawal symptoms. Use of nortriptyline, a tricyclic antidepressant, also reduces withdrawal symptoms, and selective serotonin reuptake inhibitors have been shown to eliminate the positive and negative mood swings associated with smoking cessation. Neither use of bupropion nor use of nortriptyline have been associated with adverse fetal effects. In small studies, the use of selective serotonin reuptake inhibitors has been associated with an increased risk of cardiac defects, and use after 20 weeks of gestation has been associated with an increased risk of neonatal pulmonary hypertension, whereas other studies have found no such effects. Use of this drug should be avoided during pregnancy unless the benefits clearly outweigh the risks.

References

1. Substance Abuse and Mental Health Services Administration. Results from the 2008 National Survey on Drug Use and Health: national findings. Rockville (MD): SAMHSA; 2009. Available at: http://www.oas.samhsa.gov/nsduh/2k8nsduh/2k8Results.pdf. Retrieved October 15, 2009.

2. Clark KA, Dawson S, Martin SL. The effect of implementing a more comprehensive screening for substance use among pregnant women in North Carolina. Matern Child Health J 1999;3:161–6.

3. Coelho R, Rangel R, Ramos E, Martins A, Prata J, Barros H. Depression and the severity of substance abuse. Psychopathology 2000;33:103–9.

4. Krantz MJ, Martin J, Stimmel B, Mehta D, Haigney MC. QTc interval screening in methadone treatment. Ann Intern Med 2009;150:387–95.

5. Berghella V, Lim PJ, Hill MK, Cherpes J, Chennat J, Kaltenbach K. Maternal methadone dose and neonatal withdrawal. Am J Obstet Gynecol 2003;189:312–7.

6. Dashe JS, Sheffield JS, Olscher DA, Todd SJ, Jackson GL, Wendel GD. Relationship between maternal methadone

dosage and neonatal withdrawal. Obstet Gynecol 2002; 100:1244–9.

7. Smith L, Yonekura ML, Wallace T, Berman N, Kuo J, Berkowitz C. Effects of prenatal methamphetamine exposure on fetal growth and drug withdrawal symptoms in infants born at term. J Dev Behav Pediatr 2003;24:17–23.

8. Coupey SM. Barbiturates. Pediatr Rev 1997;18:260–4; quiz 265.

9. Reinisch JM, Sanders SA, Mortensen EL, Rubin DB. In utero exposure to phenobarbital and intelligence deficits in adult men. JAMA 1995;274:1518–25.

10. Murray JB. Phencyclidine (PCP): a dangerous drug, but useful in schizophrenia research. J Psychol 2002;136:319–27.

11. Rahbar F, Fomufod A, White D, Westney LS. Impact of intrauterine exposure to phencyclidine (PCP) and cocaine on neonates. J Natl Med Assoc 1993;85:349–52.

12. Khan A, Levy P, DeHorn S, Miller W, Compton S. Predictors of mortality in patients with delirium tremens. Acad Emerg Med 2008;15:788–90.

13. McKeon A, Frye MA, Delanty N. The alcohol withdrawal syndrome. J Neurol Neurosurg Psychiatry 2008;79:854–62.

14. Aggarwal N, Sawhney H, Vasishta K, Dhiman RK, Chawla Y. Non-cirrhotic portal hypertension in pregnancy. Int J Gynaecol Obstet 2001;72:1–7.

15. Hall W, Solowij N. Adverse effects of cannabis. Lancet 1998;352:1611–6.

16. de Moraes Barros MC, Guinsburg R, de Araujo Peres C, Mitsuhiro S, Chalem E, Laranjeira RR. Exposure to marijuana during pregnancy alters neurobehavior in the early neonatal period. J Pediatr 2006;149:781–7.

17. Fried PA. Prenatal exposure to tobacco and marijuana: effects during pregnancy, infancy, and early childhood. Clin Obstet Gynecol 1993;36:319–37.

18. Abou-Saleh MT, Foley S. Prevalence and incidence of hepatitis C in drug users: a review. Addict Disord Their Treat 2008;7:190–8.

19. Halstead AC, Godolphin W, Lockitch G, Segal S. Timing of specimen collection is crucial in urine screening of drug dependent mothers and newborns. Clin Biochem 1988;21:59–61.

20. Archie C. Methadone in the management of narcotic addiction in pregnancy. Curr Opin Obstet Gynecol 1998; 10:435–40.

21. Lui S, Terplan M, Smith Erica J. Psychosocial interventions for women enrolled in alcohol treatment during pregnancy. Cochrane Database of Systematic Reviews 2008, Issue 3. Art. No.: CD006753. DOI: 10.1002/14651858. CD006753.pub2; 10.1002/14651858.CD006753.pub2.

22. Ferri M, Amato L, Davoli M. Alcoholics Anonymous and other 12-step programmes for alcohol dependence. Cochrane Database of Systematic Reviews 2006, Issue 3. Art. No.: CD005032. DOI: 10.1002/14651858.CD005032. pub2; 10.1002/14651858.CD005032.pub2.

23. Amato L, Minozzi S, Davoli M, Vecchi S, Ferri M, Mayet S. Psychosocial and pharmacological treatments versus pharmacological treatments for opioid detoxification. Cochrane Database of Systematic Reviews 2008, Issue 4. Art. No.: CD005031. DOI: 10.1002/14651858.CD005031. pub3; 10.1002/14651858.CD005031.pub3.

24. Mayet S, Farrell M, Ferri Marica MF, Amato L, Davoli M. Psychosocial treatment for opiate abuse and dependence. Cochrane Database of Systematic Reviews 2004, Issue 4. Art. No.: CD004330. DOI: 10.1002/14651858.CD004330. pub2; 10.1002/14651858.CD004330.pub2.

25. Binder T, Vavrinkova B. Prospective randomised comparative study of the effect of buprenorphine, methadone and heroin on the course of pregnancy, birthweight of newborns, early postpartum adaptation and course of the neonatal abstinence syndrome (NAS) in women followed up in the outpatient department. Neuro Endocrinol Lett 2008;29:80–6.

26. Terplan M, Lui S. Psychosocial interventions for pregnant women in outpatient illicit drug treatment programs compared to other interventions. Cochrane Database of Systematic Reviews 2007, Issue 4. Art. No.: CD006037. DOI: 10.1002/14651858.CD006037.pub2; 10.1002/14651858. CD006037.pub2.

27. Lumley J, Chamberlain C, Dowswell T, Oliver S, Oakley L, Watson L. Interventions for promoting smoking cessation during pregnancy. Cochrane Database of Systematic Reviews 2009, Issue 3. Art. No.: CD001055. DOI: 10.1002/14651858. CD001055.pub3; 10.1002/14651858.CD001055.pub3.

28. Dempsey DA, Benowitz NL. Risks and benefits of nicotine to aid smoking cessation in pregnancy. Drug Saf 2001;24:277–322.

29. Oncken C, Dornelas E, Greene J, Sankey H, Glasmann A, Feinn R, et al. Nicotine gum for pregnant smokers: a randomized controlled trial. Obstet Gynecol 2008;112:859–67.

30. Frishman WH, Mitta W, Kupersmith A, Ky T. Nicotine and non-nicotine smoking cessation pharmacotherapies. Cardiol Rev 2006;14:57–73.

Teratogenic Exposures

Katharine D. Wenstrom

Major congenital anomalies are observed in approximately 3% of all births. It is believed that 5% of these—affecting approximately 1 in 670 liveborn infants—result from maternal exposure to drugs or environmental chemicals. Only approximately 1% of teratogen-related anomalies can be attributed to the use of pharmaceutic agents; the bulk result from maternal ethanol use.

The most important determinants of the developmental toxicity of an agent are timing, dose, and fetal susceptibility. Many agents have teratogenic effects only if taken while the susceptible fetal organ system is forming. For example, thalidomide produces phocomelia only if taken between the 27th day and 33rd day after conception. Similarly, an agent suspected of causing a cardiac defect would have to be taken during the critical period of heart development, from 20 days to 50 days after fertilization, to have an adverse effect. By extension, the same drug taken 60 days after fertilization would be considered safe. Other agents are teratogenic only at certain doses. Most X-ray exposures (ambient solar radiation or diagnostic X-rays) have no effect on the fetus, whereas high-dose exposures, such as those encountered in cancer radiation therapy, might result in fetal abnormalities. Additionally, the fetal tissue must be susceptible. Radioactive iodine, I 131, can damage the fetal thyroid when the organ is fully formed and functional. Thus, I 131 given at less than 10 weeks of gestation, before thyroid development is complete, is unlikely to have an effect.

Susceptibility also is influenced by the genetic makeup of both the fetus and the mother. Genetic variability in susceptibility to developmental toxicity is attributed to differences in the absorption, biotransformation, or elimination of drugs and chemicals. These processes are controlled by enzymes with activities that differ among individuals, a difference called pharmacogenetic variation. For example, variations in the gene encoding epoxide hydrolase, an enzyme required for metabolism of the anticonvulsant phenytoin, is believed to explain why major malformations occur in some exposed fetuses but not in others.

It is now recognized that some teratogens produce functional rather than structural abnormalities. Although exposure to certain agents during first-trimester organogenesis can result in anatomic anomalies, exposure later in pregnancy may cause functional problems that are less readily identified. For example, first-trimester exposure to alcohol can result in a specific embryopathy, which includes distinct facial anomalies, microcephaly, joint contractures, and cardiac defects, whereas exposure during the second and third trimesters can result in learning and behavioral abnormalities that might not be detected before school age. Because infants exposed to potential teratogens are rarely if ever monitored throughout their lives, and exposure-related functional abnormalities are thus unlikely to be detected, the safety of any drug can never be completely ensured.

The following section discusses examples of agents that are believed to be teratogenic and is not intended to be exhaustive. For additional current information sources on these and other agents, see Appendix A.

Drugs and Chemicals

Most drugs commonly used during pregnancy (eg, aspirin, acetaminophen, metronidazole, caffeine, and aspartame) have not been associated with an increased risk of congenital anomalies at ordinary exposure levels. Some agents, however, increase the risk of congenital malformations even under ordinary dosing conditions.

Sedatives

Once marketed as a sedative–hypnotic, thalidomide was withdrawn when its use during pregnancy was associated with severe anomalies in 20% of exposed fetuses. The most striking abnormalities were severe upper and lower limb reduction defects known as phocomelia and other abnormalities involving the ears, bowel musculature, kidneys, and heart. This agent has been reintroduced for treatment of the skin manifestations of leprosy. The manufacturer has instituted an elaborate system of controls designed to prevent treatment of pregnant women. The effectiveness of these controls remains to be demonstrated.

Antidepressants

The antidepressants most commonly used by reproductive age women are the selective serotonin reuptake inhibitors (SSRIs). Although there have been reports of anatomic defects and lower birth weight or earlier birth (but not fetal growth restriction or preterm birth) in children exposed prenatally to SSRIs, there also have been many studies in which no such associations were found. This discrepancy is probably related in part to the fact that most of the studies of antenatal SSRI use have methodologic problems (1) and that the absolute risk is small (2). Fetal exposure late in pregnancy has been associated with transient neonatal abstinence symptoms, such as jitteriness, mild respiratory distress, transient tachypnea, weak cry, and poor tone. Before prescribing an SSRI during pregnancy, the relative risks should be balanced against the benefits for each patient and treatment should be individualized. Patients for whom the benefits of SSRIs outweigh the risks are those with an increased risk of relapse during pregnancy if medication is withdrawn. These include patients with a long history (longer than 5 years) of major depressive illness and a history of recurrent relapses (3).

Antihypertensive Agents

Angiotensin-converting enzyme inhibitors are used in the treatment of hypertension and other cardiovascular disorders. Their use during pregnancy can cause severe fetal hypotension and thus hypoperfusion of the fetal kidney, leading to renal ischemia, renal tubular dysgenesis, and anuria. Use in the first trimester has been associated with fetal limb shortening and with maldevelopment of the calvaria, a structure formed from membranous bone that requires extensive vascularity and high oxygen tension for growth. Exposure during the second or third trimesters can result in oligohydramnios, leading to limb contractures, pulmonary hypoplasia, and, sometimes, fetal death. Similar problems have been seen after use of angiotensin receptor blockers.

Chemotherapeutic Agents

Chemotherapeutic agents are of concern because of their mechanisms of action (Table 2) and the fact that

virtually all of them cross the placenta and reach the fetus to some extent. The malignancies most commonly associated with pregnancy are cancer of the genital tract, breast cancer, and malignant melanoma, and all of them have been treated during pregnancy. The fetal effects of most chemotherapeutic agents are related directly to gestational age, with vulnerability decreasing as gestational age increases. Although data on the first-trimester effects of specific agents are sparse because treatment at this time generally is avoided if the patient does not desire pregnancy interruption, available reports and results of some research indicate that first-trimester chemotherapy increases the risk of spontaneous abortions and fetal demise and major malformations in surviving fetuses. In the second and third trimesters, exposure to most agents usually results only in intrauterine growth restriction or leads to iatrogenic preterm delivery, although the fetal eyes, genitalia, and hematopoietic and central nervous systems remain vulnerable to drug effects (4).

Anti-infectives

Although there are a wide variety of antibiotics that have varying effects when used during pregnancy, most are not considered teratogenic. Antibiotics to be avoided during pregnancy if possible include tetracyclines, which have been associated with staining of deciduous teeth; sulfonamides, which displace bilirubin from protein binding sites and may result in hyperbilirubinemia; and

Table 2. Classes of Chemotherapeutic Agents and Their Mechanisms of Action

Class	Examples of Agents	Mechanism of Action	Use
Antimetabolites	5-fluorouracil, 6-mercatopurine, methotrexate, and cytarabine	Inhibit DNA and RNA synthesis, inhibit nucleic acid synthesis, and block folic acid	Treatment of breast cancer, gastrointestinal malignancies, leukemia, lymphoma, and trophoblastic disease
Alkylating agents	Busulfan, cyclophosphamide, and dacarbazine	Prevent cell division by cross-linking strands of DNA	Treatment of leukemia, lymphoma, breast cancer, and ovarian cancer
Antibiotics	Daunorubicin, doxorubicin, and epirubicin	Interfere with cell division by interposing between DNA strands	Treatment of leukemia, lymphoma, and breast cancer
Alkaloids	Vincristine and vinblastine	Prevent mitosis by binding protein that forms mitotic spindle	Treatment of breast cancer, lymphoma, and choriocarcinoma
Other	Cisplatin	Binds to and cross-links DNA	
	Tamoxifen	Acts as estrogen-receptor antagonist	
	Taxol	Inhibits mitosis	
	Carboplatin	Interacts with DNA (similar to alkylating agents)	
	Monoclonal antibodies	Enhance cytolytic mechanisms against tumor cells, inhibit cell cycle progression, promote apoptosis, and disrupt angiogenesis	

ciprofloxacin, which is toxic to developing cartilage in experimental animals. As with any drug, the risk–benefit ratio should be carefully considered on an individual basis before prescribing an antibiotic during pregnancy.

Anticoagulants

Warfarin and coumarin inhibit the synthesis of vitamin K-dependent coagulation factors. Their use during pregnancy can produce major and minor congenital anomalies in as many as 25% of exposed fetuses. Fetuses exposed during the first trimester can develop warfarin embryopathy, which typically includes a hypoplastic nose and midface and epiphyseal stippling. These defects occur because warfarin inhibits the posttranslational carboxylation of coagulation proteins called osteocalcins. Exposure during the second and third trimesters can cause hemorrhage that results in scarring of developing tissues, leading to uncoordinated and abnormal tissue growth. The resulting fetopathy is characterized by intrauterine growth restriction and asymmetric limb defects as well as midline central nervous system anomalies, such as agenesis of the corpus callosum, Dandy–Walker syndrome, and midline cerebellar atrophy, as well as optic atrophy and microcephaly. Use of heparin, including low molecular weight heparin, does not increase the risk of congenital anomalies because it does not cross the placenta.

Anticonvulsants

Use of most older anticonvulsant medications increases the incidence of congenital anomalies, especially cardiac defects and orofacial clefts, in exposed fetuses (see Neurologic Diseases). Fetal exposure to phenytoin can be associated with abnormal facies, cleft lip or palate, microcephaly, growth deficiency, hypoplastic nails and distal phalanges, and mild to moderate mental and developmental delay. Of exposed offspring, 10% have all these abnormalities—the full fetal hydantoin syndrome—and 30% have some feature of it. The mechanism by which phenytoin (diphenylhydantoin) use causes these defects involves its metabolism. Phenytoin is metabolized to oxidative intermediates called arene oxides or epoxides, which are then detoxified by cytoplasmic epoxide hydrolase. Because fetal epoxide hydrolase activity is weak, oxidative intermediates build up in fetal tissues where they have dose-related mutagenic and toxic effects. A mutation in the gene for epoxide hydrolase that makes it even less functional has been reported. Fetuses that inherit this mutation are at highest risk to have the full hydantoin syndrome. Valproic acid causes neural tube defects in 4–5% of exposed fetuses, usually involving the lumbosacral area. Carbamazepine use has been associated with neural tube defects in some reports and with abnormalities similar to fetal hydantoin syndrome. Use of phenobarbital and lamotrigine reduces folic acid levels, which could increase the risk of neural tube defects and other malformations associated with decreased folate, and topiramate use has caused defects or adverse pregnancy outcomes in all animals tested.

Several newer agents, however, appear to be safe for use during pregnancy. Use of gabapentin and felbamate has not been associated with the same developmental toxicity in animal experiments as has use of the older medications, and no increase in congenital anomalies has been reported in exposed offspring. However, experience with the use of these medications during pregnancy is not yet as extensive as with the older drugs.

Immunosuppressants

Pregnancy after solid organ transplantation is becoming more common because of advances in transplantation surgery and improved immunosuppressant agents. Previously, infertile women with end-stage organ failure often become fertile again after transplantation, and many children with organ transplants are now reaching childbearing age. Pregnancy is most common after renal transplantation, but pregnancies after liver, liver–kidney, pancreas–kidney, pancreas, heart, heart–lung, and bowel transplantation have also been reported (5, 6).

Immunosuppressant agents are prescribed to prevent acute rejection, to treat acute episodes of rejection, and as part of maintenance regimens to provide long-term immunosuppression. Maintenance regimens with a combination of corticosteroids (prednisone), calcineurin inhibitors (cyclosporine and tacrolimus), antimetabolites (azathioprine), or macrolide antibiotics (tacrolimus) are used most often in pregnancy; most are considered safe, and the ideal doses associated with optimal pregnancy outcome are presented in Table 3 (7–9). The exception is the use of mycophenolic mofetil, which has been associated with orofacial abnormalities and microtia. For more information on effects of immunosuppressants on pregnancy outcome, see the section "Renal Disease."

Lithium

Although case reports and small retrospective series have suggested an association between antenatal lithium use and a rare fetal cardiac malformation called Ebstein anomaly, these data have been challenged. For example, in a Canadian multicenter study of lithium exposure during pregnancy, in which women taking lithium were monitored prospectively and confounding factors were carefully detailed, no increase in the incidence of birth defects and no association between lithium and any cardiac malformation was found. Considering all data, fetuses exposed to lithium probably experience a 0.14% increase in the risk of cardiac

Table 3. Common Immunosuppressive Agents Prescribed After Transplantation

Drug	Uses (Best Dose for Pregnancy)	Fetal or Neonatal Effects*
Corticosteroids: prednisone, prednisolone, and methylprednisolone	Maintenance or antirejection (prednisone, 15 mg/kg/d)	No risk of congenital anomalies[†], but risk of impaired fetal growth
Azathioprine	Maintenance (2 mg/kg/d)	No risk of congenital anomalies[†]
Cyclosporine A	Maintenance (5 mg/kg/d)	No risk of congenital anomalies[†]
Cyclosporine capsules	Maintenance	No risk of congenital anomalies[†]
Tacrolimus	Maintenance and antirejection	No risk of congenital anomalies[†], but risk of preterm birth, hypertension, and preeclampsia
Mycophenolate mofetil	Maintenance	Risk of spontaneous abortion, preterm birth, and congenital anomalies (microtia and facial clefts)
Sirolimus	Maintenance	No data in humans

*Data from www.reprotox.org

[†]Although data regarding use in humans indicate no increased risk of anomalies, much data are in the form of case reports and small series; therefore, the safety of these agents cannot be ensured.

defects. Exposure late in pregnancy also may produce neonatal lithium intoxication; symptoms include cyanosis, hypotonia, disturbances of cardiac rhythm, nephrogenic diabetes insipidus, goiter, and hypothyroidism. Because lithium crosses the placenta, maternal and fetal serum lithium levels are similar. The risk of toxicity can therefore be reduced by monitoring maternal lithium levels at term; reducing the dose, if possible, as term approaches; and keeping the patient well hydrated during labor. Breastfeeding infants have a serum lithium level that is approximately one fourth of the maternal serum level, thus monitoring the maternal lithium dose postpartum also should be considered.

Vitamin A and Its Congeners

The two forms of vitamin A found in nature are beta-carotene, a precursor of provitamin A, and preformed vitamin A or retinol. Beta-carotene is found in fruits and vegetables and has never been shown to cause birth defects. Vitamin A is found in many foods, especially animal liver, and also is included in vitamin supplements. Although one report associated intake of more than 10,000 international units of this nutrient per day during pregnancy with a significant risk of fetal renal and craniofacial anomalies, other studies have found no increase in adverse pregnancy outcome in women taking 25,000–50,000 international units per day (10, 11). However, given that the American diet is not deficient in vitamin A, it appears prudent to limit vitamin A supplementation to no more than 5,000 international units per day.

Isotretinoin (the 13-*cis* isomer of retinoic acid), an acne medication, is a vitamin A–like compound. Miscarriage is common after exposure during pregnancy,

and serious congenital anomalies occur at a rate that is 26 times higher than the background rate, affecting at least 35% of surviving exposed fetuses. The most commonly identified abnormalities are cardiac malformations, thymic agenesis, microphthalmia, hydrocephalus, cleft palate, deafness, and blindness. Because isotretinoin also can cause anotia, a defect that is otherwise exceedingly rare, it was not difficult to determine that isotretinoin is teratogenic. Neurobehavioral abnormalities have been described among surviving children.

Although currently not available in the United States, etretinate is an oral agent used to treat psoriasis. Case reports link the use of this agent to birth defects similar to those observed after prenatal exposure to isotretinoin. In contrast to isotretinoin, however, etretinate has been detected in the sera of patients for as long as 7 years after cessation of use, and fetal anomalies similar to those observed with isotretinoin use have been reported when conception occurred 18 months after discontinuing use of the drug. If possible, this drug should only be used in women who have completed childbearing.

Tretinoin (all-trans-retinoic acid) is a topical medication. Application of tretinoin to the skin results in little detectable systemic absorption. As a result, it does not increase the incidence of congenital anomalies.

Dietary Additives, Contaminants, and Herbal Remedies

Aspartame is used as an artificial sweetener. It is metabolized to aspartic acid, which does not cross the placenta; phenylalanine, which is normally metabolized in individuals who do not have phenylketonuria; and methanol, which is produced at levels lower than those found in an equivalent amount of fruit juice. It is thus not biologically plausible that aspartame is a teratogen, and no adverse effects of aspartame have been reported in human pregnancies. Women with phenylketonuria should be advised to avoid aspartame whether or not they are pregnant.

Mercury, although not a drug, is a known teratogen. The developing nervous system is particularly susceptible. Prenatal exposure to mercury results in a variety of defects ranging from developmental delay and mild neurologic abnormalities to microcephaly and severe brain damage (12). Mercury enters the ecosystem through industrial pollution, gets into surface water, and eventually reaches the ocean where it is absorbed by fish. Several varieties of large fish, including tuna, shark, king mackerel, and tilefish not only absorb mercury from the water but ingest it when they eat smaller fish and aquatic organisms. Women who eat these large fish ingest mercury as well. Although methyl mercury is metabolized and eventually eliminated from the body, the process is slow; the elimination half-life is 45–70 days. The U.S. Food and Drug Administration currently recommends that pregnant women refrain from eating large fish or at least consume no more than 12 ounces per week (6 ounces of white tuna or tuna steaks) (13). Albacore has been shown to be more toxic than chunk light tuna.

Because herbal remedies are not regulated as prescription or over-the-counter drugs, the identity and quantity of all ingredients are unknown, and there are virtually no studies of their teratogenic potential. Because it is not possible to assess their safety, pregnant women should be counseled to avoid these substances. Remedies containing substances with pharmaceutical properties that could theoretically have adverse fetal effects include black cohosh, which contains a chemical that acts like estrogen; garlic and willow barks, which have anticoagulant properties; gingko, which can interfere with the effects of monoamine oxydase inhibitors and has anticoagulant properties; real licorice, which has hypertensive and potassium-wasting effects; valerian, which intensifies the effects of prescription sleep aids; and ginseng, which interferes with monoamine oxydase inhibitors (for sources on detailed information on specific herbs, see Appendix A). Herbal remedies used as abortifacients also should be avoided; blue and black cohosh and pennyroyal appear to stimulate uterine musculature directly, and pennyroyal also can cause liver damage, renal failure, disseminated intravascular coagulation, and maternal death.

Radiation

Ionizing radiation exposure is universal; most radiation originates from beyond the earth's atmosphere, from the land, and from endogenous radionuclides. The total radiation exposure from these sources is approximately 0.00125 Gy (125 microrad) per year. Although radiation exposure has the potential to cause gene mutations, growth impairment, chromosome damage and malignancy, or even fetal death, large doses are required to produce discernible fetal effects. During the first 2 weeks after fertilization, exposure to 0.10 Gy (10 rad) is required to produce an effect. Because this is the "all or none" period, this level of exposure will either cause death ("all") or have no effect ("none"). In the first trimester, 0.25 Gy (25 rad) are required to produce detectable damage, and 1 Gy (100 rad) are required in later pregnancy. The recommended upper limit of exposure during pregnancy, 0.05 Gy (5 rad), is thus well below the level that could actually produce damage and well below the amount of radiation exposure resulting from diagnostic radiologic studies (Table 4).

The risks of radionuclide exposure during pregnancy depend on the agent used and the amount and kind of particle or wave emitted. Of the radionuclides in common use, only I 131 exposes the fetus to dangerous levels of radiation and only if the exposure occurs after 10 weeks of gestation, when I 131 is concentrated by the fetal thyroid and then ablates the gland. Before 10 weeks of gestation, the fetus is not at risk because the fetal thyroid is immature and incapable of concentrating iodine.

Electromagnetic radiation in the nonionizing spectrum includes radiofrequency and microwave radiation as well as visible light. Electronic appliances emit nonionizing radiation, but such exposures have not been shown to adversely affect fetal development. Magnetic resonance imaging results in high-level exposure to radiofrequency radiation, and also appears to have no adverse effect on the fetus (14).

Recreational Drugs

The use of recreational drugs during pregnancy can have adverse fetal effects. Patient education about the possible deleterious effects of drug use is appropriate during preconception and prenatal visits (see the sections "Preconception Care" and "Substance Abuse").

References

1. Ter Horst PG, Jansman FG, van Lingen RA, Smit JP, de Jong-van den Berg LT, Brouwers JR. Pharmacological aspects of neonatal antidepressant withdrawal. Obstet Gynecol Surv 2008;63:267–79.

2. Use of psychiatric medications during pregnancy and lactation. ACOG Practice Bulletin No. 92. American College of Obstetricians and Gynecologists. Obstet Gynecol 2008; 111:1001–20.

3. Cohen LS, Altshuler LL, Harlow BL, Nonacs R, Newport DJ, Viguera AC, et al. Relapse of major depression during pregnancy in women who maintain or discontinue antidepressant treatment [published erratum appears in JAMA 2006;296:170]. JAMA 2006;295:499–507.

Table 4. Estimated Fetal Exposure From Some Common Radiologic Procedures

Procedure	Fetal Exposure
CT scan of abdomen and lumbar spine	3.5 rad
Barium enema or small bowel series	2–4 rad
Intravenous pyelography (5 views)	686–1,398 millirad*
CT scan of head or chest	Less than 1 rad
Spiral CT of the thorax (pitch 1 or greater)	Less than 1 rad
CT pelvimetry	250 millirad
Hip film (2 views)	103–213 millirad
Abdominal film (2 views)	122–245 millirad
Lumbo-sacral spine film (3 views)	168–359 millirad
Ventilation–perfusion scan with technetium 99m and xenon gas	50 millirad
Mammography (4 views)	7–20 millirad
Chest X-ray (2 views)	0.02–0.07 millirad
Skull films (4 views)	Less than 0.05 millirad
Magnetic resonance imaging	None

Abbreviation: CT indicates computed tomography.

*Amount of exposure depends on the number of films obtained

Data from Cunningham FG, Leveno KJ, Bloom SL, Hauth JC, Gilstrap LC 3rd, Wenstrom KD. General considerations and maternal evaluation. In: Williams obstetrics. 22nd ed. New York (NY): McGraw-Hill; 2005. p. 9788.

Adapted from Guidelines for diagnostic imaging during pregnancy. ACOG Committee Opinion No. 299. American College of Obstetricians and Gynecologists. Obstet Gynecol 2004;104:647–51.

4. Cardonick E, Iacobucci A. Use of chemotherapy during human pregnancy. Lancet Oncol 2004;5:283–91.

5. Mastrobattista JM, Gomez-Lobo V. Pregnancy after solid organ transplantation. Society for Maternal-Fetal Medicine. Obstet Gynecol 2008;112:919–32.

6. Coscia LA, Constantinescu S, Moritz MJ, Radomski JS, Gaughan WJ, McGrory CH, et al. Report from the National Transplantation Pregnancy Registry (NTPR): outcomes of pregnancy after transplantation. National Transplantation Pregnancy Registry. Clin Transpl 2007;29–42.

7. Albengres E, Le Louet H, Tillement JP. Immunosuppressive drugs and pregnancy: experimental and clinical data. Transplant Proc 1997;29:2461–6.

8. Sifontis NM, Coscia LA, Constantinescu S, Lavelanet AF, Moritz MJ, Armenti VT. Pregnancy outcomes in solid organ transplant recipients with exposure to mycophenolate mofetil or sirolimus. Transplantation 2006;82:1698–702.

9. Perez-Aytes A, Ledo A, Boso V, Saenz P, Roma E, Poveda JL, et al. In utero exposure to mycophenolate mofetil: a characteristic phenotype? Am J Med Genet A 2008;146A:1–7.

10. Miller RK, Hendrickx AG, Mills JL, Hummler H, Wiegand UW. Periconceptional vitamin A use: how much is teratogenic? Reprod Toxicol 1998;12:75–88.

11. Mastroiacovo P, Mazzone T, Addis A, Elephant E, Carlier P, Vial T, et al. High vitamin A intake in early pregnancy and major malformations: a multicenter prospective controlled study. Teratology 1999;59:7–11.

12. Clarkson TW. The three modern faces of mercury. Environ Health Perspect 2002;110 Suppl 1:11–23.

13. Food and Drug Administration. An important message for pregnant women and women of childbearing age who may become pregnant about the risks of mercury in fish. FDA CFSAN Conumer Advisory. Silver Spring (MD): FDA; 2001. Available at: http://www.fda.gov/OHRMS/DOCKETS/ac/02/briefing/3872_Advisory%203.pdf. Retrieved October 15, 2009.

14. Roberts MD, Lange RC, McCarthy SM. Fetal anatomy with magnetic resonance imaging. Magn Reson Imaging 1995;13:645–9.

Ultrasonography

William H. Barth Jr

Ultrasound examination has become an integral part of obstetric practice. Most U.S. women have at least one ultrasound examination during their pregnancies. The American College of Obstetricians and Gynecologists (the College) now suggests that the benefits and limitations of ultrasound screening should be discussed with all patients and that if an informed patient requests such an examination, it is reasonable to honor that request (1).

Types of Examinations

Collaborating with the American College of Radiology (ACR) and the American Institute of Ultrasound in Medicine (AIUM), the College has endorsed a standard set of terms to describe the types of obstetric ultrasound exam-inations. These include the terms "standard" (also called "basic"), "limited," and "specialized" (also called "detailed") (1).

Standard Obstetric Ultrasound Examination

A standard obstetric ultrasound examination in the second or third trimester includes an evaluation of the fetal presentation, amniotic fluid volume, cardiac activity, placental position, fetal biometry, and fetal number, plus an anatomic survey. The components of this anatomic survey are shown in Box 8. The maternal cervix and adnexa also should be assessed. When factors, such as fetal position, maternal body habitus or maternal abdominal scarring, preclude visualization of these components, the report of the examination should document these technical limitations.

Limited Obstetric Ultrasound Examination

A limited obstetric ultrasound examination is performed to answer a specific question. Examples include confirmation of fetal cardiac activity, determination of fetal position, amniotic fluid volume, or placental location. Ultrasound guidance for procedures, such as amniocentesis, chorionic villous biopsy or external cephalic version, also is considered a limited obstetric ultrasound examination. Brief or limited examinations may be appropriate during emergencies. Depending on the indication, a limited examination should be followed by a standard examination unless the patient previously had such an examination in the second or third trimester.

Specialized Ultrasound Obstetric Examination

A specialized examination is performed when an abnormality is suspected on the basis of medical history, laboratory test results, or the results of other ultrasound examinations. A detailed practice guideline for the conduct of antepartum obstetric ultrasound examination has been jointly developed by the AIUM, ACR, and the College.

Box 8

Essential Elements of Standard Examination of Fetal Anatomy

- Head, Face, and Neck*
  - Cerebellum
  - Choroid plexus
  - Cisterna magna
  - Lateral cerebral ventricles
  - Midline falx
  - Cavum septi pellucidi
  - Upper lip
- Chest–Heart (The basic cardiac examination includes a four-chamber view of the fetal heart. As part of the cardiac screening examination, an attempt should be made, if technically feasible, to view the outflow tracts.)
- Abdomen
  - Stomach (presence, size, and situs)
  - Kidneys
  - Bladder
  - Umbilical cord insertion side into the fetal abdomen
  - Umbilical cord vessel number
- Spine—cervical, thoracic, lumbar, and sacral spine
- Extremities—legs and arms (presence or absence)
- Sex—medically indicated in low-risk pregnancies only for evaluation of multiple gestations

*A measurement of the nuchal fold may be helpful during a specific gestational age to suggest an increased risk of aneuploidy.

American College of Radiology. Practice guideline for the performance of obstetrical ultrasound. In: ACR practice guidelines and technical standards, 2007. Reston (VA): ACR; 2007. Available at: http://www.acr.org/Secondary MainMenuCategories/quality_safety/guidelines/us/us_obstetrical.aspx. Retrieved October 15, 2009.

Specialized ultrasound examinations generally are performed by physicians with advanced training in ultrasonography, such as maternal–fetal medicine specialists or radiologists and obstetricians with similar training and experience in consultative fetal imaging. Such physicians often are referred to as sonologists in contrast with specially trained and certified technicians who are referred to as sonographers. Whereas sonographers can assist in performing the ultrasound examination, obtaining images, and documenting reports, only licensed physicians (sonologists) can independently interpret the results of these ultrasound examinations. Both, the AIUM and the ACR offer ultrasound facility accreditation. Accreditation by these bodies requires a comprehensive review of the quality of ultrasound studies, equipment, reporting, image management and archiving, and the qualifications of the sonographers and sonologists.

Coding

Coding for reimbursement is guided by the components and purpose of the specific ultrasound examination (Table 5). Although both the standard obstetric ultrasound examination (code 76805) and the detailed obstetric ultrasound examination (code 76811) include a fetal anatomic survey, the detailed examination requires an additional technological sophistication and imaging expertise and is expected to be rare outside of a consultative fetal imaging practice (2). It is intended that only one detailed examination (code 76811) is appropriate during a pregnancy unless the patient is referred to another consultative fetal imaging practice for a second opinion

or is transferred to a tertiary care center in anticipation of delivery of an anomalous fetus. Both, the College and the Society for Maternal–Fetal Medicine, offer additional guidance for coding obstetric ultrasound examinations (see Appendix A). Indications for first-trimester obstetric ultrasonography are listed in Box 9 and indications for second-trimester and third-trimester obstetric ultrasonography are listed in Box 10. First-trimester and second-trimester ultrasound screening for aneuploidy is addressed in the section "Prenatal Diagnosis of Genetic Disorders."

Current Developments

A number of important developments in the use of obstetrics ultrasonography have occurred since the previous edition of *Precis: Obstetrics*. The remainder of this section will review some of these developments, including the ultrasound diagnosis of placenta accreta, the use of transvaginal ultrasonography to assess cervical length, traditional and Doppler ultrasonography for the fetus with growth restriction or at risk for anemia, and three-dimensional and four-dimensional ultrasonography and the concept of prudent use.

Ultrasonography for the Detection of Placenta Accreta and Placenta Percreta

Especially when unanticipated, placenta accreta and placenta percreta can be life threatening for a pregnant woman. Anticipation of a placenta accreta or placenta percreta may allow advanced surgical planning or possibly transfer to a center with the personnel and blood

Table 5. Types of Ultrasound Examinations

Type of Examination	CPT Code*	Description of Use
First trimester (less than 14 weeks of gestation)	76801	Fetal and maternal evaluation, transabdominal approach, singleton gestation
Standard obstetric ultrasonography (14 weeks of gestation or more), also known as "basic obstetric ultrasonography"	76805	Fetal and maternal evaluation, transabdominal approach; includes anatomy survey, singleton gestation
Detailed obstetric ultrasonography, also known as "specialized obstetric ultrasonography" (in some centers "Level II" or "Comprehensive" obstetric ultrasonography)	76811	Includes detailed fetal anatomic examination, singleton gestation
Limited	76815	Focused brief examination of fetal heartbeat, placental location, fetal position, or qualitative amniotic fluid volume, or all of these items
Follow-up	76816	Follow-up examination for reevaluation of previously examined fetus, singleton gestation
Transvaginal	76817	Transvaginal examination of uterus during pregnancy

Abbreviation: CPT indicates *Current Procedural Terminology*.

*CPT codes and *International Classification of Diseases, Ninth Revision, Clinical Modification* codes are subject to change.

Box 9

Indications for First-Trimester Ultrasonography

- To confirm the presence of an intrauterine pregnancy
- To evaluate a suspected ectopic pregnancy
- To evaluate vaginal bleeding
- To evaluate pelvic pain
- To estimate gestational age
- To diagnose or evaluate multiple gestations
- To confirm cardiac activity
- As an adjunct to chorionic villus sampling, embryo transfer, or localization and removal of an intrauterine device
- To assess for certain fetal anomalies, such as anencephaly, in patients at high risk
- To evaluate maternal pelvic or adnexal masses or uterine abnormalities
- To screen for fetal aneuploidy
- To evaluate suspected hydatidiform mole

American College of Radiology. Practice guideline for the performance of obstetrical ultrasound. In: ACR practice guidelines and technical standards, 2007. Reston (VA): ACR; 2007. Available at: http://www.acr.org/Secondary MainMenuCategories/quality_safety/guidelines/us/us_ obstetrical.aspx. Retrieved October 15, 2009.

Box 10

Indications for Second-Trimester and Third-Trimester Ultrasonography

- Estimation of gestational age
- Evaluation of fetal growth
- Evaluation of vaginal bleeding
- Evaluation of cervical insufficiency
- Evaluation of abdominal and pelvic pain
- Determination of fetal presentation
- Evaluation of suspected multiple gestation
- Adjunct to amniocentesis or other procedure
- Significant discrepancy between uterine size and clinical dates
- Evaluation of pelvic mass
- Examination of suspected hydatidiform mole
- Adjunct to cervical cerclage placement
- Evaluation of suspected ectopic pregnancy
- Evaluation of suspected fetal death
- Evaluation of suspected uterine abnormality
- Evaluation for fetal well-being
- Evaluation of suspected amniotic fluid abnormalities
- Evaluation of suspected placental abruption
- Adjunct to external cephalic version
- Evaluation for premature rupture of membranes or premature labor
- Evaluation for abnormal biochemical markers
- Follow-up evaluation of fetal anomaly
- Follow-up placental location for suspected placenta previa
- Evaluation of patients with a history of previous congenital anomaly
- Evaluation of fetal condition in late registrants for prenatal care
- Assessment of findings that may increase the risk of aneuploidy
- Screening for fetal anomalies

American College of Radiology. Practice guideline for the performance of obstetrical ultrasound. In: ACR practice guidelines and technical standards, 2007. Reston (VA): ACR; 2007. Available at: http://www.acr.org/Secondary MainMenuCategories/quality_safety/guidelines/us/us_ obstetrical.aspx. Retrieved October 15, 2009.

---

bank resources to manage massive surgical hemorrhage. Ultrasound examination of the placenta can assist in determining a particular patient's risk for placenta accreta in two ways. First, among women with a prior cesarean delivery, the most important risk factor for placenta accreta is the presence or absence of a placenta previa in the current pregnancy (Table 6) and ultrasonography is a reliable means of detecting placenta previa (3). Second, among women thought to be at risk for placenta accreta, the ultrasound appearance of the placenta and lower uterine segment may offer further determination of the level of risk. Ultrasound findings suggestive of placenta accreta include obliteration of the bladder wall–uterine interface, with loss of hypoechoic retroplacental myometrial zone (Figure 1), adjacent placental sonolucent spaces (Figure 2), and increased vascularity proximate to the bladder wall by color Doppler ultrasonography (Figure 3). Results from retrospective cohort studies suggest the following diagnostic test characteristics for ultrasonography in the detection of placenta accreta or placenta percreta: sensitivity, 77–93%; specificity, 71–96%; positive predictive value, 65–74%; and negative predictive value, 92–98% (4, 5). Magnetic resonance imaging is not clearly superior to ultrasonography for the detection of placenta accreta or placenta percreta, but may be of value when the ultrasound findings are equivocal.

Ultrasound Assessment of Cervical Length

The cervix may be seen at any time during pregnancy through transabdominal or transvaginal ultrasonography. In general, the most accurate information about cervical length is obtained through transvaginal ultrasonography because transabdominal ultrasound assessment of cervical length can be misleading (6). The length

Table 6. Risk of Placenta Accreta by Number of Cesarean Deliveries and Presence or Absence of Placenta Previa

Order of Cesarean Delivery	With Placenta Previa (%)	Without Placenta Previa (%)
First	3	0.03
Second	11	0.2
Third	40	0.1
Fourth	61	0.8
Fifth	67	0.4
Sixth and Greater	67	4.7

Silver RM, Landon MB, Leveno KJ, Spong CY, Thom EA, Moawad AH, et al. Maternal morbidity associated with multiple repeat cesarean deliveries. National Institute of Child and Human Development Maternal–Fetal Medicine Units Network. Obstet Gynecol 2006; 107:1226–32.

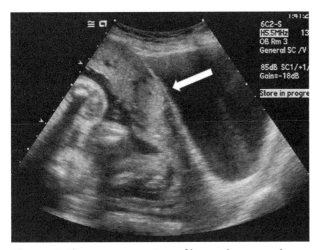

Figure 1. Placenta accreta. Loss of hypoechoic retroplacental myometrial zone.

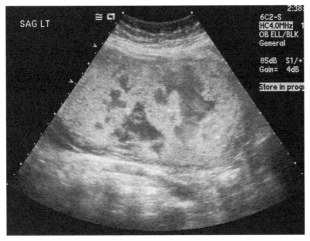

Figure 2. Placenta accreta. Adjacent placental sonolucent spaces.

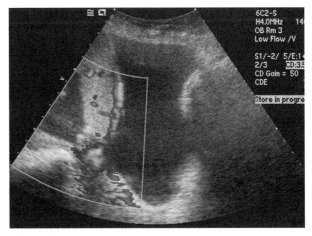

Figure 3. Placenta accreta. Increased vascularity proximate to the bladder wall by color Doppler ultrasonography.

of the endocervical canal and the contour of the internal os can be seen easily with transvaginal ultrasonography. The technique for transvaginal ultrasound assessment of cervical length is important. The maternal bladder should be empty to avoid compression of the lower uterine segment, which can falsely increase measurements of cervical length. Similarly, in order to avoid excessive pressure from the transvaginal transducer, the probe should be inserted and advanced until the endocervical canal is seen clearly, withdrawn just to the point of degradation of that image and then gently advanced again only until the endocervical canal is seen (Figure 4). Finally, this image should be repeated while applying transabdominal pressure to the fundus for 30 seconds in order to elicit dynamic cervical shortening or funneling (Figure 5). Cervical length obtained with this type of ultrasound examination has been shown to correlate with the risk of preterm delivery (7). Although both shortening of the cervix and the presence of funneling of the internal os have been correlated with preterm delivery, cervical length is the most important measurement. Contrary to earlier reports, recent evidence suggests that transabdominal ultrasound imaging of the cervix of a patient with an empty bladder may provide accurate assessment of cervical length comparable with that obtained with transvaginal ultrasonography (8). However, this technique is operator dependent and until these findings are confirmed by larger studies, the transvaginal approach should remain the standard for cervical length assessment among patients at high risk for cervical insufficiency or preterm birth.

The clinical application of ultrasonography for cervical length assessment remains an area of active research. At present, there is no compelling evidence that routine screening with ultrasonography is of value in a low-risk obstetric population. However, serial transvaginal cervical length ultrasound assessment among patients at risk for preterm birth may allow identification of those who are at particularly high risk and who might

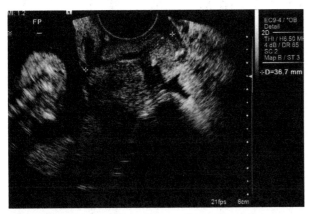

Figure 4. Transvaginal ultrasound image of the uterine cervix with normal (greater than 3 cm) cervical length.

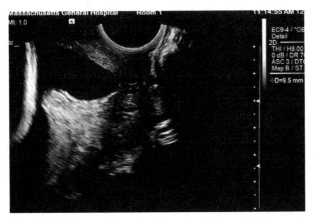

Figure 5. Shortened cervical length with funneling.

benefit from therapies such as cerclage or progesterone. In one study, the authors performed transvaginal ultrasound assessment of cervical length for all patients who had been referred for a detailed second trimester ultrasonography and randomized those found to have a cervical length of 1.5 cm or less to 200 mg of vaginal progesterone nightly or placebo (9). Women assigned to the progesterone group were less likely to have a spontaneous preterm birth before 34 completed weeks of gestation (19.2% versus 34.4%; relative risk, 0.56; 95% confidence interval, 0.36–0.86). In another study, the authors performed serial transvaginal ultrasound assessment of cervical length in a large cohort of women with prior preterm birth (10). Women found to have a cervical length less than 2.5 cm were then randomized to cerclage or no cerclage. Although there was a reduction in the risk of preterm birth at less than 35 completed weeks of gestation, the effect was most pronounced for women whose cervical lengths were less than 1.5 cm at the time of randomization (adjusted odds ratio [95% confidence interval] for preterm birth at less than 35 weeks of gestation was 0.23 [0.08–0.66]). Other clinical trials are ongoing and additional information is available (see Appendix A).

Fetal Echocardiography

The amount of attention and detail involved in ultrasound examination of the fetal heart depends on the type of ultrasound examination. At a minimum, a four-chamber view of the heart during a standard ultrasound examination in the second or third trimester should be obtained (1). Results from most studies suggest that a standard four-chamber view of the heart will detect approximately 50% of major fetal cardiac malformations. The previously mentioned joint guidelines for the conduct of antepartum obstetric ultrasound examination also suggest that, if technically feasible, an attempt should be made to view the cardiac outflow tracts. Adding an assessment of the fetal cardiac right and left outflow tracts increases the detection of major congenital cardiac malformations to 60–70%. For a specialized or detailed obstetric ultrasound examination performed by maternal–fetal medicine specialists or others with special training and experience in fetal sonology, an assessment of the outflow tracts is expected. An examination in even greater detail may be indicated for patients at particular risk for fetal cardiac malformations or arrhythmias. Examples of such patients include those with type I diabetes mellitus, a personal history or prior child with congenital heart disease, cardiac malformations suspected on a previous ultrasound examination, or suspected fetal arrhythmias. The additional attention to the fetal heart during a specialized or detailed obstetric ultrasound examination is sometimes referred to as a screening fetal echocardiogram and may be appropriate for some of these patients. However, when a fetal cardiac abnormality is confirmed or when a patient is at very high risk, referral to a pediatric cardiologist or maternal–fetal medicine specialist with special training and experience in comprehensive diagnostic fetal echocardiography is more appropriate. These fetal echocardiograms are more detailed, lengthy examinations performed in specialized centers in which multiple aspects of intracardiac anatomy and function are assessed through the use of two-dimensional imaging and color flow Doppler imaging.

Fetal Doppler Studies

At present, there is no role for fetal Doppler examinations in detecting fetal compromise in the general obstetric population. The value of fetal umbilical artery Doppler velocimetry is most established in pregnancies with fetal growth restriction. In these cases, an abnormal pattern of blood flow is associated with a poor outcome and warrants close surveillance or intervention. After 24 weeks of gestation, measurement of the relationship of peak systolic-to-diastolic flow velocities, with the systolic–diastolic ratio, pulsatility index, or resistance index, is a useful predictor of fetal compromise (Figure 6). Absent or reversed diastolic flow is an ominous finding that is associated with high perinatal mortality (Figure 7).

However, this finding may occur weeks before actual fetal compromise, and the decision to deliver should not be based on the result of the umbilical artery Doppler velocimetry alone, especially when remote from term. Several investigators have studied a more comprehensive evaluation of Doppler imaging of the growth restricted fetus in hopes of gaining information that might better inform decisions regarding the timing of delivery. These

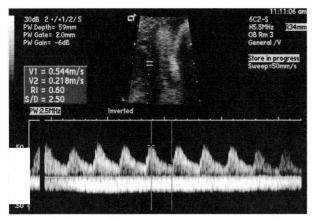

Figure 6. Normal umbilical artery Doppler flow velocity waveform.

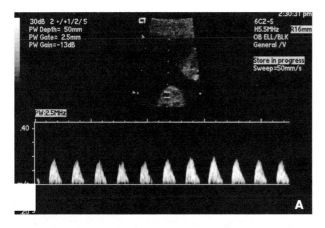

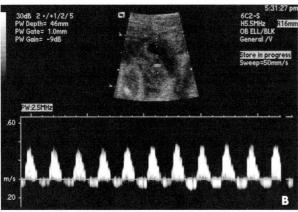

Figure 7. Examples of absent end-diastolic flow **(A)** and reversed diastolic flow **(B)** on umbilical artery Doppler flow velocity waveform.

studies often include analyses of Doppler waveforms in additional fetal blood vessels, including the middle cerebral artery, ductus venosus, and umbilical vein (11, 12). These extended Doppler imaging evaluations are technically difficult and require special experience in order to minimize interobserver and intraobserver variability. Furthermore, the sequence of abnormalities among these different blood vessels detected on Doppler imaging may vary between patients and with the underlying cause of fetal growth restriction (13). These and other challenges must be addressed with additional research before such studies are routinely recommended for the management of growth-restricted fetuses. Noninvasive monitoring of alloimmunized pregnancy has largely replaced invasive diagnosis. Doppler measurement of the peak systolic velocity in the fetal middle cerebral artery (Figure 8) has become the standard for the detection of fetal anemia at many referral centers (14). Serial testing is undertaken every 1–2 weeks, starting at 18–20 weeks of gestation once a critical maternal antibody titer has been reached. A value greater than 1.5 multiples of the median indicates a high likelihood for fetal anemia with a false-positive rate of approximately 12%. This strategy virtually eliminates the need for amniocentesis for ΔOD_{450}. Importantly, assessment of the peak systolic velocity in the fetal middle cerebral artery is less reliable for the detection of fetal anemia after 35 weeks of gestation or when hydrops fetalis is present.

Three-Dimensional and Four-Dimensional Ultrasound Imaging

Three-dimensional ultrasound imaging is now clinically available in many centers and is frequently sought by patients. Some ultrasound systems are able to construct these images in real time allowing one to view fetal movements in three dimensions. These ultrasound systems often are referred to as four-dimensional ultrasound systems. Despite the remarkable images of structures, such as the fetal face, that these systems can generate, the clini-

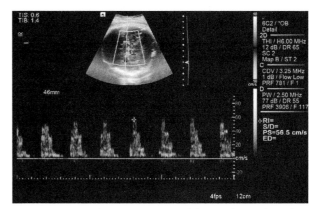

Figure 8. Doppler measurement of the peak systolic velocity in the fetal middle cerebral artery.

cal utility of three-dimensional or four-dimensional ultrasound systems remains to be established in obstetrics.

Prudent Use of Ultrasonography in Obstetric Practice

Obstetric ultrasonography should be performed only for valid medical indications. Even though there is no evidence at this time to suggest that ultrasound exposure of the fetus is harmful, clinicians should take care to use the lowest power settings available consistent with the policy of "as low as reasonably achievable." Some ultrasound systems, such as those used in cardiovascular laboratories, may deliver higher energies to the fetus than standard obstetric ultrasound systems and should not be used for fetal imaging. The promotion, sale, and lease of ultrasound equipment for nonmedical use, such as the production of keepsake videos or "fetal portraits" have been condemned by the U.S. Food and Drug Administration. Indeed, the use of ultrasound equipment without a physician's order may be in violation of state and local laws and regulations concerning nonprescribed use of a medical device (1).

References

1. Ultrasonography in pregnancy. ACOG Practice Bulletin No. 101. American College of Obstetricians and Gynecologists. Obstet Gynecol 2009;113:451–61.

2. Society for Maternal Fetal Medicine. White paper on ultrasound code 76811. 2nd ed. Washington, DC: SMFM; 2009. Available at: https://www.smfm.org/CodingNews PageDetail.cfm?one = coding&nav = viewnews&newsID = 461&codeon = yes. Retrieved October 15, 2009.

3. Silver RM, Landon MB, Rouse DJ, Leveno KJ, Spong CY, Thom EA, et al. Maternal morbidity associated with multiple repeat cesarean deliveries. National Institute of Child Health and Human Development Maternal-Fetal Medicine Units Network. Obstet Gynecol 2006;107:1226–32.

4. Warshak CR, Eskander R, Hull AD, Scioscia AL, Mattrey RF, Benirschke K, et al. Accuracy of ultrasonography and magnetic resonance imaging in the diagnosis of placenta accreta. Obstet Gynecol 2006;108:573–81.

5. Dwyer BK, Belogolovkin V, Tran L, Rao A, Carroll I, Barth R, et al. Prenatal diagnosis of placenta accreta: sonography or magnetic resonance imaging? J Ultrasound Med 2008;27:1275–81.

6. To MS, Skentou C, Cicero S, Nicolaides KH. Cervical assessment at the routine 23-weeks' scan: problems with transabdominal sonography. Ultrasound Obstet Gynecol 2000;15:292–6.

7. Iams JD, Goldenberg RL, Meis PJ, Mercer BM, Moawad A, Das A, et al. The length of the cervix and the risk of spontaneous premature delivery. National Institute of Child Health and Human Development Maternal Fetal Medicine Unit Network. N Engl J Med 1996;334:567–72.

8. Saul LL, Kurtzman JT, Hagemann C, Ghamsary M, Wing DA. Is transabdominal sonography of the cervix after voiding a reliable method of cervical length assessment? J Ultrasound Med 2008;27:1305–11.

9. Fonseca EB, Celik E, Parra M, Singh M, Nicolaides KH. Progesterone and the risk of preterm birth among women with a short cervix. Fetal Medicine Foundation Second Trimester Screening Group. N Engl J Med 2007;357:462–9.

10. Owen J, Hankins G, Iams JD, Berghella V, Sheffield JS, Perez-Delboy A, et al. Multicenter randomized trial of cerclage for preterm birth prevention in high-risk women with shortened midtrimester cervical length. Am J Obstet Gynecol 2009;201:375.e1–375.e8.

11. Baschat AA, Gembruch U, Harman CR. The sequence of changes in Doppler and biophysical parameters as severe fetal growth restriction worsens. Ultrasound Obstet Gynecol 2001;18:571–7.

12. Ferrazzi E, Bozzo M, Rigano S, Bellotti M, Morabito A, Pardi G, et al. Temporal sequence of abnormal Doppler changes in the peripheral and central circulatory systems of the severely growth-restricted fetus. Ultrasound Obstet Gynecol 2002;19:140–6.

13. Mari G. Doppler ultrasonography in obstetrics: from the diagnosis of fetal anemia to the treatment of intrauterine growth-restricted fetuses. Am J Obstet Gynecol 2009; 200:613.e1–613.e9.

14. Management of alloimmunization. ACOG Practice Bulletin No. 75. American College of Obstetricians and Gynecologists. Obstet Gynecol 2006;108:457–64.

Prenatal Diagnosis of Genetic Disorders

Katharine D. Wenstrom

Genetic disorders can result in considerable morbidity and mortality for reproductive-age women and their families. Eight percent (1/13) of conceptuses are chromosomally abnormal, accounting for 50% of all first-trimester abortions and 6–11% of all stillbirths and neonatal deaths. By grade school, a major or minor structural birth defect will be recognized in 8% of all children, and another 8% will have developmental delay. Additionally, it is estimated that 60% of diseases in adults (eg, hypertension, diabetes mellitus, or cancer) has a genetic basis. Specific knowledge of the genetic etiology of these conditions is expanding rapidly. The indications for preconception counseling and prenatal diagnosis also are expanding because more women request counseling and testing. Counseling by a genetic counselor, geneticist, or physician with special expertise in prenatal diagnosis can assist patients in making an informed decision, and should be considered for all but the most straightforward counseling issues.

Ethnic Groups at High Risk of Selected Disorders

Although single-gene disorders generally are rare, some ethnic groups are at higher risk of having certain diseases than the general population and should be counseled and offered genetic screening accordingly (Table 7 and Box 11). If only one person in a couple is a member of the high-risk group, that person can be tested first. If it is determined that he or she is not a carrier, the partner may not need to be screened.

Sickle Cell Disease

African Americans are at increased risk of having sickle cell disease, the most common hemoglobin (Hb) disorder in the United States. Hemoglobin is a tetrameric protein composed of two α and two β polypeptide

Table 7. Ethnic Groups at Risk for Single-Gene Disorders

Ethnic Group	Disease	Heterozygote (Carrier) Rate	Incidence of Disease
African American	Hemoglobin SS (sickle cell disease)	1 in 12	1 in 576
	Hemoglobin CC	1 in 40	1 in 4,790
	Hemoglobin SC	Variable	1 in 757
	Hemoglobin S–β-thalassemia	1 in 22	1 in 1,672
Mediterranean (also Asian)	β-thalassemia	1 in 10 to 1 in 20	1 in 10 to 1 in 20 (β-thalassemia minor)*
Asian (also Mediterranean)	α-thalassemia	1 in 5	1 in 50 (α-thalassemia minor)†
Jewish	Tay–Sachs disease	1 in 30	1 in 3,600
	Canavan disease	1 in 40	1 in 6,400
	Gaucher disease	1 in 12 to 1 in 25	1 in 576 to 1 in 2,500
	Cystic fibrosis	1 in 24 to 1 in 90	1 in 2,304 to 1 in 32,400
North European Caucasians	Cystic fibrosis	1 in 20 to 1 in 25	1 in 2,500
Native Americans	Cystic fibrosis	1 in 20 to 1 in 31	1 in 1,580 to 1 in 3,970
Southeast Asians	Hemoglobin EE	1 in 1,000	1 in 400
	Hemoglobin E and β-thalassemia	Variable	1 in 400 to 1 in 800
	Hemoglobin E and α-thalassemia	Variable	1 in 200

*Deletion of both chain genes results in Cooley anemia and is usually lethal.

†Deletion of three-chain genes results in hemoglobin H, which is transfusion dependent and often lethal; deletion of four-chain genes results in hemoglobin Bart and hydrops fetalis and is lethal.

Box 11

Clinical Features of Autosomal Recessive Genetic Diseases Frequent Among Individuals of Eastern European Jewish Descent

Bloom syndrome is a genetic condition associated with increased chromosome breakage, a predisposition to infections and malignancies, prenatal and postnatal growth deficiency, skin findings (such as facial telangiectasias, abnormal pigmentation), and in some cases learning difficulties and mental retardation. The mean age of death is 27 years and usually is related to cancer. No effective treatment currently is available.

Canavan disease is a disorder of the central nervous system characterized by developmental delay, hypotonia, large head, seizures, blindness, and gastrointestinal reflux. Most children die within the first several years of life. Canavan disease is caused by a deficiency of the aspartoacylase enzyme. No treatment currently is available.

Familial dysautonomia is a neurologic disorder characterized by abnormal suck and feeding difficulties, episodic vomiting, abnormal sweating, pain and temperature insensitivity, labile blood pressure levels, absent tearing, and scoliosis. There currently is no cure for familial dysautonomia, but some treatments are available that can improve the length and quality of a patient's life.

Fanconi anemia group C usually presents with severe anemia that progresses to pancytopenia, developmental delay, and failure to thrive. Congenital anomalies are not uncommon, including limb, cardiac, and genital–urinary defects. Microcephaly and mental retardation may be present. Children are at increased risk for leukemia. Some children have been successfully treated with bone marrow transplantation. Life expectancy is 8–12 years.

Gaucher disease is a genetic disorder that mainly affects the spleen, liver, and bones; it occasionally affects the lungs, kidneys, and brain. It may develop at any age. Some individuals are chronically ill, some are moderately affected, and others are so mildly affected that they may not know that they have Gaucher disease. The most common symptom is chronic fatigue caused by anemia. Patients may experience easy bruising, nosebleeds, bleeding gums, and prolonged and heavy bleeding with their menses and after childbirth. Other symptoms include an enlarged liver and spleen, osteoporosis, and bone and joint pain. Gaucher disease is caused by the deficiency of the β-glucosidase enzyme. Treatment is available through enzyme therapy, which results in a vastly improved quality of life.

Mucolipidosis IV is a neurodegenerative lysosomal storage disorder characterized by growth and psychomotor retardation, corneal clouding, progressive retinal degeneration, and strabismus. Most affected infants never speak, walk, or develop beyond the level of a 1–2 year old. Life expectancy may be normal, and there currently is no effective treatment.

Niemann–Pick disease type A is a lysosomal storage disorder typically diagnosed in infancy and marked by a rapid neurodegenerative course similar to Tay–Sachs disease. Affected children die by age 3–5 years. Niemann–Pick disease type A is caused by a deficiency of the sphingomyelinase enzyme. There currently is no treatment.

Tay–Sachs disease is a severe, progressive disorder of the central nervous system leading to death within the first few years of life. Infants with Tay–Sachs disease appear normal at birth but by age 5–6 months develop poor muscle tone, delayed development, loss of developmental milestones, and mental retardation. Children with Tay–Sachs disease lose their eyesight at age 12–18 months. This condition usually is fatal by age 6 years. Tay–Sachs disease is caused by a deficiency of the hexosaminidase A enzyme. No effective treatment currently is available.

Prenatal and preconceptional carrier screening for genetic diseases in individuals of Eastern European Jewish descent. ACOG Committee Opinion No. 298. American College of Obstetricians and Gynecologists. Obstet Gynecol 2004;104:425–8.

---

chains. Hemoglobin S results from the alteration of a single peptide in the β chain—the substitution of valine for glutamic acid at the sixth position of the polypeptide. Approximately 8% of African Americans carry the sickle Hb gene, which also is found with increased frequency in those of Mediterranean, Caribbean, Latin American, or Middle Eastern descent.

Hemoglobin E Mutation

Southeast Asians are at increased risk of carrying Hb E, the second most common abnormal Hb in the world. The homozygous state results in microcytosis but not marked anemia, whereas individuals with Hb E–β-thalassemia can have severe hemolytic anemia requiring transfusion during pregnancy. Women whose ancestors came from high-risk areas should be offered hemoglobinopathy screening. Hemoglobin electrophoresis is the test of choice because it will identify all abnormal Hbs, not just Hb S. If the patient is a hemoglobinopathy carrier, the partner should be screened as well so that the couple's risk of having an affected child can be determined.

Thalassemias

Individuals of Mediterranean or Asian origin are at increased risk of having α-thalassemia or β-thalassemia. The thalassemias occur as the result of a functional deletion of one or more of the two β genes or two or more of the four α genes. The loss of these genes leads to decreased production of the Hb chain in question, reduced production of the intact Hb molecule, hemolysis, and anemia that can be severe. Carrier testing begins with determination of red blood cell indices; a mean erythrocyte volume of less than 79 cubic micrometers indicates increased risk (Figure 9). Because the most common explanation for a reduced mean corpuscular volume (MCV) is iron deficiency, the patient with a low MCV should first be evaluated with iron studies or begin iron therapy presumptively. If iron study results are normal or there is no response to therapy, Hb electrophoresis should be performed.

If the patient has a functional deletion of a β gene and thus makes reduced quantities of the β chain, the excess α chains will combine with δ chains instead to make Hb A_2. An Hb A_2 level of at least 3.5% (determined by Hb electrophoresis) confirms the diagnosis of β-thalasse-

mia. Prenatal diagnosis of all forms of β-thalassemia can be accomplished by molecular testing.

In α-thalassemia, two or more α chain genes must be deleted before the MCV is decreased. In contrast to β-thalassemia, α-thalassemia does not result in the production of an alternate Hb molecule because there is no protein that can substitute for the α chain. The loss of two or more genes encoding the α chain thus results only in reduced production of normal Hb A. As a result, α-thalassemia cannot be diagnosed by Hb electrophoresis. However, most α-thalassemia cases can be identified by molecular genetic testing. Patients with two or more α chain genes deleted will have normal iron study results as well as normal levels of Hb A_2. Thus, the patient with a low MCV, normal iron study results, and normal hemoglobin electrophoresis results should be referred for genetic counseling and molecular genetic testing. Prenatal diagnosis of α-thalassemia by molecular testing usually is possible.

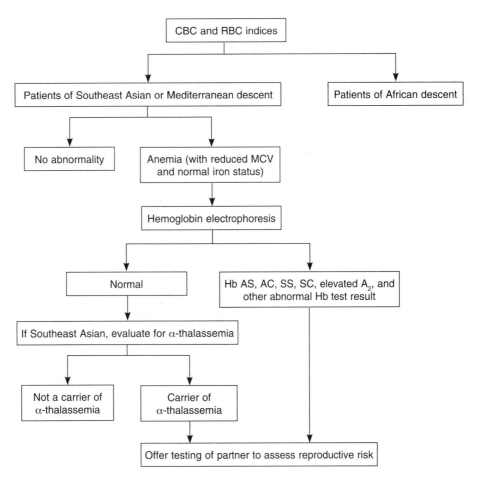

Figure 9. Specialized antepartum evaluation for hematologic assessment of patients of African, Southeast Asian, or Mediterranean descent. Patients of Southeast Asian or Mediterranean descent should undergo electrophoresis if their blood test results reveal anemia. Abbreviations: CBC indicates complete blood count; Hb, hemoglobin; MCV, mean corpuscular volume; RBC, red blood cell. (Hemoglobinopathies in pregnancy. ACOG Practice Bulletin No. 78. American College of Obstetricians and Gynecologists. Obstet Gynecol 2007;109:229–37.)

Cystic Fibrosis

White individuals of North European descent, individuals of Ashkenazi Jewish heritage, and Native Americans are at increased risk of cystic fibrosis. A chronic pulmonary and exocrine pancreatic disease, cystic fibrosis is the most common monogenic disorder in this population. It is transmitted in autosomal recessive fashion and has a carrier frequency of 1 in 22 in Caucasian individuals of North European heritage and 1 in 24 in those with Ashkenazi Jewish heritage. The carrier rate and the most common cystic fibrosis mutations in Native Americans are incompletely known. Ethnic groups at low risk of cystic fibrosis include African Americans (carrier rate 1 in 65), Hispanic Americans (1 in 46), and Asian Americans (1 in 94). More than 1,300 different gene mutations that cause cystic fibrosis have been identified. The most common cystic fibrosis mutation in Caucasian individuals, ΔF508, accounts for 75% of cystic fibrosis cases in this group.

If a specific gene mutation has been identified in an affected family, individuals at risk can be tested for that particular mutation. In a family with no history of cystic fibrosis, the laboratory receives no specific guidance regarding the gene deletions for which it should screen. Because it is not possible to screen for all 1,300 known mutations during carrier testing, most laboratories now screen for a panel of 23 mutations that each have a frequency of at least 0.1% in North American cystic fibrosis patients as well as one or more of seven second-tier mutations if certain specific mutations are identified in the first mutation panel.

Because the current screening test identifies only 23 of the 1,300 known cystic fibrosis mutations, an individual who has a negative cystic fibrosis screening test result cannot be told that she does not carry the cystic fibrosis gene. However, because the 23 mutations being evaluated account for most of cystic fibrosis cases in this country, the patient can be informed that the negative test significantly reduces her risk of carrying a cystic fibrosis mutation—from 1 in 22 (the a priori risk based solely on ethnic origin) to 1 in 246. If both members of the couple test negative, their risk of having a child with cystic fibrosis is reduced to 1 in 242,100. The National Institutes of Health and the American College of Obstetricians and Gynecologists (the College) have recommended that cystic fibrosis screening be offered to all pregnant Caucasian women of North European descent or Ashkenazi Jewish heritage, and made available to pregnant women of other ethnic groups.

Tay–Sachs Disease, Canavan Disease, and Gaucher Disease

In addition to being at increased risk of having a child with cystic fibrosis, individuals with Jewish heritage are at increased risk of having a child with Tay–Sachs disease, familial dysautonomia, Canavan disease, or Gaucher disease, each of which is caused by a different enzyme deficiency (hexosaminidase A, IKAP protein, aspartoacylase, and glucocerebrosidase, respectively) as well as several other less common diseases. Individuals with these autosomal recessive disorders all have in common the inability to degrade certain byproducts of normal catabolism, leading to a neurovisceral storage abnormality and a rapidly progressive neurodegenerative course. The carrier rate among individuals of Jewish descent is 1 in 30 for Tay–Sachs disease, 1 in 32 for familial dysautonomia, 1 in 40 for Canavan disease, and 1 in 12 to 1 in 25 for Gaucher disease. The College recommends that counseling and carrier screening for Tay–Sachs disease, familial dysautonomia, Canavan disease, and cystic fibrosis be offered to all patients of Jewish heritage, and prenatal diagnosis of all four diseases is possible (1). Molecular testing for four additional disorders, Fanconi anemia group C, Niemann–Pick disease type A, Bloom syndrome, and mucolipidosis type IV, also is available. Although these disorders are much less common than the four previously mentioned, with an average incidence of 1 in 32,000 or less, each is caused by only one to four mutations, making molecular testing relatively easy. Some authorities therefore recommend that individuals of Ashkenazi Jewish heritage be offered screening for all eight of these diseases.

Gaucher disease is different from the eight diseases just discussed in two important ways. First, there are three clinical forms of Gaucher disease, representing different degrees of enzyme deficiency and, thus, a wide range of severity. Whereas types 2 and 3 are associated with hepatosplenomegaly and progressive brain damage, Type 1 is much less severe and usually is characterized by the adult onset of mild symptoms (ie, easy bruising, fatigue, and mild splenomegaly). Second, carriers can be identified by molecular testing, which determines whether they carry any of the known Gaucher mutations, but phenotype–genotype correlation is poor, and prediction of the homozygous fetus's phenotype is difficult if there are no other affected family members (ie, if the parents underwent genetic testing only because of their ethnic origin). At the present time it is possible to provide accurate prenatal diagnosis only of type 1 Gaucher disease, and because this is the mildest form, prenatal diagnosis rarely alters pregnancy management. It is not currently possible to accurately determine if a fetus inheriting two Gaucher mutations will have type 2 or type 3 disease. For these reasons, prenatal screening for Gaucher disease remains controversial.

Spinal Muscular Atrophy

Spinal muscular atrophy is an autosomal recessive neurodegenerative disease characterized by atrophy of skeletal muscle and generalized weakness. There are three forms of the disease. Type I spinal muscular atrophy

(Werdnig–Hoffman disease) is the most severe form, with onset before 6 months of age and death from respiratory failure by age 2 years. Type II spinal muscular atrophy, the most common, has onset by age 2 years and intermediate symptomology. Although affected children usually cannot stand or walk unaided and have some degree of respiratory insufficiency, some survive into their twenties. Type III spinal muscular atrophy (Kugelberg–Welander disease) has onset after age 18 months and highly variable symptomology, ranging from being wheelchair-bound to being able to walk unaided with only minor muscle weakness. There is no effective therapy. Spinal muscular atrophy is caused by a deletion in the *SMN1* gene, and the carrier rate is estimated to be 1 in 40 to 1 in 60. Molecular diagnosis in patients with symptoms is 95% sensitive, and carrier testing identifies 98% of carriers. However, the severity of the disease is determined by how many copies of a second gene, the *SNM2* gene, the individual has, with more copies meaning less severe disease. Most of the population has one to three copies, but 15% of individuals have none. Unfortunately, at present it is not possible to accurately determine the number of copies of *SMN2*, and, thus, accurate phenotype prediction in fetuses inheriting the *SMN1* deletion may not be possible. At present, screening for spinal muscular atrophy should be offered to couples with a family history of the disease and made available to those who request it after appropriate genetic counseling.

Nonmendelian Inheritance

Certain single-gene disorders are transmitted in nonclassical (nonmendelian) ways. For example, some inherited diseases occur as a result of a mutation in mitochondrial DNA (ie, Leber hereditary optic atrophy, Kearns–Sayre syndrome, and myoclonic epilepsy with ragged red fibers). Because mitochondria are passed to the ovum exclusively by the mother, mitochondrial disorders are characterized by maternal inheritance.

Another nonclassical inheritance pattern involves germline mosaicism. Although it was previously understood that conditions caused by new autosomal dominant mutations (ie, osteogenesis imperfecta type II or achondroplasia) occurred sporadically and had no recurrence risk, it is now believed that some individuals carry two or more populations of germ cells, one of which contains the new mutation. Because of the possibility of germline mosaicism, the risk of having another child with the same condition caused by a new autosomal dominant mutation is therefore not zero but somewhere between 1% and 7%.

Hereditary unstable DNA is the name for certain genes that can change in size and, thus, change the phenotype as they are passed from parent to child. Most of these genes contain a series of trinucleotide repeats (for example, 100 copies of CGG) that can increase or decrease in size as the gene is transmitted. Once a region of repeats reaches a critical size, the gene usually is turned off and the protein it encodes is no longer produced. *Fragile X syndrome*, the most common inherited form of mental retardation, is caused by a region of CGG repeats in the *FMR1* gene on the X chromosome. Most people carry an *FMR1* gene containing fewer than 50 repeats; women who carry a gene with 60–100 repeats have a "premutation" because once the region reaches this size it can expand further as it is transmitted (2). When the region expands to more than 200 repeats, it will be methylated, thus turning the *FMR1* gene off; the fragile X phenotype is caused by the lack of *FMR1* protein. The *FMR1* gene can only expand when it is transmitted through a female. Male offspring are preferentially affected because they have only one X chromosome. However, not all males who inherit an expanded *FMR1* gene are affected to the same degree because of mosaicism for methylation and for the number of repeats. Females who inherit an expanded *FMR1* gene usually are phenotypically normal because they have a normal *FMR1* gene on their second X chromosome that directs the production of a normal amount of FMR1 protein. However, females can be affected as the result of unfavorable lyonization (the normal X is preferentially turned off and the abnormal X is active in most cells).

Women with a family history of fragile X syndrome or unexplained mental retardation or autism should be offered genetic counseling and, if appropriate, testing to determine if they are premutation carriers. Prenatal diagnosis is possible with amniocentesis. However, phenotype prediction may be difficult in cases in which there is no family history because it is not possible to identify mosaicism for either methylation or for the number of repeats (which could alter the phenotype in males) or to assess lionization (which could alter the phenotype in females). Chorionic villus sampling (CVS) is less accurate than amniocentesis because it may not allow accurate determination of the methylation status of the *FMR1* gene. Other diseases caused by trinucleotide repeats include myotonic dystrophy and Huntington disease.

Genomic imprinting results in gene expression that differs according to the gender of the parent who transmitted the gene (3). The differential expression is caused by gender-specific differences in DNA methylation; because methylation turns genes off, imprinting results in altered gene dosing. Imprinting is not permanent across generations. Although somatic cells retain the genomic methylation patterns inherited from each parent, they are erased in the germ cells of the fetus and replaced with a methylation pattern that reflects the fetus's gender. Thus the fetus will eventually pass on its own imprinting pattern to its offspring. This situation, in which the function of a gene can be reversibly changed without a permanent mutation, is called *epigenetic modification*. The function of the gene and, thus, the course of certain diseases may be altered by genomic imprinting. For example, when the gene for Huntington disease is transmitted by the father, the symptoms have a much earlier onset than when the gene is transmitted by the mother.

Uniparental disomy occurs when both copies of a chromosome are transmitted by one parent. A person with uniparental disomy therefore has two copies of certain genes from one parent and no copies of the same genes from the other parent. Because of genomic imprinting and resulting differential gene expression, uniparental disomy may cause phenotypic abnormalities. Additionally, if the two copies of the gene inherited from one parent are abnormal, the individual may express features of an autosomal recessive disease even though only one parent carries the abnormal gene.

Structural Disorders of Multifactorial Etiology

The discovery of a structural malformation of a major fetal organ or structure or the finding of two or more minor malformations or dysmorphisms (ie, choroid plexus cyst, extra digit, or single umbilical artery), increases the risk of aneuploidy sufficiently to warrant genetic testing of the fetus, regardless of maternal age or parental karyotypes. An exception to this dictum is a fetal defect known to be familial and not associated with aneuploidy (eg, fetal cleft lip discovered during an ultrasound examination ordered because the mother has a cleft lip).

Multifactorial disorders are caused by a combination of factors, some genetic and some nongenetic (ie, environmental). Multifactorial disorders tend to recur in families but are not transmitted in any distinctive pattern. Many congenital single organ system structural abnormalities are multifactorial, with an incidence in the general population of approximately 1 in 1,000. Some examples of multifactorial traits that might have a genetic component are listed in Box 12.

Because most of the defects listed in Box 12 also may occur as a result of a genetic syndrome, a single-gene disorder, or a chromosome abnormality, a thorough evaluation by a geneticist or fetal pathologist (in the case of pregnancy loss) may be necessary before multifactorial inheritance can be assumed. When multifactorial inheritance has been ascertained, the patient can be counseled regarding her risks (4) (Box 13).

Screening Techniques

Currently, several screening techniques are available for detection of specific genetic disorders. This section will briefly review the different uses of maternal serum screening, nuchal translucency screening, and ultrasonography.

Box 12

Examples of Multifactorial Traits

- Cleft lip, with or without cleft palate
- Congenital cardiac defects
- Diaphragmatic hernia
- Hydrocephalus
- Müllerian fusion defects
- Neural tube defects
- Posterior urethral valves
- Pyloric stenosis
- Renal agenesis
- Talipes equinovarus

Box 13

Genetic Counseling for a Patient With Multifactorial Inheritance

Once a multifactorial inheritance has been diagnosed, the patient can be counseled regarding the following factors:

- The risk to first-degree relatives of the affected individual (mother, father, brother, or sister) is higher than in the general population. The most commonly quoted risk is an empirical risk based on experience with similar families (1–5% in most cases).
- The risk is sharply lower (less than 1%) for second-degree and more distant relatives.
- The recurrence risk is higher when more than one family member is affected and when the defect is more severe (indicating the presence of more abnormal genes or environmental influences).
- If the trait is more common in one gender than in the other, the risk is higher if the affected individual is of the less susceptible gender (indicating the presence of more abnormal genes).

Maternal Serum Screening for Down Syndrome

Most women at increased risk of having a child with Down syndrome can now be identified in the first or second trimesters by any of several multiple-marker screening tests. The most widely used second-trimester screening test, the quadruple screen, is based on the levels of maternal serum alpha-fetoprotein (MSAFP), unconjugated estriol, human chorionic gonadotropin (hCG), and inhibin. It identifies approximately 81% of all pregnancies affected by Down syndrome and 75% of all pregnancies affected by trisomy 18, at a screen positive rate of 5%.

For women who seek prenatal care in the first few months of pregnancy, first-trimester Down syndrome screening is possible using maternal serum analytes, either alone or in combination with a ultrasound marker. The most discriminatory first-trimester maternal serum analytes are either free β-hCG or intact hCG and pregnancy-associated plasma protein A (PAPP-A). The most predictive ultrasound marker is the nuchal translucency, an echolucent area seen in longitudinal midsagittal views of the back of the fetal neck between 10 weeks of gestation and 14 weeks of gestation. Fetuses with Down syndrome tend to have larger nuchal translucency than euploid fetuses of the same age. Because the nuchal translucency increases in size as the fetus grows, using a specific size cut off to define an abnormal result leads to decreased test sensitivity. Expressing the nuchal translucency as a multiple of the normal median accounts for gestational age-related size changes and also allows it to be used in the algorithm along with maternal serum analyte levels to determine a composite risk. Because the nuchal translucency is a very small area, accurate and reproducible measurements are difficult to obtain, and minor measurement inaccuracies can lead to major changes in risk estimation, specific training in standardized measurement techniques is required and adherence to specific guidelines for measuring the nuchal translucency is imperative. In addition, because nuchal translucency medians vary not only from center to center but also from operator to operator, and the medians gradually change or "drift" over time, each center's or operator's medians should be monitored carefully and adjusted as necessary (5).

Four large trials of combined first trimester ultrasound and serum screening, including 103,856 patients and 328 cases of Down syndrome, have been completed and yielded similar results. The BUN (6), FASTER (7), SURUSS (8), and OSCAR (9) trials enrolled women who underwent screening between 10 weeks 4 days of gestation and 13 weeks 6 days of gestation and determined the risks of Down syndrome and trisomy 18 based on maternal age, free β-hCG, PAPP-A, and nuchal translucency measurement. When the screen-positive rates were held at 5% or less, the Down syndrome detection rate in these four trials averaged 84%. For women of all ages, the detection rate for trisomy 18 was 90% at a screen-positive rate of 2% (6).

The sensitivity of the screening test can be further improved by combining the screening tests for the first-trimester and the second-trimester. In this integrated screening test, both first-trimester analyte levels and nuchal translucency and second-trimester analyte levels are measured, and one composite screening test result is provided after completion of the second-trimester portion of the test. The advantage of this strategy is that a detection rate of 90–96% can be achieved at a screen positive rate of 5% (10). The disadvantage is that no result is provided until the second trimes-

ter, all analytes must be assayed in the same laboratory, and the patient must complete the entire two-part test or else does not receive a result. An alternative is the sequential screening test, in which the first-trimester screening test is performed, the woman is informed of the result, and then the woman may or may not go on to have the second-trimester screening test. In stepwise sequential screening, women with a very high first-trimester risk, above a certain cutoff, are offered diagnostic testing by CVS or amniocentesis, and only those whose risk is below the cutoff go on to second-trimester screening. This strategy results in a 95% detection rate at a 5% screen-positive rate. In contingent sequential screening, the first trimester result is placed in one of three categories—patients with the highest risk are offered immediate diagnostic testing, patients with the lowest risk need no further screening, and patients with intermediate risk go on to have the second-trimester screening test. This strategy appears to be optimal because it has an 85–94% detection rate at a screen-positive rate on the order of 1–2%.

One advantage of both forms of sequential screening is that the woman learns the result of her first-trimester test and can act accordingly. The woman whose risk is very low may decide not to proceed to the second-trimester test, whereas the woman whose risk is very high may choose to have CVS rather than wait for the second part of the test. Another advantage is that the Down syndrome detection rates are still high—88–95%—but fewer second-trimester tests are done, and fewer women need to undergo invasive testing; thus, the screening process is less expensive and fewer unaffected fetuses are lost as the result of an invasive diagnostic procedure. Disadvantages include the necessity of doing both tests in the same laboratory, and the need to provide test results and counseling twice. One important rule to remember is that when either form of sequential screening is chosen, it is essential that both tests be done in the same laboratory. The laboratory then will be able to incorporate the risk estimate determined by the first-trimester test into the second-trimester test, yielding the most accurate ultimate risk estimate at the lowest screen-positive rate. By contrast, if the tests are done separately, the final screen-positive rate will be the sum of the rates of the first-trimester and second-trimester test results and, thus, twice as high.

Current College guidelines regarding screening for fetal Down syndrome recommend that screening and invasive testing for fetal aneuploidy should be made available to all women who seek prenatal care before 20 weeks of gestation, regardless of maternal age. Although the ability to choose from among a variety of screening strategies may be attractive to some patients, others may find it confusing. Therefore, it is reasonable for practitioners to choose a limited number of strategies to routinely offer patients, such as first-trimester screening or sequential screening for women who seek prenatal care in the first few months of pregnancy and the quadruple screen for women who seek prenatal care after that period. In areas where nuchal translucency measurement is not available, both first-trimester screening and combined first-trimester and second-trimester screening can be done using only maternal serum analytes; the detection rates are somewhat lower than when nuchal translucency is included but still acceptable. The woman who chooses first-trimester screening should be informed that because the first-trimester test does not include a screen for fetal neural tube defects, she will need to return in the second trimester for the MSAFP test, a targeted ultrasound examination, or both.

Follow-up of an Increase in Nuchal Translucency

Data from a variety of sources indicate that the fetus with an increased nuchal translucency (defined as thickness of 3.5 mm or greater) but a normal karyotype is at an increased risk of having a cardiac defect, an abdominal wall defect, a diaphragmatic hernia, or a genetic syndrome (11, 12). Women with such fetuses should be offered a targeted ultrasound examination, fetal echocardiography, or both at 18–22 weeks of gestation.

Maternal Serum Screening for Neural Tube Defects

Prenatal screening started with the measurement of maternal serum alpha-fetoprotein (AFP); in the second trimester, MSAFP levels are elevated when there is a fetal neural tube defect (NTD). Because 95% of all NTDs occur in families with no previous affected children or relatives, all pregnant women should be offered NTD screening, regardless of their family history. Maternal serum AFP screening identifies 90% of fetuses with open spina bifida or anencephaly and at least one half of all fetuses with a ventral wall defect. The likelihood of a fetal defect increases along with the AFP level; levels of 3.5 or greater multiples of the median are unlikely to be false positive. All variations of the second-trimester Down syndrome screening test include MSAFP. However, because the measurement of AFP is not included in any first-trimester screening protocols, it is important that women who undergo first-trimester Down syndrome screening have a second-trimester MSAFP test or a targeted ultrasound examination to screen for NTDs. The MSAFP level may be decreased in the setting of maternal diabetes mellitus, which requires altered interpretation. Therefore, the laboratory performing the test should be informed of the woman's diabetic status.

All pregnancies characterized by confirmed elevated MSAFP should be evaluated ultrasonographically. In the second trimester, 90–99% of open NTDs can be diagnosed by ultrasound examination. Most spinal defects can be directly visualized, and 99% of fetuses with an open spina bifida have at least one of five ultrasound cranial signs: 1) lemon sign (frontal scalloping or notching), 2) obliteration of the posterior fossa, 3) banana sign (Chiari deformation), 4) ventriculomegaly, and 5) small biparietal diameter (13). When a fetal defect is identified by ultrasonography, amniocentesis can be performed to confirm the diagnosis. An elevated amniotic fluid AFP level and the presence of acetylcholinesterase, which indicates direct exposure of neural tissue to amniotic fluid, identify all NTDs except those in the 3–5% of fetuses whose spinal defects are covered by skin. If an amniocentesis is performed, a fetal karyotype should be obtained. In the setting of an elevated MSAFP level, 16% of abnormal fetuses and 0.61% of normal appearing fetuses will have chromosome abnormalities (14).

Amniocentesis also can be performed to rule out a fetal defect when there is an elevated AFP level but no fetal abnormalities are seen on ultrasound examination. However, given the excellent resolution of current ultrasound equipment, some clinicians believe that amniocentesis is not necessary in this situation.

Ultrasound Screening

A structural abnormality involving a major organ or structure or the presence of two or more minor structural abnormalities or dysmorphisms in the same fetus indicate a high risk of fetal aneuploidy. The presence of a major anomaly increases the risk enough that invasive testing is justified regardless of the patient's age, family history, or maternal serum screening results. As noted earlier, an exception to this dictum is a fetal defect known to be familial and not associated with aneuploidy (eg, fetal cleft lip discovered during an ultrasound examination ordered because the mother has a cleft lip). The specific risk associated with each of several major anomalies is listed in Table 8.

Major structural fetal anomalies may be discovered serendipitously in otherwise low-risk pregnancies during an ultrasound examination performed for other indications, such as pregnancy dating, evaluation of size and growth, or as part of a workup of complications, such as vaginal bleeding. However, it is a matter of controversy whether early second-trimester ultrasound examinations should be performed routinely to screen for fetal structural abnormalities in pregnancies at low risk for such abnormalities. Before this issue can be resolved, the detection and false-negative rates for such examinations need to be improved. Data from several large studies indicate that only 16–50% of major structural defects are typically identified during a second-trimester ultrasound examination.

Minor dysmorphisms, by definition, are not major structural abnormalities and commonly are found in many normal individuals. Certain dysmorphisms arouse interest because they are found with greater frequency in aneuploid fetuses. The risks of dysmorphism associated with Down syndrome are listed in Table 9. Whether an ultrasound examination performed specifically to screen for such dysmorphisms should be offered as the sole Down syndrome screening test to low-risk women is controversial. This is because much of the research concerning ultrasound evaluation of fetal dysmorphisms as a screening test for fetal chromosome abnormalities has

Table 8. Aneuploid Risk of Most Common Major Anomalies

Structural Defect	Population Incidence	Aneuploidy Risk	Aneuploidy (Trisomy)
Cystic hygroma	1 in 120 (EU) at 1 in 6,000 (B)	60 at 75%	45X (80%); 21,18,13, XXY
Hydrops	1 in 1,500 at 1 in 4,000 (B)	30 at 80%.*	13, 21,18, 45X
Hydrocephalus	3 in 10,000 at 8 in 10,000 (LB)	3 at 8%	13, 18, triploidy
Hydranencephaly	2 in 1,000 (IA)	Minimal	Not available
Holoprosencephaly	1 in 16,000 (LB)	40 at 60%	13, 18, 18p
Cardiac defects	7 in 1,000 at 9 in 1,000 (LB)	5 at 30%	21, 18, 13, 22, 8, 9
Complete audiovisual canal		40 at 70%	21
Diaphragmatic hernia	1 in 3,500 at 1 in 4,000 (LB)	20 at 25%	13, 18, 21, 45X
Omphalocele	1 in 5,800 (LB)	30 at 40%	13,18
Gastroschisis	1 in 10,000 at 1 in 15,000 (LB)	Minimal	Not available
Duodenal atresia	1 in 10,000 (LB)	20 at 30%	21
Bowel obstruction	1 in 2,500 at 5,000 (LB)	Minimal	Not available
Bladder outlet obstruction	1 in 1,000 at 2 in 1,000 (LB)	20 at 25%	13, 18
Prune belly syndrome	1 in 35,000 at 1 in 50,000 (LB)	Low	18, 13, 45X
Facial cleft	1 in 700 (LB)	1%	13, 18, deletions
Limb reduction	4 in 10,000 at 6 in 10,000 (LB)	8%	18
Club foot	1.2 in 1,000 (LB)	20 at 30%	18, 13, 4p-,18q-
Single umbilical artery	1%	Minimal	Not available

Abbreviations: B indicates birth; EU, early ultrasonography; IA, infant autopsy; LB live birth.
*30% if diagnosed by 24 weeks of gestation; 80% if diagnosed by 17 weeks of gestation

Table 9. Down Syndrome Risk of Dysmorphism

Ultrasound Marker	Number of Studies	Down Syndrome Detection Rate (%)	False-Positive Rate (%)
Nuchal fold, 6 mm	16	38	1.3
Femur length (observed versus expected)	10	34	5.9
Femur length (biparietal diameter–femur length)	4	22	5.9
Humerus length (observed versus expected)	6	37	5.3
Femur plus humerus (observed versus expected)	3	36	3.7
Pyelectasis	4	19	2.4
Hyperechogenic bowel	3	11	0.7
Cerebral ventricular dilatation	1	6	0.0
Choroid plexus cyst	1	0	1.8
Ear length	1	78	8.0
Fifth-digit midphalanx hypoplasia	1	75	18.0
Increased iliac length	1	50	2.0
Short frontal lobe	1	21	4.8

been performed on high-risk women, primarily women who are aged 35 years and older, who have a history of a previous aneuploidy, or who have a positive Down syndrome screening test result and are already scheduled to undergo invasive genetic testing. Because the predictive value of a screening test is determined by the prevalence of the abnormality in the population studied and the predictive value increases as the prevalence increases, a screening test will perform better in a population with a high prevalence than in one with a low prevalence. Thus, data from studies of high-risk women may not be applicable to a population of younger low-risk women. Another area of controversy is whether the woman with a positive Down syndrome screening test result should undergo an ultrasound examination to screen for dysmorphisms instead of having diagnostic testing. This is because such an ultrasound examination cannot be considered diagnostic because it cannot confirm or rule out fetal aneuploidy and is in effect another screening test. Performing a second screening test reduces the sensitivity of the initial screening test. Other concerns include the transient nature of many dysmorphisms (eg, choroid plexus cysts), the difficulty in clearly visualizing all dysmorphisms (eg, absence of the middle phalanx of the little finger), and variations in both measurement technique and the methods used to classify the size of a structure as abnormal (eg, short femur). The utility and appropriateness of both ultrasound screening for major structural malformations and ultrasound screening for dysmorphisms as a Down syndrome screening test in low-risk women remain unresolved.

Current Strategies for Fetal Aneuploidy Detection

The remainder of this section will review the methods for prenatal diagnosis of aneuploidy, including amniocentesis, fluorescent in situ hybridization (FISH), CVS, and preimplantation diagnosis. Newer techniques also will be described.

Amniocentesis

Traditional amniocentesis for prenatal diagnosis of aneuploidy or genetic disease usually is offered between 14 weeks of gestation and 20 weeks of gestation. Early amniocentesis, performed between 11 weeks of gestation and 13 weeks and 6 days of gestation, is not recommended and no longer offered by many centers. It has been associated with a spontaneous pregnancy loss rate three to four times that of traditional amniocentesis, an increased incidence of positional foot deformities, and in some reports an increased incidence of neonatal respiratory distress (15) . In addition, amniocyte culture failure is more likely after early amniocentesis, necessitating an additional invasive diagnostic procedure in these patients.

Fluorescent in Situ Hybridization

One disadvantage of amniocentesis is the need to culture cells for several days before a karyotype analysis; a high-resolution karyotype usually takes at least 8 days to complete. Fluorescent in situ hybridization, which can be performed on uncultured amniocytes using fluorescently tagged DNA probes specific for chromosomes 13, 18, 21, X, and Y, now allows the ploidy of these chromosomes to be determined in 24–48 hours. Fluorescent in situ hybridization may not detect mosaicism and does not detect structural chromosomal abnormalities or aneuploidies in other chromosomes unless specific probes are used (ie, a probe for a deletion on chromosome 22 can identify Di George syndrome). It typically is used to obtain preliminary results only as an adjunct to and not as a replacement for a traditional cytogenetic analysis with high resolution banding.

Chorionic Villus Sampling

The primary advantage of CVS is that results are available earlier in pregnancy. Early reports of an association between CVS and limb reduction and oromandibular defects virtually all involved cases in which the procedure was performed before 10 weeks of gestation. Subsequent research indicated that CVS does not increase the risk of these anomalies above the background risk when the procedure is performed at or beyond 10 weeks of gestation. Chorionic villus sampling at this gestational age is believed to be as safe as second-trimester amniocentesis; in some reports, the transabdominal approach is even safer than the transvaginal method.

Chorionic villus sampling and amniocentesis entail a similar low risk of pregnancy loss. The safety of both procedures is most directly related to the gestational age at which they are performed and the skill and experience of the operator. Research has shown that the safety of both CVS and amniocentesis increases along with the number of procedures performed by the operator, and that ongoing performance of a minimum number of procedures each month is necessary to maintain operator skill. In most experienced centers, patients are counseled that the procedure-induced miscarriage rates for CVS and second-trimester amniocentesis are equivalent and in the range of 1 in 200 to 1 in 400.

Preimplantation Diagnosis (Embryo Biopsy)

Preimplantation diagnosis is now available in many urban centers. After in vitro fertilization, a biopsy of the blastomere (at the 8–16 cell stage) or the polar body is performed, followed by genetic testing using polymerase chain reaction, FISH, or both and intrauterine transfer of the embryo once it is confirmed that the embryo is unaffected (16, 17). The benefits of preimplantation diagnosis are obvious. The drawbacks include having to conceive by using reproductive technology, the fact that only a limited number of FISH probes can be applied to a single cell, and the possibility of misdiagnosis because of "allele dropout" or failure to correctly identify an abnormal allele because one of the parental alleles in a heterozygous cell fails to amplify. In addition, many authorities strongly recommend that the preimplantation diagnosis be confirmed by CVS or amniocentesis, thus incurring the risk and expense of an invasive diagnostic procedure (18, 19).

Special Considerations

Trisomy 21 has been diagnosed in fetal cells isolated from maternal blood during the first trimester using FISH. However, fetal cells in the maternal circulation are rare (with only one to six fetal cells per milliliter of maternal blood), there are few fetus-specific cell surface markers that can be used to separate fetal cells from maternal cells, and fetal cell enrichment and cell sorting techniques are complex and cumbersome.

However, maternal blood also contains free fetal DNA, from shed fetal cells or in the form of apoptotic bodies, nucleosomes, or free DNA fragments. Because of apoptosis, there is a significant turnover of fetal cells each day, releasing increasing quantities of fetal DNA into the maternal circulation as gestational age increases. The half-life of free fetal DNA is short, with no fetal DNA detected in the maternal circulation within hours of delivery; thus, there is no possibility of misdiagnosis because the recovered fetal DNA is actually from a previous pregnancy (as can occur with certain types of whole fetal cells). Free fetal DNA fragments can be recovered from maternal blood by centrifugation and amplified using polymerase chain reaction, and then used for genetic testing. Free fetal DNA has been used to diagnose fetal aneuploidy, to determine fetal gender, and to identify paternally inherited alleles in the fetus. The presence of increased quantities of free fetal DNA in maternal plasma also may be a marker for certain obstetric complications, such as preeclampsia, preterm labor, or placenta increta or percreta. Although at present this technique is used for research purposes only, it has more clinical promise that the isolation of whole fetal cells from the maternal circulation.

Array-based comparative genome hybridization is a relatively new technique that detects very small DNA deletions and duplications—an increase or decrease in the number of base pairs or "copy number variation" —that would not be recognized with standard high-resolution karyotyping. It uses a microarray constructed of small segments of DNA (oligonucleotides), representing thousands of discrete genomic locations, fixed to a slide. A microarray could be designed to represent a complete normal genome or could be composed of selected DNA sequences that correspond to a single chromosome or chromosome region, known genes, or multiple loci of interest. The patient's DNA and a sample of normal reference DNA are fragmented and labeled differentially, using two different color fluorophores, and allowed to hybridize to the oligonucleotides on the microarray slide. A fluorescent scanner determines the relative amounts of the two fluorophores bound to each oligonucleotide. Equal binding of the two fluorophores indicates that the patient's DNA is identical to the reference DNA, whereas unequal binding indicates copy number variation, or a very small duplication or deletion in that region. Computer software converts the scanner information into data showing the size and location of the copy number changes within the genome.

Array-based comparative genome hybridization could be used to complement a high-resolution karyotype. For example, array-based comparative genome hybridization has been used to evaluate apparently balanced chromosome translocations, and microdeletions have been identified that were not detected with a standard high-resolution karyotype. In a small series of neonates with specific structural anomalies, dysmorphisms, or developmental delay who had been evaluated by array-based comparative genome hybridization, approximately 11–12 % were found to have previously unrecognized copy number abnormalities. The potential utility of array-based comparative genome hybridization for the prenatal evaluation of anomalous fetuses is beginning to be explored (20). It is possible that array-based comparative genome hybridization might eventually obviate the need for a standard karyotype. Because array-based comparative genome hybridization identifies copy number abnormalities, it could identify trisomies, such as Down syndrome, and other numerical aneuploidies; marker chromosomes; unbalanced translocations; and deletions and duplications.

References

1. Preconception and prenatal carrier screening for genetic diseases in individuals of Eastern European Jewish descent. ACOG Committee Opinion No. 442. American College of Obstetricians and Gynecologists. Obstet Gynecol 2009;114: 950–3.

2. Rousseau F, Rouillard P, Morel ML, Khandjian EW, Morgan K. Prevalence of carriers of premutation-size alleles of the FMRI gene--and implications for the population genetics of the fragile X syndrome. Am J Hum Genet 1995; 57:1006–18.

3. Langlois S. Genomic imprinting: a new mechanism for disease. Pediatr Pathol 1994;14:161–5.

4. Nussbaum RL, McInnes RR, Willard HF, Thompson MW, editors. Thompson & Thompson Genetics in Medicine. 6th ed. Philadelphia: Saunders; 2001.

5. D'Alton ME, Cleary-Goldman J, Lambert-Messerlian G, Ball RH, Nyberg DA, Comstock CH, et al. Maintaining quality assurance for sonographic nuchal translucency measurement: lessons from the FASTER Trial. Ultrasound Obstet Gynecol 2009;33:142–6.

6. Wapner R, Thom E, Simpson JL, Pergament E, Silver R, Filkins K, et al. First-trimester screening for trisomies 21 and 18. First Trimester Maternal Serum Biochemistry and Fetal Nuchal Translucency Screening (BUN) Study Group. N Engl J Med 2003;349:1405–13.

7. Malone FD, Wald NJ, Canick JA, Ball RH, Nyberg DA, Comstock CH, et al. First- and Second-Trimester Evaluation of Risk (FASTER) Trial: principal results of the NICHD multicenter Down Sydrome screening study [abstract]. Am J Obstet Gynecol 2003;189 (suppl):S56.

8. Wald NJ, Rodeck C, Hackshaw AK, Walters J, Chitty L, Mackinson AM. First and second trimester antenatal screening for Down's syndrome: the results of the Serum, Urine and Ultrasound Screening Study (SURUSS) [published erratum appears in J Med Screen 2006;13:51–2]. J Med Screen 2003;10:56–104.

9. Spencer K, Spencer CE, Power M, Dawson C, Nicolaides KH. Screening for chromosomal abnormalities in the first trimester using ultrasound and maternal serum biochemistry in a one-stop clinic: a review of three years prospective experience. BJOG 2003;110:281–6.

10. Wald NJ, Watt HC, Hackshaw AK. Integrated screening for Down's syndrome on the basis of tests performed during the first and second trimesters. N Engl J Med 1999; 341:461–7.

11. Hyett J, Perdu M, Sharland G, Snijders R, Nicolaides KH. Using fetal nuchal translucency to screen for major congenital cardiac defects at 10-14 weeks of gestation: population based cohort study. BMJ 1999;318:81–5.

12. Souka AP, Von Kaisenberg CS, Hyett JA, Sonek JD, Nicolaides KH. Increased nuchal translucency with normal karyotype [published erratum appears in Am J Obstet Gynecol 2005;192:2096]. Am J Obstet Gynecol 2005;192: 1005–21.

13. Campbell J, Gilbert WM, Nicolaides KH, Campbell S. Ultrasound screening for spina bifida: cranial and cerebellar signs in a high-risk population. Obstet Gynecol 1987; 70:247–50.

14. Watson WJ, Chescheir NC, Katz VL, Seeds JW. The role of ultrasound in evaluation of patients with elevated maternal serum alpha-fetoprotein: a review. Obstet Gynecol 1991; 78:123–8.

15. Tredwell SJ, Wilson D, Wilmink MA. Review of the effect of early amniocentesis on foot deformity in the neonate. Canadian Early and Mid-Trimester Amniocentesis Trial Group (CEMAT), and the Canadian Pediatric Orthopedic Review Group. J Pediatr Orthop 2001;21:636–41.

16. Mastenbroek S, Twisk M, van Echten-Arends J, Sikkema-Raddatz B, Korevaar JC, Verhoeve HR, et al. In vitro fertilization with preimplantation genetic screening. N Engl J Med 2007;357:9–17.

17. Swanson A, Strawn E, Lau E, Bick D. Preimplantation genetic diagnosis: technology and clinical applications. WMJ 2007;106:145–51.

18. Thornhill AR, deDie-Smulders CE, Geraedts JP, Harper JC, Harton GL, Lavery SA, et al. ESHRE PGD Consortium 'Best practice guidelines for clinical preimplantation genetic diagnosis (PGD) and preimplantation genetic screening (PGS)'. ESHRE PGD Consortium. Hum Reprod 2005;20:35–48.

19. Preimplantation genetic testing: a Practice Committee opinion. American Society for Reproductive Medicine. Fertil Steril 2007;88:1497–504.

20. Van den Veyver IB, Patel A, Shaw CA, Pursley AN, Kang SH, Simovich MJ, et al. Clinical use of array comparative genomic hybridization (aCGH) for prenatal diagnosis in 300 cases. Prenat Diagn 2009;29:29–39.

Fetal Therapy

Kenneth J. Moise Jr

The advent of fetal therapy occurred in the early 1960s with reports of successful intrauterine transfusion for severe hemolytic disease of the fetus and newborn. Subsequent experience with various procedures for other fetal indications has taught us that understanding the natural course of a fetal disease is paramount to proper patient selection. Although initial attempts at fetal therapy were billed as innovative, many of the more recently adopted therapies have been evaluated through randomized clinical trials. Establishment of centers of excellence would appear prudent in order to forward research, training, and the development of new therapies.

Conditions Treated Noninvasively

Congenital Adrenal Hyperplasia

Neonates with congenital adrenal hyperplasia can present with a clinical spectrum of no symptoms to ambiguous genitalia and cardiovascular collapse. Typically, a genetic defect in one of two enzymes (21-hydroxylase or 11-hydroxylase) involved in the production of adrenal steroids creates a block in these metabolic pathways, with a resulting increase in adrenal androgens. Virilization of a female fetus can then occur. Because the disease is inherited in an autosomal recessive fashion, one of four subsequent offspring will be affected. In such cases, maternal oral dexamethasone therapy is initiated after biochemical confirmation of pregnancy. Early suppression of the fetal adrenal axis is important because development of the external genitalia is complete by 7–12 weeks of gestation. A maternal blood sample can be obtained at 8–10 weeks of gestation to assess fetal gender using free fetal DNA. If the result of the analysis indicates a male fetus (*SRY* gene present), maternal steroids can be discontinued. A tapering dose schedule should be used. If a free fetal DNA sample is not obtained or the result of the analysis indicates a female fetus, then a chorionic villus sampling is undertaken at 10–12 weeks of gestation. Steroids are discontinued if a male fetus or an unaffected female fetus is identified through karyotype and DNA analysis. If an affected female fetus is identified, maternal dexamethasone is continued until delivery. Stress doses of steroids should be given to the pregnant woman at the time of delivery to prevent addisonian crisis in labor. If the fetus has not been previously tested for the genetic mutation, DNA testing and a 17-hydroxyprogesterone assay should be drawn on the first day of life and empiric hydrocortisone and fluorinated steroid therapy initiated until the mutation analysis returns. Mixed results in the neonate have been reported with prenatal therapy: one third of fetuses were still completely virilized and an additional one third exhibited partial virilization. This may result from inadequate dosing or late entry into therapy (1).

Fetal Arrhythmias

Although all fetal tachyarrhythmias are not supraventricular in origin, a sustained rate in excess of 200 beats per minute should result in an urgent referral to a maternal–fetal medicine specialist or pediatric cardiologist. If this arrhythmia is sustained, hydrops fetalis can result. Fetal echocardiography rarely reveals structural abnormalities. In gestations of 35 or more weeks, delivery with subsequent cardioversion in the nursery would appear prudent. In a preterm gestation, in utero therapy is aimed at decreasing the conduction time of the fetal atrioventricular node to allow adequate time for ventricular filling. This usually is accomplished by the administration of digoxin to the mother. In most cases, hospitalization with monitoring of maternal digoxin levels is indicated. In addition, larger doses of digoxin than typically are used in the nonpregnant patient are needed secondary to increased maternal glomerular filtration. If fetal supraventricular tachycardia persists, oral flecainide or sotalol is added as second-line therapy (2). Because many of these agents increase digoxin levels, the maternal digoxin dose should be reduced appropriately. In cases of recalcitrant fetal tachycardia or severe fetal hydrops, medications can be administered directly to the fetus through intramuscular injection performed under ultrasound guidance. Maternal administration of oral sotalol appears to be the therapy of choice in cases of fetal atrial flutter. A reversal of hydrops can be expected once the fetal supraventricular tachycardia resolves. Maternal medications should be continued until delivery.

Fetal bradyarrhythmias can occur for a variety of reasons. More than 50% of cases of congenital heart block result from structural cardiac abnormalities. Most remaining cases are secondary to immune destruction of the fetal cardiac conduction system in response to maternal autoantibodies (anti-SS-A and anti-SS-B).

Maternal administration of steroids (dexamethasone) that cross the placenta has been attempted in an effort to ameliorate the inflammatory action on fetal conduction. Steroid therapy after the detection of fetal bradycardia has not proved beneficial. The disease tends to recur in subsequent offspring because of the persistence of maternal antibodies. Steroid therapy before 14 weeks of gestation may prevent recurrence.

Fetal Thyroid Disorders

Small amounts of maternal thyroxine (T_4) cross the human placenta. By 12 weeks of gestation, however, the fetal thyroid begins to produce T_4, and by 20 weeks of gestation the fetal pituitary–thyroid axis is functionally mature and independent of the maternal endocrine system. Fetal thyroid disorders usually are unrecognized until after birth, when they are detected through mandated neonatal screening programs. Fetal goiter on routine antenatal ultrasonography is sometimes detected; however, this finding can be associated with both hypothyroidism and hyperthyroidism in the fetus as well as a euthyroid state. It often is associated with polyhydramnios caused by external compression of the fetal esophagus. Intrauterine growth restriction has been reported in fetal hypothyroidism and hyperthyroidism. Congenital heart block and cardiac failure are noted in some cases of fetal hypothyroidism; tachycardia, hydrops fetalis, and craniosynostosis can be seen in hyperthyroid cases.

Although neonatal supplementation will avert most cases of delayed neurologic development when the fetus is hypothyroid, language, motor, and spatial visual development still may be impaired. Most cases of fetal goiter and hypothyroidism are related to overzealous use of maternal propylthiouracil or methimazole, which readily enter the fetal compartment. Direct fetal causes include dysgenesis of the thyroid gland or enzymatic defects in the formation of thyroid hormones.

In cases of maternal thyrotoxicosis, antithyroid medications should be adjusted to maintain serum thyroid hormone levels in the upper limits of the normal range. If a fetal goiter is noted in the euthyroid pregnant patient or in the hyperthyroid patient receiving appropriate doses of antithyroid medications, cordocentesis should be undertaken to determine the fetal free T_4 and thyrotropin levels (3). Amniotic fluid levels of these hormones are not indicative of the fetal status. If hypothyroidism is detected, the fetus can be treated with weekly intraamniotic injections of T_4. Fetal blood sampling should be repeated 4–6 weeks later to confirm the fetal response.

Maternal Graves disease is associated with fetal hyperthyroidism in 2–10% of cases. High levels of maternal thyroid-stimulating antibody can stimulate the fetal thyroid gland after transplacental passage. Maternal thyroid-stimulating antibody levels should be measured in women who are euthyroid but previously have been treated with I 131 ablation. Cordocentesis at 20–24 weeks of gestation is undertaken to measure fetal thyroid function in the pregnant patient with previous or current Graves disease and with any of the following conditions (4):

- History of a previously affected infant
- Elevated thyroid-stimulating antibody level (greater than 160% of normal)

- Ultrasound findings suggestive of fetal hyperthyroidism—goiter, tachycardia, growth restriction, hydrops, or cardiomegaly

Maternal treatment with propylthiouracil (with thyroxine supplementation, if necessary) can be implemented if the fetus is found to be hyperthyroid. Repeat cordocentesis should be undertaken in 4–6 weeks to confirm fetal response. Close supervision of the neonate by pediatricians is warranted in cases of fetal hypothyroidism or hyperthyroidism requiring in utero treatment.

Management of Fetal Anemia and Thrombocytopenia

Red Cell Alloimmunization

Maternal sensitization or alloimmunization to erythrocyte antigens can produce hemolytic disease of the fetus and newborn. More than 40 erythrocyte antigens can cause the disorder; however, the three major antigens that often lead to the need for in utero therapy include Rh D, Rh c, and Kell.

PREVENTION OF RH ALLOIMMUNIZATION

Most cases of spontaneous fetomaternal hemorrhage occur late in pregnancy. In the United States, the use of 300 micrograms of intramuscularly administered anti-D immune globulin (formerly referred to as Rh [D] immune globulin) at 28 weeks of gestation has produced a 10-fold reduction in cases of antepartum sensitization to the Rh D antigen. Whether a maternal antibody screen is needed before administering antenatal anti-D immune globulin is controversial, and it may not be cost-effective. At delivery, approximately 15–20% of patients are found to have a positive indirect Coombs test result for Rh D antibody secondary to the persistence of antenatal anti-D immune globulin. Titers in this situation are four or less and should not prevent the use of postpartum prophylaxis. However, in situations where a high titer is noted at delivery, indicating maternal sensitization, anti-D immune globulin has not been shown to be advantageous (5).

Anti-D immune globulin should be administered in a dose of 300 micrograms within 72 hours of delivery if cord blood indicates that the neonate of an Rh D-negative, nonsensitized patient is Rh D positive. Because some protective effects have been reported with the use of anti-D immune globulin for up to 28 days after delivery, inadvertent omission of anti-D immune globulin within 72 hours of delivery should not preclude the use of anti-D immune globulin after this time. All Rh D-negative, nonsensitized patients giving birth to Rh D-positive infants should be screened for excessive fetomaternal hemorrhage in the immediate postpartum period. This usually entails an initial qualitative rosette test performed on maternal blood. Negative results warrant the administration of one vial of anti-D immune globulin (300 micrograms). If the rosette test result is positive, quantification of the amount of fetomaternal hemorrhage is undertaken using either the Kleihauer–Betke test or flow cytometry. The calculated volume of the fetomaternal hemorrhage then is divided by 30 to determine the number of vials of anti-D immune globulin needed. If the calculation indicates that a fraction of a vial is needed, the fraction usually is rounded to the nearest whole number (ie, less than 0.5 would result in the addition of one more vial). In cases of large fetomaternal hemorrhage, the administration of an additional vial of anti-D globulin in excess of the calculated amount may be advised by the blood bank. Four different Rh immune globulin products are now available in the United States to prevent Rh D alloimmunization. The original product approved for clinical use as well as a second product must be given by intramuscular injection because of minimal contamination with immunoglobulin (Ig) A antibodies and other plasma proteins. Two intravenous anti-D preparations are now available for use. Because these formulations are prepared by sepharose column and ion-exchange chromatography, they contain only IgG. Both can be administered by the intramuscular route as well.

Patients with a weak D-positive type (once termed Du positive) are not candidates for anti-D immune globulin. In these patients, Rh D antigens are expressed on the surface of the erythrocytes in a weaker concentration than in most Rh D-positive individuals. Patients with a weak D-positive type therefore are not at risk for sensitization. However, an error can occur when a weak D-positive type patient undergoes her first blood typing at delivery. If a significant fetomaternal hemorrhage occurred after delivery, a mixed field agglutination reaction will result from the Rh D-positive fetal cells in the maternal circulation, yielding an erroneous weak D-positive type. Such confusing cases can be prevented by routine screening for fetomaternal hemorrhage at delivery.

If delivery occurs within 3 weeks of antenatal anti-D immune globulin administration, the dose need not be repeated if there is no evidence of excessive fetomaternal hemorrhage. This recommendation would apply also to the use of anti-D immune globulin after late third-trimester amniocentesis or external cephalic version.

Monitoring of the Sensitized Pregnancy

In the first sensitized pregnancy, once a patient's antibody screening result is positive for an antibody associated with hemolytic disease of the fetus and newborn, a titer should be obtained. Serial maternal titers are then monitored on a monthly basis until a critical titer is noted (16 for anti-D immune globulin or other anti-red cell antibodies; 8 for anti-Kell antibodies). Paternal blood should be eval-

uated for the presence of the putative antigen. If present, molecular techniques can be used in the case of the Rh D antigen to determine paternal zygosity. Serology can be used with paternal blood to determine zygosity for other involved antigens.

Once a critical titer is noted, the patient should be referred to a maternal–fetal medicine specialist. Free fetal DNA testing is now available to determine the fetal Rh D status in cases of paternal heterozygosity. The fetal antigen status can be determined through amniocentesis for other red cell antigens that cause hemolytic disease of the fetus and newborn (6).

Once the fetus is determined to be antigen positive, serial middle cerebral artery Doppler velocimetry should be undertaken every 1–2 weeks. Recent studies have indicated that a value for the peak systolic velocity of greater than 1.5 multiples of the median is more accurate than ΔOD_{450} measurements on amniotic fluid (7). If an elevated middle cerebral artery value is present, cordocentesis with blood readied for intrauterine transfusion is the next step in management. Antenatal testing should be initiated at 32 weeks gestation. If serial middle cerebral artery Doppler velocimetry results remain normal, the fetus should be delivered by 38 weeks of gestation. A cross match for one unit of packed red blood cells should be performed at the time of delivery—this unit can be used for neonatal transfusion in the rare instance where the newborn is noted to have an unexpected anemia.

In a subsequent sensitized pregnancy, maternal titers are less useful to predict fetal disease. Early referral for serial middle cerebral artery Doppler velocimetry starting at 18 weeks of gestation is appropriate.

Intrauterine Transfusion

Typically, an intrauterine transfusion involves targeting the umbilical cord at its insertion into the placenta using continuous ultrasound guidance. On some occasions, the intrahepatic portion of the umbilical vein can be used. An initial fetal hematocrit value is obtained; a value of less than 30% warrants transfusion. Standardized formulas based on fetal weight estimated by ultrasonography are then used to calculate the volume of erythrocytes to be given. In many instances, neuromuscular blocking agents, such as pancuronium or vecuronium, are administered into the umbilical cord to prevent fetal movement. Maternal packed erythrocytes can be used as the source of red cells after extensive washing to remove the antibody-containing plasma. Leukoreduction and irradiation with 25 Gy are performed to prevent graft-versus-host reaction. If donor red cells are used, a fresh source that tests negative for cytomegalovirus should be identified. These cells also should be leukoreduced and irradiated. Intrauterine transfusions are continued at 1–3-week intervals until approximately 35 weeks of gestation, when delivery of the fetus probably represents a safer alternative than continued in utero therapy. Induction of labor is undertaken 2–3 weeks later. An overall survival rate of 85% can be expected, with slightly lower rates of survival if the fetus is hydropic at the first procedure.

Although the need for neonatal exchange transfusion has become less frequent with aggressive in utero therapy, many of these infants require simple transfusions in the first few months of life because of persistent bone marrow suppression. These children, therefore, should be monitored with weekly hematocrit determinations and reticulocyte counts. Data to date have indicated normal developmental outcomes in infants who survive intrauterine transfusion.

Kell Alloimmunization

Clinical and basic laboratory data suggest that unlike Rh disease, the Kell antibody causes both hemolysis and suppression of erythropoiesis (8). Bilirubin levels in fetal serum and amniotic fluid are lower in Kell-positive fetuses that exhibit signs of hemolytic disease of the fetus and newborn. For this reason, serial middle cerebral artery Doppler imaging is indicated for the detection of fetal anemia.

Fetomaternal Hemorrhage

A limited number of cases of fetal hydrops secondary to fetomaternal hemorrhage have been reported in which the intrauterine transfusion of erythrocytes resulted in a successful outcome. In these cases, a presentation of decreased fetal movement led to ultrasound detection of the hydrops. Kleihauer–Betke tests performed on maternal blood can confirm the diagnosis of fetomaternal hemorrhage. Although intrauterine transfusion prolongs most pregnancies, pregnancies that are greater than 32 weeks of gestation may benefit from premature delivery secondary to continued fetomaternal hemorrhage.

Alloimmune Thrombocytopenia

Alloimmune thrombocytopenia affects approximately 1 in 1,200 pregnancies. Similar to red cell alloimmunization, maternal antibodies to platelet-specific antigens are actively transported across the placenta, resulting in profound fetal thrombocytopenia. Platelet function also appears to be affected as spontaneous intracranial bleeding can occur in 10–20% of cases, with 25–50% of these occurring in utero. Important differences between alloimmune thrombocytopenia and hemolytic disease of the newborn include the possibility of an affected fetus or infant in the patient's first pregnancy (50% of cases) and the inability of the maternal antiplatelet antibody titer to predict perinatal disease. The HPA-la

(PLA[1]) platelet antigen is involved in more than 80% of cases in white individuals. The HPA-3a (Bak[a]) and HPA-5b (Br[a]) antigens comprise most of the remaining cases. In Asians, antibodies to the HPA-4 (Pen, Yuk) antigen system are the most common etiology.

Typically, alloimmune thrombocytopenia is first diagnosed after the birth of an affected infant who exhibits clinical manifestations of severe thrombocytopenia. Platelet typing of the parents will reveal an antigen incompatibility with evidence of maternal antibodies against both neonatal and paternal platelets. Once there is an antecedent history, subsequent offspring have more than a 90% chance of recurrent disease. A previous sibling with antenatal intracranial bleeding is useful in determining the severity of perinatal disease in the next pregnancy (Table 10).

Treatment strategies involve the use of maternal immunomodulation with intravenous immunoglobulin (IVIG), oral prednisone, or both. Potential risks of IVIG, a plasma product, include a local reaction at the administration site, fever, rash, headache, altered immunity, and transmission of infectious diseases. Risks for prednisone include osteoporosis, glucose intolerance and gestational diabetes mellitus, depressed immunity, mood swings, and gastrointestinal irritation.

Several randomized clinical trials have been undertaken to determine the correct dosing of IVIG and prednisone for optimal perinatal results. Many of the initial protocols involved cordocentesis to see if fetal thrombocytopenia was not responding with institution of salvage therapy if a low platelet count persisted. However, a 1–2% rate of fetal loss with an additional 5% of patients experiencing other complications, such as preterm premature rupture of the membranes and fetal bradycardia with the need for emergent cesarean delivery, have been reported. This has led to considerations to forego invasive testing and institute empiric therapy (9). Patients with standard risk usually start the treatment by 20 weeks of gestation, consisting of either 2 g/kg/week of IVIG (given in two doses) or 1 g/kg/week of IVIG with 0.5-mg/kg/day oral prednisone.

Table 10. History of Fetal Intracranial Bleeding and Risk Categories for Subsequent Pregnancies

Risk Category	History
Standard	The previous sibling was thrombocytopenic at birth, but did not experience an intracranial bleeding.
High	The previous sibling experienced an intracranial bleeding between 28 weeks of gestation and the neonatal period.
Very High	The previous sibling experienced an intracranial bleeding before 28 weeks of gestation.

Cordocentesis can be considered at 32 weeks of gestation to evaluate the fetal platelet response, or therapy can be empirically increased at this point in pregnancy by increasing the dose of IVIG or adding prednisone. Patients with high risk or very high risk should have therapy instituted by 12 weeks of gestation with higher doses of IVIG and prednisone as follows: 2 g/kg/week and 1 mg/kg/day, respectively. Further studies are underway to better delineate the optimal treatment strategy in these latter two groups of patients.

Fetal blood sampling can be used near term to decide on the route of delivery. The procedure should be performed by experienced maternal–fetal medicine specialists and with the availability of direct infusion of maternal-derived platelets. In utero transfusion of maternal-derived platelets should occur if the fetal platelet count is less than 50×10^9/L to prevent exsanguination from the needle site of cordocentesis. Cesarean delivery is recommended; vaginal delivery should be considered only if the fetal platelet count is greater than 50×10^9/L at cordocentesis before delivery.

Fetal Surgery

Since the first reported case of open fetal surgery in 1983, such surgery has been restricted to fetal conditions such as diaphragmatic hernia, which are considered likely to be lethal in neonatal life (10). More recently, spina bifida, a fetal condition associated with life-long morbidity, has become the most common indication for this procedure. Proposed requirements to consider invasive intervention for fetal conditions include the following situations:

- The morbidity (both maternal and fetal) of the antenatal intervention is acceptable.
- The diagnosis of the condition can be made accurately.
- The condition can be differentiated from other non-surgical anomalies.
- The natural evolution of the disease, if left untreated, should be predictable and the condition should be lethal or severely debilitating.
- Adequate postnatal treatment should not exist.
- The proposed in utero intervention should be technically feasible.

Minimally Invasive Techniques

Percutaneous Shunting

Ultrasound-guided placement of a double-pigtail polymeric silicone shunt has been successfully employed to drain excessive collections of intracavitary fluid that might compromise fetal renal or pulmonary function. The most common indication for this technique is the treatment of severe oligohydramnios in cases of bladder outlet obstruction (urethral atresia or posterior urethral valves). Serial bladder aspirations are undertaken initially to evaluate the fetal karyotype and urinary electrolyte levels. An abnormal karyotype or evidence of poor renal reserve based on elevated electrolyte levels and β_2 microglobulin precludes placement of the shunt. Percutaneous shunts also have been used to drain large collections of thoracic fluid associated with fetal hydrops secondary to lateral displacement of the fetal heart. Such cases include unilateral pleural effusions and type I cystic adenomatoid malformations of the lung.

Laser Therapy

Twin–twin transfusion is a major contributor to perinatal morbidity and mortality in monochorionic multiple gestations. Although initially thought to be caused by simple transfusion of excessive blood volume from one fetus to another, more recent insight suggests that the pathophysiology is more complex and involves derangements in the renin–angiotensin system. The severity of the disease is graded using a staging system of ultrasound criteria (11):

- *Stage 1*—There is polyhydramnios (greater than 8 cm deepest vertical pocket by ultrasonography at less than 20 weeks of gestation and greater than 10 cm after 20 weeks of gestation) in association with the recipient twin and severe oligohydramnios (less than 2 cm) associated with the donor or "stuck" twin. The bladder of the donor twin is still seen; Doppler imaging results are normal.
- *Stage 2*—The bladder of the donor twin is absent; Doppler imaging results are normal.
- *Stage 3*—Abnormal Doppler imaging results, such as absent or reversed end-diastolic flow in the umbilical artery or reversed diastolic flow in the ductus venosus or pulsatile venous flow in the umbilical vein, are noted in one or both twins.
- *Stage 4*—Ascites, pleural effusions, scalp edema, or overt hydrops is present in one or both twins.
- *Stage 5*—One or both twins are dead.

Stage I disease at gestational ages of less than 27 weeks should be observed with serial ultrasonography on a weekly basis. Many of these cases regress spontaneously without treatment. Observation is favored over amnioreduction because an invasive procedure may result in intraamniotic bleeding or chorion–amnion separation, complications that can preclude a successful laser therapy if the disease progresses.

In the case of stage II disease or severely symptomatic hydramnios in stage I disease at less than 27 weeks of gestation, referral to an experienced center for laser photocoagulation of placental anastomoses is the treatment of choice. Patients typically undergo fetoscopy (introduction of a 2–3 mm laparoscopiclike device into the amniotic cavity of the recipient twin) under local anesthesia with intravenous sedation. Light energy from an yttrium–aluminum–garnet or diode laser is directed down a quartz fiber and used to selectively coagulate aberrant connections between the circulations of the twins. The presence of a significant structural anomaly in one of a twin pair with twin–twin transfusion syndrome is a relative contraindication to laser therapy. Possible treatment options include selective reduction of the anomalous fetus using radiofrequency ablation or bipolar cautery in an effort to reverse the twin–twin transfusion syndrome in the normal twin. In the setting of a twin with a lethal malformation, such as anencephaly, this would be the treatment of choice. In the case of a nonlethal abnormality, the decision for selective reduction may be more difficult and should be considered within the context of state laws that govern termination of pregnancy.

Both a randomized clinical trial and a meta-analysis have indicated that perinatal outcome is improved with laser therapy over amnioreduction (12, 13). In cases of twin–twin transfusion syndrome that present after 27 weeks of gestation, amnioreduction or septostomy (intentional perforation of the intervening membrane with a small gauge needle) is probably the current treatment of choice.

Open Maternal–Fetal Surgery

The ultrasound finding of right-sided displacement of the fetal heart should lead to a suspicion of a fetal diaphragmatic hernia. When a hernia is present, lesions are predominantly left sided, and the stomach or liver often can be herniated into the thoracic cavity. Direct compression of the ipsilateral lung and deviation of the heart with compression of the contralateral lung can lead to pulmonary hypoplasia. Kinking of the gastroesophageal junction produces polyhydramnios. Initial efforts to correct this lesion with open maternal–fetal surgery met with poor success because of preterm premature rupture of membranes and preterm labor after maternal hysterotomy (14). In addition, high rates of fetal loss were noted when hepatic herniation into the chest was present. Results from a small, randomized clinical trial revealed equivalent neonatal rates of survival between prenatal surgical repair and standard neonatal repair (15). These data led to the abandonment of open maternal–fetal surgery for the direct repair of diaphragmatic hernia.

Investigations into animal models for diaphragmatic hernia revealed that occlusion of the fetal trachea prevented the egress of pulmonary fluid, leading to enlargement of the fetal lungs and displacement of the

abdominal viscera from the thorax. Clinical trials in humans were initiated with surgical clips placed on the trachea first by open hysterotomy and later by fetoscopy. Subsequently, the procedure was modified to use a detachable balloon placed inside the trachea through a fetoscope. Results to date from European trials have indicated a marked improvement in perinatal survival in cases of extreme fetal lung hypoplasia (16). Randomized trials of tracheal occlusion for fetuses with diaphragm hernia and moderate pulmonary hypoplasia are ongoing in Europe. The procedure currently is only available in the United States at select centers on a compassionate basis.

Large and predominantly solid fetal sacrococcygeal teratomas can cause the development of nonimmune hydrops because of high-output cardiac failure. Open maternal–fetal surgery has been employed in such cases with mixed success (17). In many cases, the pregnant patient develops mirror syndrome, consisting of maternal fluid retention and respiratory compromise secondary to adult respiratory distress syndrome, and the fetus must be delivered. Minimally invasive techniques for the in utero treatment of sacrococcygeal teratomas have been of limited success to date (18).

Hamartomas of the fetal lungs can be readily detected with ultrasonography. Previously called pulmonary sequestrations or cystic adenomatoid malformations, they are currently classified as with or without a systemic arterial blood supply. Although many of the predominantly solid lesions can regress, some can increase in size, particularly before 26 weeks of gestation. Displacement of the fetal mediastinum can lead to decreased venous return and hydrops. Weekly ultrasound surveillance until 26 weeks of gestation would, therefore, appear prudent. Open maternal–fetal surgery can be offered for in utero resection of the lesion should hydrops develop. Minimally invasive procedures have been undertaken in some cases with successful occlusion of the blood supply and regression of the lesion.

Maternal–fetal surgery for meningomyelocele originally was attempted laparoscopically through the use of maternal skin grafts; success was limited. Centers turned to open hysterotomy for definitive repair of the lesion. Initial results in the infants who underwent these repairs revealed a decrease in the incidence of neonatal ventriculoperitoneal shunting by 30–50% for lumbosacral lesions. The greatest effect was associated with lesions below L-2, moderate ventriculomegaly, and repair before 25 weeks of gestation. The Chiari II malformation associated with meningomyelocele was noted to reverse in utero in virtually all cases of fetal repair. Neonatal urodynamic follow-up has not revealed clear improvement in function. Developmental studies regarding lower extremity function have revealed conflicting results (19). In 2000, the National Institutes of Health held a consensus conference that called for a randomized clinical trial to study open hysterotomy for the correction of meningomyelocele. The MOMS study was initiated in January 2003. Entry criteria include the following conditions:

- Myelomeningocele defect between T-1 and S-1, inclusive
- Hindbrain herniation (Chiari II malformation) identified by fetal magnetic resonance imaging
- Maternal age 18 years or older
- Normal fetal karyotype
- Gestational age of 19–25 weeks at randomization

A moratorium on open maternal–fetal surgery for spina bifida has been called until the trial is completed.

Stem Cell Transplantation

The human fetus is thought to be immunologically tolerant in early gestation. This has led several investigators to attempt hematopoietic or mesenchymal stem cell transfusions early in gestation for a variety of conditions. Both maternal and paternal bone marrow as well as frozen banked cells from abortuses have been used as sources. The cells are typically placed into the fetal peritoneal cavity. Detectable engraftment has been documented in 12 of 44 cases, however the level of chimerism has been low, with no impact on the clinical course of disease. Only in X-linked severe combined immunodeficiency syndrome has long-term outcome revealed a favorable clinical response (20).

References

1. Nimkarn S, New MI. Prenatal diagnosis and treatment of congenital adrenal hyperplasia. Pediatr Endocrinol Rev 2006;4:99–105.

2. Oudijk MA, Ruskamp JM, Ambachtsheer BE, Ververs TF, Stoutenbeek P, Visser GH, et al. Drug treatment of fetal tachycardias. Paediatr Drugs 2002;4:49–63.

3. Abuhamad AZ, Fisher DA, Warsof SL, Slotnick RN, Pyle PG, Wu SY, et al. Antenatal diagnosis and treatment of fetal goitrous hypothyroidism: case report and review of the literature. Ultrasound Obstet Gynecol 1995;6:368–71.

4. Kilpatrick S. Umbilical blood sampling in women with thyroid disease in pregnancy: Is it necessary [editorial]? Am J Obstet Gynecol 2003;189:1–2.

5. American College of Obstetricians and Gynecologists. Prevention of RhD alloimmunization. ACOG Practice Bulletin 4. Washington, DC: ACOG; 1999.

6. Moise KJ Jr. Management of rhesus alloimmunization in pregnancy. Obstet Gynecol 2008;112:164–76.

7. Oepkes D, Seaward PG, Vandenbussche FP, Windrim R, Kingdom J, Beyene J, et al. Doppler ultrasonography versus amniocentesis to predict fetal anemia. DIAMOND Study Group. N Engl J Med 2006;355:156–64.

8. Vaughan JI, Manning M, Warwick RM, Letsky EA, Murray NA, Roberts IA. Inhibition of erythroid progenitor cells by anti-Kell antibodies in fetal alloimmune anemia. N Engl J Med 1998;338:798–803.

9. Bussel JB, Primiani A. Fetal and neonatal alloimmune thrombocytopenia: progress and ongoing debates. Blood Rev 2008;22:33–52.

10. Albanese CT, Harrison MR. Surgical treatment for fetal disease. The state of the art. Ann N Y Acad Sci 1998;847:74–85.

11. Quintero RA, Morales WJ, Allen MH, Bornick PW, Johnson PK, Kruger M. Staging of twin-twin transfusion syndrome. J Perinatol 1999;19:550–5.

12. Senat MV, Deprest J, Boulvain M, Paupe A, Winer N, Ville Y. Endoscopic laser surgery versus serial amnioreduction for severe twin-to-twin transfusion syndrome. N Engl J Med 2004;351:136–44.

13. Rossi AC, D'Addario V. Laser therapy and serial amnioreduction as treatment for twin-twin transfusion syndrome: a metaanalysis and review of literature. Am J Obstet Gynecol 2008;198:147–52.

14. Harrison MR, Langer JC, Adzick NS, Golbus MS, Filly RA, Anderson RL, et al. Correction of congenital diaphragmatic hernia in utero, V. Initial clinical experience. J Pediatr Surg 1990;25:47–55; discussion 56–7.

15. Harrison MR, Adzick NS, Bullard KM, Farrell JA, Howell LJ, Rosen MA, et al. Correction of congenital diaphragmatic hernia in utero VII: a prospective trial. J Pediatr Surg 1997;32:1637–42.

16. Deprest J, Jani J, Gratacos E, Vandecruys H, Naulaers G, Delgado J, et al. Fetal intervention for congenital diaphragmatic hernia: the European experience. FETO Task Group. Semin Perinatol 2005;29:94–103.

17. Hedrick HL, Flake AW, Crombleholme TM, Howell LJ, Johnson MP, Wilson RD, et al. Sacrococcygeal teratoma: prenatal assessment, fetal intervention, and outcome. J Pediatr Surg 2004;39:430–8; discussion 430–8.

18. Paek BW, Jennings RW, Harrison MR, Filly RA, Tacy TA, Farmer DL, et al. Radiofrequency ablation of human fetal sacrococcygeal teratoma. Am J Obstet Gynecol 2001;184:503–7.

19. Wilson RD, Johnson MP, Bebbington M, Flake AW, Hedrick HL, Sutton LN, et al. Does a myelomeningocele sac compared to no sac result in decreased postnatal leg function following maternal fetal surgery for spina bifida aperta? Fetal Diagn Ther 2007;22:348–51.

20. Westgren M. In utero stem cell transplantation. Semin Reprod Med 2006;24:348–57.

COMPLICATIONS OF PREGNANCY

Preeclampsia and Gestational Hypertension

Susan M. Ramin

Hypertension is the most common medical risk factor among women who give birth to live babies. It affects as many as 8% of all pregnant women and remains a significant cause of maternal and neonatal morbidity and mortality (1).

Terminology and Clinical Manifestations

The report of the National High Blood Pressure Education Program Working Group on High Blood Pressure in Pregnancy has classified hypertensive disorders in pregnancy as follows (2):

- Chronic hypertension
- Preeclampsia and eclampsia
- Gestational hypertension
- Chronic hypertension with superimposed preeclampsia

This classification also has been adopted by the American College of Obstetricians and Gynecologists (3). Both the Working Group and the American College of Obstetricians and Gynecologists have provided criteria and definitions for diagnosing the various hypertensive disorders during pregnancy. Chronic hypertension is preexisting hypertension that is present before 20 weeks of gestation (see the section "Chronic Hypertension").

Gestational hypertension is presumed after 20 weeks of gestation in the absence of proteinuria or other signs and symptoms of preeclampsia and when the blood pressure returns to normal by 12 weeks postpartum. Many patients with this condition will develop actual preeclampsia as pregnancy progresses. If not, they receive the designation of transient hypertension. The term gestational hypertension has replaced the older term, pregnancy-induced hypertension.

Preeclampsia is defined as a pregnancy-specific syndrome that occurs after 20 weeks of gestation and is characterized by systolic pressure of 140 mm Hg or higher or diastolic pressure of 90 mm Hg or higher occurring with proteinuria (300 mg of protein or greater over 24 hours or a random dipstick urine determination of 1+ or greater protein or 30 mg/dL or greater).

Preeclampsia is considered severe when systolic blood pressure levels are equal to or greater than 160 mm Hg or diastolic blood pressure levels are equal to or greater than 110 mm Hg (Box 14). Blood pressure should be elevated on two occasions at least 6 hours apart. From a clinical standpoint, it is not necessary to wait for repeat elevation of blood pressure to confirm the diagnosis of preeclampsia (especially near term) when the patient has hypertension in the 180 mm Hg/120 mm Hg range.

Edema is no longer used as a diagnostic criterion for preeclampsia. Moreover, the incremental increase of 30 mm Hg (systolic blood pressure) or 15 mm Hg (diastolic blood pressure) above the baseline blood pressure is not used as a diagnostic criterion. Although not diagnostic and not risk factors for adverse outcomes (4), such changes in blood pressure should not be ignored and warrant close observation (2).

Superimposed preeclampsia in women with chronic hypertension often is difficult to diagnose but includes new-onset proteinuria, a sudden increase in proteinuria, a sudden sustained increase in hypertension, or the development of any component of hemolysis, elevated liver enzymes, and low platelet count (HELLP) syndrome, or symptoms of severe preeclampsia (2, 3).

Eclampsia is defined as new-onset grand mal seizures in women with preeclampsia or gestational hypertension. Other etiologies, such as arteriovenous malformations, ruptured aneurysm, or idiopathic seizures, should be considered when seizures occur after 48–72 hours postpartum (2, 3). However, eclamptic seizures may occur up to 2 weeks postpartum.

A subclassification of preeclampsia into early-onset preeclampsia (occurring before 34 weeks of gestation) and late-onset preeclampsia (occurring at 34 weeks of gestation or later) has been proposed (5). This subclassification makes sense from both a clinical standpoint and a research standpoint and is of paramount importance in trying to establish evidence-based protocols for the management of women with preeclampsia remote from term.

Epidemiology and Risk Factors

Numerous risk factors are associated with preeclampsia and gestational hypertension (6). These include first pregnancies, multifetal gestations, the presence of certain vascular disorders, such as those seen with diabetes mellitus (types 1 and 2), lupus erythematosus, renal disease, antiphospholipid antibody syndrome, obesity, advanced maternal age, African-American race, and chronic hypertension (2, 3). Other less common conditions associated with preeclampsia include fetal hydrops and gestational trophoblastic disease.

Box 14

Diagnosis of Preeclampsia

Criteria for Diagnosis of Preeclampsia

- Blood pressure of 140 mm Hg systolic or higher or 90 mm Hg diastolic or higher that occurs after 20 weeks of gestation in a woman with previously normal blood pressure
- *Proteinuria,* defined as urinary excretion of 0.3 g protein or higher in a 24-hour urine specimen

Criteria for Diagnosis of Severe Preeclampsia *

- Systolic blood pressure of 160 mm Hg or higher or diastolic blood pressure of 110 mm Hg or higher on two occasions 6 hours apart[†]
- Proteinuria of more than 5 g in 24 hours (normal less than 300 mg/24 h) or 3 g or greater on two random urine samples collected 4 hours apart
- Elevated serum creatinine level (greater than 1.2 mg/dL)
- Grand mal seizures (eclampsia)
- Pulmonary edema
- Oliguria of less than 500 mL in 24 hours
- Microangiopathic hemolysis (fragmented red blood cells, schizocytosis, spherocytosis, reticulocytosis, anemia, and elevated lactate dehydrogenase level)
- Thrombocytopenia (platelet count less than 100,000/mL, for overt severe disease)
- Hepatocellular dysfunction (elevated alanine aminotransferase and aspartase levels)
- Intrauterine growth restriction or oligohydramnios
- Symptoms suggesting significant end organ involvement: headache, visual disturbances, epigastric pain, or pain in the right upper quadrant

*Women with any one of the noted additional findings are categorized as having severe preeclampsia.

[†]The diastolic blood pressure is the pressure at which the cardiac cycle sounds disappear (Korotkoff phase V). Moreover, blood pressure should be taken with the woman in a sitting or left lateral recumbent position with her arm at the level of the heart. (Report of the National High Blood Pressure Education Program Working Group on High Blood Pressure in Pregnancy. Am J Obstet Gynecol 2000;183:S1–22.)

Diagnosis and management of preeclampsia and eclampsia. ACOG Practice Bulletin No. 33. American College of Obstetricians and Gynecologists. Obstet Gynecol 2002;99:159–67.

Pathophysiology

The major pathophysiologic derangements are focal vasospasm and a transfer of fluid from the intravascular space to extravascular spaces (a "porous" vascular tree). The exact cause of vasospasm is unclear, but research has focused on an interaction of various vasodilators and vasoconstrictors, such as prostacyclin, nitric oxide, endothelin 1, angiotensin II, and thromboxane. The literature regarding etiology and pathophysiology of preeclampsia has focused on the role played by angiogenic factors and their inhibitors (eg, soluble fms-like tyrosine kinase 1) as well as the degree of endovascular trophoblastic invasion, which appears to be incomplete (2, 3). Oxidative stress and an intense inflammatory response appear to play a role (1, 2).

The physiologic maternal consequences of preeclampsia include cardiovascular and hematologic effects (eg, hemolysis and thrombocytopenia) and regional perfusion abnormalities. The porous vascular tree is related primarily to an increase in vascular permeability and a decrease in colloid osmotic pressure, which usually is decreased in pregnant women with normal blood pressure but is decreased further in women with preeclampsia. The most frequently cited hemodynamic consequence of preeclampsia is constriction of plasma volume and focal vasospasm, which results in decreased perfusion of certain specific organs. Women with preeclampsia are volume constricted but not hypovolemic in the usual sense of the word (2, 3). Peripheral resistance and cardiac output are increased in women with preeclampsia. In fact, before hydration, cardiac output actually is in a hyperdynamic state in women with preeclampsia.

Thrombocytopenia is the most frequently observed coagulation abnormality in women with preeclampsia, and disseminated intravascular coagulation rarely develops. Microangiopathic hemolytic anemia probably is the consequence of endothelial damage resulting from the arteriolar spasm that accompanies preeclampsia. Abnormalities of hepatic function tests often are found and are elevated in association with thrombocytopenia in HELLP syndrome. The serum uric acid level has not proved to be a clinically useful aid in diagnosing preeclampsia (2, 3, 7).

Women with early-onset (before 34 weeks of gestation) severe preeclampsia may be tested for lupus erythematosus and antiphospholipid antibodies. There is considerable controversy about the role of maternal inherited thrombophilia in the genesis of early-onset, severe preeclampsia. The clinical utility and cost-effectiveness of testing for these factors are unclear and await further study.

Clinical Management

There is no known cure for preeclampsia other than fetal delivery. With rare exceptions, delivery is appropriate regardless of gestational age in a woman with eclampsia, renal failure, or rapidly worsening maternal manifestations, such as HELLP syndrome. The urgency for delivery can be evaluated on the basis of the severity of maternal manifestations and an assessment of fetal status.

For women with severe preeclampsia before viability, pregnancy termination, preferably performed at a tertiary-care center, is recommended because fetal survival is very unlikely, and the likelihood of maternal complications is great. Testing for antiphospholipid antibody syndrome may help explain this occurrence and lead to therapy for subsequent pregnancies. Women should be counseled that they are at increased risk for repeat preterm preeclampsia, insulin resistance, and chronic hypertension.

Women with severe preeclampsia at 23–34 weeks of gestation should be admitted for intensive assessment of maternal and fetal disease status at a tertiary-care center. Initial therapy includes administration of corticosteroids (at 24–34 weeks of gestation) and magnesium sulfate and control of blood pressure during the first 24–48 hours of hospitalization. Under optimal conditions, the pregnancy can be continued under intensive daily surveillance unless there is evidence of HELLP syndrome, maternal disease progression, or nonreassuring fetal status. As long as blood pressure is neither excessive nor trending upward, maternal laboratory values are stable, oliguria and symptoms of worsening disease (headache, scotomata, or epigastric pain) are absent, and fetal monitoring and assessments remain reassuring, delivery can be postponed to maximize the chance for fetal survival.

Women with mild preeclampsia or worsening chronic hypertension but without criteria for severe disease may benefit from brief hospitalization to evaluate maternal–fetal status thoroughly and develop a management plan. Some form of regular antepartum fetal surveillance, such as a weekly biophysical profile, should begin between 32 weeks of gestation and 34 weeks of gestation for pregnant women with a hypertensive disorder or earlier if there are concerns about reduced fetal growth or amniotic fluid volume. Blood pressure, urinary protein levels, and laboratory values should be monitored.

At term (37 weeks of gestation and greater), delivery should be strongly considered for all women with hypertensive disorders of pregnancy. Once gestational age reaches 32–34 weeks, depending on the capability of the nursery, the neonatal unit, or both, delivery is indicated for any woman with severe preeclampsia and is an option for women with mild preeclampsia because disease progression is likely. The rationale is that risks posed to the fetus by increasing placental compromise or sudden abruption may exceed those posed to the neonate by prematurity. When the diagnosis of preeclampsia is questionable, outpatient management may be appropriate if frequent maternal–fetal assessments are continued. When prompt delivery is not clearly mandated by severe disease but is chosen as a preference, documentation of fetal lung maturity by amniocentesis should be considered.

Management of Labor

Induction of labor (preceded by cervical ripening, if necessary) is preferred to elective cesarean delivery for women with hypertensive disorders unless there are obstetric indications, such as malpresentation, or there is clear evidence of nonreassuring fetal status. The type of anesthesia used depends on the clinical circumstances, the expertise of the anesthesiologist, and the patient's preference after informed consent has been obtained.

It is now well established that magnesium sulfate is the anticonvulsant of choice for the prevention or treatment of eclamptic seizures (2, 3, 8). When induction of labor is indicated for a woman with preeclampsia, magnesium sulfate to prevent seizures generally is given intravenously as a 4–6-g loading bolus over 15–20 minutes, followed by a controlled infusion at 1.5–2 g/h. Discontinuation of therapy and determination of serum magnesium levels are indicated whenever there is a loss of deep tendon reflexes, the respiratory rate is less than 12 respirations per minute, diplopia is present, or urinary output is less than 25 mL/h. The therapeutic range for serum magnesium is 4.8–8.4 mg/dL. The effects of an overdose of magnesium can be reversed by administering calcium, such as 1 g intravenous calcium gluconate given slowly. If necessary, respiration should be supported mechanically until recovery occurs. In rare cases when a woman is not a candidate for magnesium sulfate administration (eg, has myasthenia gravis), phenytoin sodium is an alternative drug for seizure prophylaxis. If the creatinine level is elevated (greater than 1.2 mg/dL), or urine output is low, the dosage may need to be adjusted. Phenytoin is not used routinely because it is less effective than magnesium in this situation.

Antihypertensive agents are used to maintain systolic blood pressures below 170–180 mm Hg and diastolic blood pressure at less than 110 mm Hg (target range, 90–99 mm Hg. Hydralazine hydrochloride, labetalol, or both are the preferred antihypertensive agents.

Invasive hemodynamic monitoring rarely is indicated in women with preeclampsia and may be associated with serious complications. However, it may help guide therapy in rare cases of persistent severe oliguria unresponsive to a fluid challenge. Although dexamethasone administered intravenously (10 mg every 12 hours) to a woman with worsening HELLP syndrome has been shown to improve some of the laboratory abnormalities, the answer to whether it affects the actual disease process has not been determined.

Management in the Postpartum Period

Although delivery is recognized as the most definitive event in the cure of preeclampsia, the manifestations of this disorder may continue well into the postpartum period but not longer than 12 weeks. Hypertension persisting beyond 12 weeks is consistent with chronic hypertension. Most patients are free of clinical manifestations within the first postpartum week. Occasionally, hypertensive disease may not become evident until after delivery. Postpartum eclampsia occurs most often in the first 72 hours postpartum but has been reported up to several weeks after delivery. The use of magnesium sulfate usually is indicated for up to 24 hours after delivery.

Prevention

Use of low-dose aspirin and calcium supplements has not been found to reduce the incidence of preeclampsia (2, 3, 9, 10). Current evidence suggests that women at high risk for preeclampsia because of antiphospholipid antibodies may benefit from therapy with heparin and low-dose aspirin (60–80 mg/d) (11). Research focusing on the use of antioxidant therapy for the prevention of preeclampsia is underway in the National Institute of Child Health and Human Development Network of Maternal–Fetal Medicine Units.

References

1. Roberts JM, Pearson GD, Cutler JA, Lindheimer MD. Summary of the NHLBI Working Group on Research on Hypertension During Pregnancy. National Heart Lung and Blood Institute. Hypertens Pregnancy 2003;22:109–27.

2. Report of the National High Blood Pressure Education Program Working Group on High Blood Pressure in Pregnancy. Am J Obstet Gynecol 2000;183:S1–S22.

3. Diagnosis and management of preeclampsia and eclampsia. ACOG Practice Bulletin No. 33. American College of Obstetricians and Gynecologists. Obstet Gynecol 2002;99:159–67.

4. Ohkuchi A, Iwasaki R, Ojima T, Matsubara S, Sato I, Suzuki M, et al. Increase in systolic blood pressure of > or = 30 mm Hg and/or diastolic blood pressure of > or = 15 mm Hg during pregnancy: is it pathologic? Hypertens Pregnancy 2003;22:275–85.

5. von Dadelszen P, Ornstein MP, Bull SB, Logan AG, Koren G, Magee LA. Fall in mean arterial pressure and fetal growth restriction in pregnancy hypertension: a meta-analysis. Lancet 2000;355:87–92.

6. Dekker GA, Sibai BM. Etiology and pathogenesis of preeclampsia: current concepts. Am J Obstet Gynecol 1998;179:1359–75.

7. Lim KH, Friedman SA, Ecker JL, Kao L, Kilpatrick SJ. The clinical utility of serum uric acid measurements in hypertensive diseases of pregnancy. Am J Obstet Gynecol 1998;178:1067–71.

8. Which anticonvulsant for women with eclampsia? Evidence from the Collaborative Eclampsia Trial [published erratum appears in Lancet 1995;346:258]. Lancet 1995;345:1455–63.

9. Levine RJ, Hauth JC, Curet LB, Sibai BM, Catalano PM, Morris CD, et al. Trial of calcium to prevent preeclampsia. N Engl J Med 1997;337:69–76.

10. Sibai BM, Ewell M, Levine RJ, Klebanoff MA, Esterlitz J, Catalano PM, et al. Risk factors associated with preeclampsia in healthy nulliparous women. The Calcium for Preeclampsia Prevention (CPEP) Study Group. Am J Obstet Gynecol 1997;177:1003–10.

11. Caritis S, Sibai B, Hauth J, Lindheimer MD, Klebanoff M, Thom E, et al. Low-dose aspirin to prevent preeclampsia in women at high risk. National Institute of Child Health and Human Development Network of Maternal-Fetal Medicine Units. N Engl J Med 1998;338:701–5.

Pregnancy-Related Hemorrhage

Michael A. Belfort

When a pregnant woman presents with uterine bleeding during pregnancy, initial steps are directed towards establishing a diagnosis, evaluating the severity of the bleeding, and stabilizing maternal hemodynamic status. The health care provider must anticipate the potential for ongoing blood loss and then respond expeditiously to establish a differential diagnosis and institute definitive therapy to ensure maternal cardiovascular stability. A logical, sequential, and aggressive treatment algorithm will usually result in a good outcome for both the mother and the fetus (Figure 10). Clinicians always should stabilize and treat the mother before directing attention to the fetus.

Diagnosis

Common causes of significant pregnancy-related bleeding include placental abruption and placenta previa in the antepartum period as well as uterine atony and morbidly adherent placenta in the postpartum period. A careful history usually will allow differentiation of placenta previa from placental abruption, but the two can coexist. Placenta previa generally is associated with painless vaginal bleeding in the third trimester. It occurs in 1 in 200 pregnancies and decreases with gestational age. Risk factors for placenta previa include prior uterine surgery, multiparity, and advanced maternal age. Acute placental abruption usually has a more dramatic presentation than placenta previa and may include vaginal bleeding, a hypertonic uterus, maternal coagulopathy, fetal distress, or even fetal death. The magnitude of these signs and symptoms depends on the degree of placental separation. Some of the most dramatic presentations may be seen with a massive concealed abruption with very little vaginal bleeding.

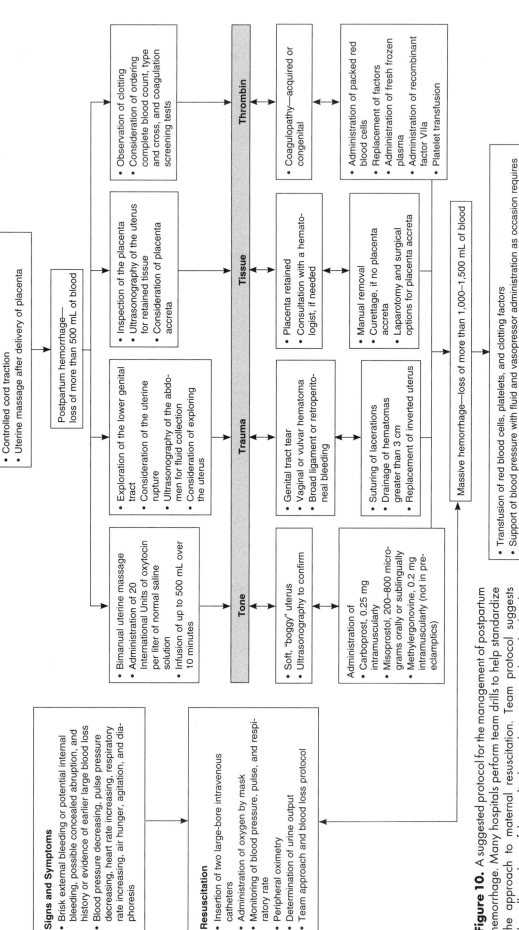

Signs and Symptoms
- Brisk external bleeding or potential internal bleeding, possible concealed abruption, and history or evidence of earlier large blood loss
- Blood pressure decreasing, pulse pressure decreasing, heart rate increasing, respiratory rate increasing, air hunger, agitation, and diaphoresis

Resuscitation
- Insertion of two large-bore intravenous catheters
- Administration of oxygen by mask
- Monitoring of blood pressure, pulse, and respiratory rate
- Peripheral oximetry
- Determination of urine output
- Team approach and blood loss protocol

Active Management of the Third Stage of Labor
- Oxytocin administered with or after delivery
- Controlled cord traction
- Uterine massage after delivery of placenta

Postpartum hemorrhage—loss of more than 500 mL of blood

Tone
- Soft, "boggy" uterus
- Ultrasonography to confirm

Administration of
- Carboprost, 0.25 mg intramuscularly
- Misoprostol, 200–800 micrograms orally or sublingually
- Methylergonovine, 0.2 mg intramuscularly (not in pre-eclamptics)

- Bimanual uterine massage
- Administration of 20 International Units of oxytocin per liter of normal saline solution
- Infusion of up to 500 mL over 10 minutes

Trauma
- Genital tract tear
- Vaginal or vulvar hematoma
- Broad ligament or retroperitoneal bleeding

- Suturing of lacerations
- Drainage of hematomas greater than 3 cm
- Replacement of inverted uterus

- Exploration of the lower genital tract
- Consideration of the uterine rupture
- Ultrasonography of the abdomen for fluid collection
- Consideration of exploring the uterus

Tissue
- Placenta retained
- Consultation with a hematologist, if needed

- Manual removal
- Curettage, if no placenta accreta
- Laparotomy and surgical options for placenta accreta

- Inspection of the placenta
- Ultrasonography of the uterus for retained tissue
- Consideration of placenta accreta

Thrombin
- Coagulopathy—acquired or congenital

- Administration of packed red blood cells
- Replacement of factors
- Administration of fresh frozen plasma
- Administration of recombinant factor VIIa
- Platelet transfusion

- Observation of clotting
- Consideration of ordering complete blood count, type and cross, and coagulation screening tests

Massive hemorrhage—loss of more than 1,000–1,500 mL of blood

- Transfusion of red blood cells, platelets, and clotting factors
- Support of blood pressure with fluid and vasopressor administration as occasion requires
- Uterine packing and tamponade
- Arterial ligation and compression suture procedures
- Hysterectomy
- Pelvic packing, if necessary
- Selective arterial embolization
- Transport to intensive care unit, if necessary

Figure 10. A suggested protocol for the management of postpartum hemorrhage. Many hospitals perform team drills to help standardize the approach to maternal resuscitation. Team protocol suggests that all members of the medical team be aware and involved in the situation. Residents, attending staff, nursing staff, anesthesiologists, obstetric backup, and critical care staff may be included. [Data from Anderson JM, Etches D. Prevention and management of postpartum hemorrhage. Am Fam Physician 2007;75:875–82 and World Health Organization. WHO statement regarding the use of misoprostol for postpartum hemorrhage prevention and treatment. Geneva: WHO; 2009. Available at http://whqlibdoc.who.int/hq/2009/WHO_RHR_09.22_eng.pdf. Retrieved January 27, 2010.]

Recognized risk factors include maternal hypertension, large myomas and uterine anomalies, folate deficiency, prior abruption, cigarette smoking, abdominal trauma, and cocaine or amphetamine abuse (1, 2). Postpartum atony may follow prolonged labor (spontaneous or pharmacologically induced), obstructed labor, or both; precipitous labor; maternal infection, such as chorioamnionitis; uterine distention (multiple pregnancy or polyhydramnios); and general anesthesia, but commonly has no antecedent risk factors. It is more common in women of high parity. Morbidly adherent placentation (accreta, increta, and percreta) is increasingly the cause of massive postpartum hemorrhage.

After initial maternal assessment in an antepartum patient with vaginal bleeding, if the location of the placenta is unknown, transvaginal ultrasound evaluation of placental location should be performed before pelvic examination. The improved resolution of modern transvaginal ultrasonography has made the double set-up virtually obsolete when placenta previa is suspected. The diagnosis of placental abruption is a clinical one, and ultrasonography and tests such as the Kleihauer–Betke test are of limited value (3). Diagnosis of a placental abruption with ultrasonography is more difficult because the acoustic characteristics of a fresh retroplacental clot often are indistinguishable from the placenta (4).

The patient with a morbidly adherent placenta can frequently be detected antepartum using a combination of careful history and ultrasound examination (5). During labor and delivery, women with prior uterine surgery and the placental insertion over this site, and those with placenta previa, are at increased risk for placenta accreta, increta, or percreta and, if the diagnosis is confirmed, should be managed by a team with adequate experience and facilities to treat massive bleeding (5). In those cases where morbid adherence of the placenta is discovered at the time of delivery, rapid diagnosis and appropriate resuscitative measures may be lifesaving. If the lower uterine segment appears distorted and highly vascular in a patient undergoing a repeat cesarean delivery, the uterine incision should be made well away from the lower segment (ie, classical incision) and if the placenta appears adherent, no attempt at placental removal should be made. In such a case, the uterus should be closed and hysterectomy performed once all preparations have been made for dealing with massive blood loss, if possible.

Initial Evaluation

Because the uterus of a pregnant woman receives 20% of maternal cardiac output, obstetric hemorrhage in the second half of pregnancy can be catastrophic for mother and fetus. Close observation of maternal vital signs in situations of actual and potential blood loss is essential. Despite stable blood pressure, increasing or persistently elevated maternal heart rate (greater than 120 beats per minute) and respiratory rate (greater than 18–20 breaths per minute) in the face of significant hemorrhage (even if it appears to have been controlled) are usually indicative of currently compensated (and reversible) shock. Such a situation demands urgent volume expansion and increase in oxygen delivery by optimizing hematocrit, oxygen saturation, and cardiac output. The clinician should not be reassured that the situation has resolved in compensated shock simply because the blood pressure appears stable. A low pulse pressure (even one that appears to be stable) in the face of tachycardia may indicate impending decompensation (6). A heart rate greater than 120 beats per minute may be associated with as much as a 30–40% loss of total blood volume (7), but hemorrhagic shock can occur in the face of a normal heart rate or bradycardia (8). Concerning hemodynamic signs of compensated shock progressing to cardiovascular collapse include increasing tachycardia, decreasing systolic blood pressure, and narrowing of the pulse pressure.

Initial laboratory work includes blood type and cross-match, complete blood count, platelet count, prothrombin time, partial thromboplastin time, fibrinogen measurement, and arterial blood gas measurement. Metabolic acidosis in this setting often indicates shock. To rapidly assess the patient for a coagulopathy a red-topped tube of blood can be observed for a firm clot to form within 7 minutes. If it does not, a coagulopathy should be suspected and a transfusion of platelets and fresh frozen plasma should be considered (9).

Treatment

Initial Management of Acute Antepartum Hemorrhage

Pregnant women or those who recently gave birth with vaginal or suspected intraabdominal bleeding are best treated using a team approach. By having a tried and practiced procedure and team members familiar with their role in management of hemorrhage, evaluation and management can progress in an orderly way to contain the situation. The availability of specifically designed surgical packs for postpartum hemorrhage, with appropriate numbers and types of abdominal and vaginal retractors, long handled pelvic instruments, and selected instruments that vascular, urologic, and general surgical consultants might use, can be very helpful in an emergency.

In cases where cesarean hysterectomy is planned in a case of known placenta percreta a team approach is important. In general, such a team should include the obstetrician, anesthesiology providers, as well as blood bank, operating room, and newborn care personnel. Particularly if involvement of surrounding organs is suspected, it is important to consider consultation of a general surgeon; urologic surgeon, vascular surgeon, or both;

or a gynecologic oncologist to be available for intraoperative assistance as needed. Preoperative discussion of the proposed surgery and responsibilities of each participant will allow identification of potential obstacles and solutions to streamline the procedure.

Bleeding patients should have adequate intravenous access to allow rapid transfusion of large fluid volumes. Although crystalloid and colloid fluids provide volume expansion and can improve tissue perfusion, neither improves oxygen-carrying capacity. Intravenous bolus doses of oxytocin should be avoided because of the deleterious hemodynamic effects. Initial maternal stabilization includes supplemental oxygen (10 L/min through nonrebreathing face mask). If cross-matched blood is unavailable, type-specific blood can be administered to a patient with a negative antibody screen result. Clinical experience has shown that type-specific therapy carries approximately the same low risk of a major transfusion reaction as cross-matched blood. Where massive bleeding is suspected (ie, abruptio placentae with fetal demise or active bleeding with shock) empiric use of fresh frozen plasma, cryoprecipitate, and platelets at the time of packed red blood cell transfusion may be lifesaving. In more controlled situations, blood product use should be tailored to the coagulation profile (9).

Management of the Fetus

The physician should focus on maternal stabilization initially, and only after this has been addressed should the physician turn to intervention based on fetal well-being. This approach will prevent the unnecessary delivery of the fetus because of transient jeopardy, and reduce the risk of surgery on a hemodynamically unstable patient. In most cases, the fetus will recover once the maternal condition is stabilized.

When a woman with placenta previa presents with antepartum bleeding, the timing of delivery depends on a number of factors including gestational age, amount of bleeding, maternal stability, and fetal well-being (10). Cesarean delivery typically is pursued once the mother is stabilized unless there is a significant risk of newborn complications because of preterm birth with delivery. Conservative management may be appropriate if the patient is hemodynamically stable with minimal bleeding. In carefully selected and individualized cases, this may include outpatient management after initial inpatient observation (4).

As with placenta previa, the timing of delivery for placental abruption depends on gestational age, volume of hemorrhage, maternal hemodynamic stability, degree of coagulopathy, and fetal well-being. Again, delivery typically is pursued unless the newborn would be at high risk for complications of prematurity. In many cases, vaginal delivery can be accomplished with volume replacement and blood component therapy. A cesarean delivery should be performed for uncontrolled

bleeding and nonreassuring fetal status, and for traditional obstetric indications, such as labor dystocia and malpresentation (1). In some cases, a small placental abruption will stabilize or bleed intermittently. If the pregnancy is remote from term and without evidence of coagulopathy or fetal jeopardy, conservative management with concurrent betamethasone therapy may be considered. Beta-mimetic and calcium channel blocker tocolytics should be used judiciously and selectively because of their potential cardiovascular effects (1). Indomethacin use may interfere with platelet function, thereby contributing to bleeding problems.

Treatment of Postpartum Hemorrhage

In addition to traditional methods for hemodynamic stabilization, evaluation of the cause of postpartum hemorrhage and treatment (uterotonics, arterial ligation, and hysterectomy), techniques for uterine tamponade and compression have received increasing attention recently.

Uterine Tamponade

Several intrauterine balloon devices are available for tamponade in cases of atony (11, 12). Placement of a balloon catheter usually can be accomplished rapidly and is easy to perform, and its effect can be quickly and reliably evaluated. Balloon tamponade may actually work by compression of the vascular structures supplying the uterus (13). Tamponading in this way may allow for correction of coagulopathy in anticipation of surgical intervention. A continuous oxytocin infusion and prophylactic antibiotic coverage are recommended while the balloon is in place.

Uterine Brace (Compression) Suture

B-Lynch and similar sutures are designed to vertically compress the uterine body in cases of diffuse bleeding caused by uterine atony (14, 15). The advantages of this method are its surgical simplicity and the fact that adequate hemostasis can be assessed immediately after its completion. In order to assess whether the suture will be effective, bimanual compression is applied to the uterus. If bleeding stops, compression with a brace suture should be equally successful. Normal uterine anatomy and resumption of normal menses has been demonstrated on follow-up (16), but unexpected occlusion of the uterine cavity with subsequent development of infection (pyometra) also has been reported with the occlusive square stitch (17).

Treatment of Placenta Previa Complicated by Placenta Accreta

The physician should be particularly aware of the risk of placenta accreta when the placenta is located over the surgical uterine scar in a patient with prior uterine surgery or prior cesarean delivery with an anterior or complete placenta previa. The risk of placenta accreta has been reported to range from 5–25% with one prior cesarean delivery and increases to more than 60% after four prior cesarean deliveries (18, 19). The condition is most commonly diagnosed with the aid of ultrasonography. Magnetic resonance imaging is reserved and may be helpful for those cases where diagnosis is uncertain or the extent of placenta percreta unclear (20).

The management of the morbidly adherent placenta can be divided into two categories: 1) the known placenta accreta and 2) the placenta accreta discovered at delivery or because of sudden onset obstetric hemorrhage (4, 9). With a placenta accreta and percreta diagnosed before labor, there is time to make arrangements for controlled delivery and management of potential hemorrhage (5). When the diagnosis is not anticipated prenatally, massive hemorrhage may already be underway with little time to take effective action. Mindful of the fact that planned cesarean hysterectomy still carries a 7% maternal mortality rate even under the best of circumstances (21), most deaths caused by placenta accreta or percreta occur in the previously unrecognized case.

As mentioned earlier, cesarean hysterectomy for placenta percreta is best managed by a coordinated team if time allows. Most cases of known placenta accreta will be managed with elective cesarean hysterectomy. The fetus can be delivered through a transfundal uterine incision and the placenta left in situ. The uterine incision is then closed to control bleeding from the uterine incision while the hysterectomy is performed. Management of massive intraoperative hemorrhage associated with placenta previa complicated by accreta is covered in detail in the section "Cesarean and Puerperal Hysterectomy."

BLOOD BANK ISSUES

When massive hemorrhage is anticipated, adequate amounts of packed red blood cells, fresh frozen plasma, platelets and cryoprecipitate should be made available to prevent (or treat) coagulopathy (5). Military surgical experience with massive trauma or hemorrhage has resulted in set protocols for massive hemorrhage. One standardized protocol includes the availability of 6 units of packed red blood cells, 6 units of fresh frozen plasma, 6 packs of platelets, and 10 units of cryoprecipitate in separate coolers. Recent data from the battlefield and civilian life suggest that patients with massive hemorrhage from trauma benefit from early and aggressive administration of fresh frozen plasma and platelets in a 1:1:1 ratio with packed red blood cells. This results in speedier correction of coagulopathy, a decreased need for packed red blood cell transfusion, and reduced mortality (22–24). There are no comparable data for use of this ratio in obstetrics. Because coagulopathy frequently accompanies massive obstetric hemorrhage,

the empiric use of early fresh frozen plasma in a 1:1 ratio with packed red blood cells makes some sense. Recombinant factor VIIa also has been proven useful in the management of coagulopathy (25). In 2008, a multidisciplinary group of Australian and New Zealand clinicians (obstetricians, anesthesiologists, and hematologists) produced a guideline recommending its use (26). However, the administration of recombinant factor VIIa has been associated with vascular thrombosis and should be reserved for refractory coagulopathy.

PREOPERATIVE PELVIC ARTERY OCCLUSION

Preoperative pelvic artery occlusion has been proposed as an adjunct to minimize blood loss at the time of hysterectomy for placenta accreta and percreta (27). Some experts have found internal iliac artery balloon placement not to be helpful and that it may actually result in opening of collateral vessels deeper in the pelvis that are more difficult to access for control of hemorrhage (28). Balloon catheter placement also may result in insertion site hematoma, abscess formation, and tissue infarction and necrosis. Because of these reasons, intraoperative internal iliac artery ligation, reserved for those cases where necessary, may be a preferable approach.

SUPRACERVICAL HYSTERECTOMY

Supracervical hysterectomy generally is discouraged in cases of placenta previa because attempts to remove the corpus of the uterus from the cervix disrupts the vascular supply to the placenta in this area. When refractory bleeding persists after removal of the uterus, placement of a pelvic pressure pack should be considered. This temporizing step can allow time for hemodynamic stabilization and correction of coagulopathy (29). Persistent efforts to stop oozing from difficult to locate bleeding points may be counterproductive and lead to hypothermia, worsening coagulopathy, and hemodynamic collapse. In extreme cases when bleeding persists, temporary cessation of the hysterectomy with pelvic packing and infrarenal aortic clamping, closure of the skin with towel clips for tamponade, and aggressive blood product resuscitation and patient warming can be lifesaving. If the bleeding can be slowed to a point where resuscitation is effective and coagulopathy can be corrected before resuming surgery, this may ultimately improve hemostasis and facilitate completion of the surgery. Placement of wide bore pelvic drains is important under this circumstance to allow monitoring for recurrent or persistent significant bleeding.

References

1. Hiippala S. Replacement of massive blood loss. Vox Sang 1998;74 Suppl 2:399–407.

2. Zaki ZM, Bahar AM, Ali ME, Albar HA, Gerais MA. Risk factors and morbidity in patients with placenta previa

accreta compared to placenta previa non-accreta. Acta Obstet Gynecol Scand 1998;77:391–4.

3. Oyelese Y, Ananth CV. Placental abruption. Obstet Gynecol 2006;108:1005–16.

4. Baron F, Hill WC. Placenta previa, placenta abruptio. Clin Obstet Gynecol 1998;41:527–32.

5. Hudon L, Belfort MA, Broome DR. Diagnosis and management of placenta percreta: a review. Obstet Gynecol Surv 1998;53:509–17.

6. Ardagh MW, Hodgson T, Shaw L, Turner D. Pulse rate over pressure evaluation (ROPE) is useful in the assessment of compensated haemorrhagic shock. Emerg Med (Fremantle) 2001;13:43–6.

7. American College of Surgeons. ATLS, advanced trauma life support program for doctors. 7th ed. Chicago, IL: ACS; 2004.

8. Brasel KJ, Guse C, Gentilello LM, Nirula R. Heart rate: is it truly a vital sign? J Trauma 2007;62:812–7.

9. Hiippala S. Replacement of massive blood loss. Vox Sang 1998;74 Suppl 2:399–407.

10. Neilson JP. Interventions for suspected placenta praevia. Cochrane Database of Systematic Reviews 2003, Issue 2. Art. No.: CD001998. DOI: 10.1002/14651858.CD001998; 10.1002/14651858.CD001998.

11. Bakri YN, Amri A, Abdul Jabbar F. Tamponade-balloon for obstetrical bleeding. Int J Gynaecol Obstet 2001;74:139–42.

12. Johanson R, Kumar M, Obhrai M, Young P. Management of massive postpartum haemorrhage: use of a hydrostatic balloon catheter to avoid laparotomy. BJOG 2001;108:420–2.

13. Cho Y, Rizvi C, Uppal T, Condous G. Ultrasonographic visualization of balloon placement for uterine tamponade in massive primary postpartum hemorrhage. Ultrasound Obstet Gynecol 2008;32:711–3.

14. B-Lynch C, Coker A, Lawal AH, Abu J, Cowen MJ. The B-Lynch surgical technique for the control of massive postpartum haemorrhage: an alternative to hysterectomy? Five cases reported. Br J Obstet Gynaecol 1997;104:372–5.

15. Hayman RG, Arulkumaran S, Steer PJ. Uterine compression sutures: surgical management of postpartum hemorrhage. Obstet Gynecol 2002;99:502–6.

16. Habek D, Kulas T, Bobic-Vukovic M, Selthofer R, Vujic B, Ugljarevic M. Successful of the B-Lynch compression suture in the management of massive postpartum hemorrhage: case reports and review. Arch Gynecol Obstet 2006;273:307–9.

17. Ochoa M, Allaire AD, Stitely ML. Pyometria after hemostatic square suture technique. Obstet Gynecol 2002;99:506–9.

18. Clark SL, Koonings PP, Phelan JP. Placenta previa/accreta and prior cesarean section. Obstet Gynecol 1985;66:89–92.

19. Silver RM, Landon MB, Rouse DJ, Leveno KJ, Spong CY, Thom EA, et al. Maternal morbidity associated with multiple repeat cesarean deliveries. National Institute of Child Health and Human Development Maternal-Fetal Medicine Units Network. Obstet Gynecol 2006;107:1226–32.

20. Warshak CR, Eskander R, Hull AD, Scioscia AL, Mattrey RF, Benirschke K, et al. Accuracy of ultrasonography and magnetic resonance imaging in the diagnosis of placenta accreta. Obstet Gynecol 2006;108:573–81.

21. O'Brien JM, Barton JR, Donaldson ES. The management of placenta percreta: conservative and operative strategies. Am J Obstet Gynecol 1996;175:1632–8.

22. Gonzalez EA, Moore FA, Holcomb JB, Miller CC, Kozar RA, Todd SR, et al. Fresh frozen plasma should be given earlier to patients requiring massive transfusion. J Trauma 2007;62:112–9.

23. Holcomb JB, Wade CE, Michalek JE, Chisholm GB, Zarzabal LA, Schreiber MA, et al. Increased plasma and platelet to red blood cell ratios improves outcome in 466 massively transfused civilian trauma patients. Ann Surg 2008;248:447–58.

24. Gunter OL Jr, Au BK, Isbell JM, Mowery NT, Young PP, Cotton BA. Optimizing outcomes in damage control resuscitation: identifying blood product ratios associated with improved survival. J Trauma 2008;65:527–34.

25. Franchini M, Franchi M, Bergamini V, Salvagno GL, Montagnana M, Lippi G. A critical review on the use of recombinant factor VIIa in life-threatening obstetric postpartum hemorrhage. Semin Thromb Hemost 2008;34:104–12.

26. Welsh A, McLintock C, Gatt S, Somerset D, Popham P, Ogle R. Guidelines for the use of recombinant activated factor VII in massive obstetric haemorrhage. Aust N Z J Obstet Gynaecol 2008;48:12–6.

27. Bodner LJ, Nosher JL, Gribbin C, Siegel RL, Beale S, Scorza W. Balloon-assisted occlusion of the internal iliac arteries in patients with placenta accreta/percreta. Cardiovasc Intervent Radiol 2006;29:354–61.

28. Mok M, Heidemann B, Dundas K, Gillespie I, Clark V. Interventional radiology in women with suspected placenta accreta undergoing caesarean section. Int J Obstet Anesth 2008;17:255–61.

29. Dildy GA, Scott JR, Saffer CS, Belfort MA. An effective pressure pack for severe pelvic hemorrhage. Obstet Gynecol 2006;108:1222–6.

Multiple Gestation

Roger B. Newman

Epidemiology

Multiple births comprise more than 3% of all live births, and they result in approximately 10% of all stillbirths, 14% of all neonates affected by respiratory distress syndrome, 12% of all cases of grade 3 or 4 intraventricular hemorrhage, and 10% of all neonatal sepsis in the United States (1). Infants of multiple gestations account for 20% of all neonatal intensive care unit admissions and 16% of neonatal deaths.

Zygosity and Chorionicity

Zygosity refers to the genetic makeup of the pregnancy. Dizygotic pregnancies result from the fertilization of two ova. Monozygotic twins result from the splitting of one zygote arising from the fertilization of one ovum by one sperm. These offspring have identical genotypes and similar phenotypes. The incidence of dizygous twins is influenced by various factors, including race, ethnicity, maternal age, ovulation induction, and use of assisted reproductive technologies (ART). It is now known that the use of ART can result in monozygous twinning and that the rate of monozygotic twinning of about 1% after the treatment with ART is increased more than twofold over the background rate (2). Although the highest rates were seen with in vitro fertilization associated with intracytoplasmic sperm injection or assisted hatching, the rate of monozygotic twinning consistently is increased with all ART treatment modalities regardless of micromanipulation. The mechanism is unclear but may be secondary to zona pellucida trauma during micromanipulation or embryo transfer, or related to increased gonadotropin levels (2, 3).

Chorionicity indicates the membrane composition of the pregnancy—the chorion from which the placenta develops and the amnion. All monochorionic gestations are monozygous, whereas dichorionic gestations may be monozygous or dizygous depending on how early splitting of the zygote occurs. Splitting before day three will result in each monozygotic embryos having their own amnion and chorion (dichorionic placentation). Approximately one third of monozygous twins are dichorionic, whereas two thirds are monochorionic and diamniotic. Monoamniotic–monochorionic gestations are rare, occurring in only approximately 3% of monozygous twins.

Chorionicity plays a substantial role in the increased perinatal morbidity and mortality associated with multiple gestations. Monochorionic gestations account for approximately 20% of twin pregnancies and have a worse prognosis than their dichorionic counterparts in part because of the presence of a single placenta (ie, twin–twin transfusion syndrome and certain structural malformations) (4, 5). The effect of zygosity on outcomes is less clear. In the absence of fetal malformations, dichorionic monozygotic pregnancies seem to have similar outcomes to those of dizygotic dichorionic pregnancies (6).

The ultrasound characteristics of chorionicity are most accurately assessed in the first trimester. Ultrasound markers of dichorionicity include separate placentas, the twin-peak sign (also called the lambda sign) in which the placenta appears to extend a short distance above the placental disc between the gestational sacs, an intertwin membrane thicker than 1.5–2 mm, and gender discordance. The presence of two yolk sacs is diagnostic of a diamniotic twin gestation while two embryos with a single yolk sac would suggest a monoamniotic, monochorionic twin gestation. Using a composite of available ultrasonographic findings, chorionicity and amnionicity can be accurately determined in 90–100% of cases between 10 weeks of gestation and 14 weeks of gestation. DNA zygosity studies on amniocytes have been used successfully to help with the management of complex cases requiring a definitive diagnosis.

Complications

The risk of maternal (Table 11) and perinatal complications (Table 12) increase in direct proportion to the number of fetuses in the gestation (1). Women with multiple fetuses have a 3.6-fold higher risk of pregnancy-related death compared with those having a singleton gestation (20.8 compared with 5.8 per 100,000 pregnancies resulting in a liveborn neonate) (7). The leading causes of death are similar for women with singleton and multiple gestations, and these include embolism, hypertensive complications of pregnancy, hemorrhage, and infection.

Preterm Labor and Birth

Preterm labor and birth is the most common complication of multiple pregnancy. The prophylactic use of cerclage, bed rest, tocolytics, and home uterine activity monitoring have not been shown to prolong pregnancies when routinely applied (8). Patient education regarding the signs and symptoms of preterm labor is important. Frequent cervical examination may help identify incipient preterm birth. A cervical score based on digital examination (cervical length minus internal os dilation in centimeters) has been studied. In results of one study, it was found that when the cervical score

Table 11. Maternal Complications in Multiple Gestation

Maternal Complications by Plurality			
	Twins	Triplets	Quadruplets and Higher Order
Number of Pregnancies	2,000	1,014	165
Antepartum Complications (%)			
Hospital admission	27	53	75
Preterm labor	35	70	94
Anemia	21	36	24
Preeclampsia	14	21	40
Preterm premature rupture of membranes	15	20	14
Cerclage	4	13	26
Gestational diabetes mellitus	7	9	11
Urinary tract infection	9	6	20
Acute fatty liver	No data	5	No data
Pulmonary edema	1	8	6
Postpartum Complications (%)			
Hemorrhage	6	12	21
Transfusion	No data	8	13
Endometritis	8	19	11
Readmission	No data	11	No data

Table 12. Fetal and Neonatal Complications in Multiple Gestation

Perinatal Complications by Plurality*				
	Singletons	Twins	Triplets	Quadruplets and higher order
Mean gestational age (weeks)	39	35.8	32.5	30.5
Mean birth weight (g)	3,357	2,389	1,735	1,455
Preterm status (less than 37 weeks of gestation) (%)	9.4	50.7	91.0	97.5
Very preterm status (less than 33 weeks of gestation) (%)	1.7	13.9	41.3	60
Low birth weight (less than 2,500 g) (%)	6.1	52.2	91.5	98.6
Very low birth weight (less than 1,500 g) (%)	1.1	10.1	31.9	68.6
Small for gestational age status (%)	9.4	35.6	36.6	62
Average neonatal intensive care unit length of stay (d)	Less than 1	18	30	58
Neonatal death (per 1,000 live births)	7.8	55.9	168.8	89.7
Infant death (per 1,000 live births)	11.2	66.4	190.4	186.7

*Results are expressed per fetus.

was 0 or less before 38 weeks of gestation, there was a 75% risk of preterm delivery and that preterm birth occurred within a week in only 3% of twin pregnancies when the cervical score was greater than 0 (9). In a separate series, none of 223 twins were born within 1 week of a cervical score greater than 0 (10).

Ultrasound evaluation of cervical length and cervicovaginal fetal fibronectin sampling also may help predict preterm labor and delivery in twin and multifetal gestations. In twins, a cervical length of 25 mm or less at 24 weeks of gestation was associated with a 6.9-fold increased risk of preterm delivery before 32 weeks of gestation (11). Conversely, a cervical length greater than 35 mm obtained between 24 weeks of gestation and 26 weeks of gestation is associated with only a 3% chance of a twin delivery before 34 weeks of gestation (12).

The presence of fetal fibronectin in cervicovaginal secretions between 22 weeks of gestation and 37 weeks of gestation has been associated with spontaneous preterm delivery. At 28 weeks of gestation and 30 weeks of gestation, a positive cervicovaginal fetal fibronectin is significantly associated with preterm delivery before 32 weeks of gestation (odds ratios, 9.4 and 46.1, respectively), although not with preterm delivery before 35 weeks of gestation or 37 weeks of gestation (11). However, the association of fetal fibronectin with preterm delivery in twins was no longer significant after controlling for cervical length. Positive predictive values for twins with a positive midtrimester fetal fibronectin ranged from 38% to 53%.

Improved efficiency in identifying twins at increased risk for preterm delivery results in enhanced surveillance and selective use of potential interventions to prevent preterm birth, prolong gestation, or improve neonatal outcomes. One possible algorithm for integrating these risk assessment techniques into clinical management is presented in Figure 11.

When preterm labor is diagnosed, tocolysis may be warranted to achieve antenatal corticosteroid benefit, allow tertiary-care transport, and possibly prolong the pregnancy. Antenatal corticosteroids should be administered to women with preterm labor before 35 weeks of gestation and to women with preterm premature rupture of membranes at less than 30–32 weeks of gestation. The physiologic adaptations to multiple gestations may predispose these women to cardiopulmonary complications when they are treated with these therapies (1, 8). When additional cardiovascular stresses are imposed, such as tocolytic therapy, iatrogenic fluid overload, and occult or overt maternal infection, serious complications can occur. Tocolytic therapy in multiples, especially with β-adrenergic agonists, is associated with an increased risk for pulmonary edema, myocardial ischemia, and tachyarrhythmias. The increasing frequency of multiple gestation, especially among older women undergoing ART, also has been associated with a small but growing risk of peripartum cardiomyopathy. These cardiovascular risks appear to be highest when prolonged tocolytic therapy, corticosteroids, and intravenous fluids are administered together. Beta-mimetic tocolytics as well as corticosteroids also increase maternal glucose levels, which can destabilize either gestational or pregestational diabetes mellitus.

Congenital Malformations

A review of more than 100,000 twin gestations from 14 series demonstrated that congenital anomalies are 1.2–2 times more frequent among twin fetuses compared with singletons. A higher prevalence occurred among like-sex or monochorionic twins, suggesting a greater risk among monozygous twins. The fetuses are discordant for the anomaly in 80–90% of the cases, which persists regardless of zygosity, although the concordance rate is slightly higher among monozygotic twins. The most common anomalies are cardiac, holoprosencephaly, neural tube defects, facial clefting, gastrointestinal anomalies, clubfoot, and anterior abdominal wall defects, including cloacal and bladder exstrophy. Most of these malformations can be accurately identified by antenatal ultrasonography with a sensitivity of almost 90% and a specificity and positive predictive value of approximately 100% (13). Of note, twins discordant for fetal anatomic abnormalities also may be at increased risk for preterm labor and delivery.

Gestational Diabetes Mellitus

Gestational diabetes mellitus is more common in multiples because of the elevated levels of anti-insulin placental hormones, notably human placental lactogen, in proportion to the increased placental volume. The incidence of gestational diabetes mellitus is increased twofold to threefold in twins compared with singletons, and it has been estimated that each additional fetus increases the risk by a factor of 1.8.

The appropriate management of gestational diabetes mellitus in a multiple pregnancy is not as straightforward as it is in a singleton pregnancy because of the need to balance this against the enhanced nutritional demands of a multifetal pregnancy. Current recommendations for the fasting and postprandial blood glucose targets, additional fetal surveillance, and the timing of delivery are similar to singleton gestations.

Preeclampsia and Gestational Hypertension

Twins are at approximately 2.5-fold higher risk of either gestational hypertension or preeclampsia, with frequencies of 13–37%. In a population-based study from Washington State, the fourfold higher risk of preeclampsia among twins was increased to 14-fold higher if the woman was also primigravid (14). In addition to being more common, preeclampsia in multiple gesta-

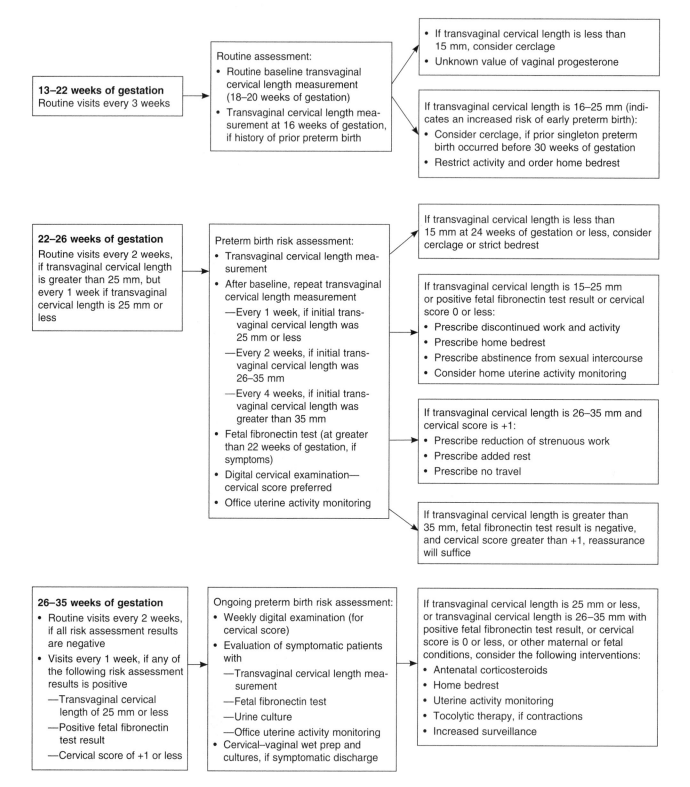

13–22 weeks of gestation
Routine visits every 3 weeks

Routine assessment:
- Routine baseline transvaginal cervical length measurement (18–20 weeks of gestation)
- Transvaginal cervical length measurement at 16 weeks of gestation, if history of prior preterm birth

- If transvaginal cervical length is less than 15 mm, consider cerclage
- Unknown value of vaginal progesterone

If transvaginal cervical length is 16–25 mm (indicates an increased risk of early preterm birth):
- Consider cerclage, if prior singleton preterm birth occurred before 30 weeks of gestation
- Restrict activity and order home bedrest

22–26 weeks of gestation
Routine visits every 2 weeks, if transvaginal cervical length is greater than 25 mm, but every 1 week if transvaginal cervical length is 25 mm or less

Preterm birth risk assessment:
- Transvaginal cervical length measurement
- After baseline, repeat transvaginal cervical length measurement
  —Every 1 week, if initial transvaginal cervical length was 25 mm or less
  —Every 2 weeks, if initial transvaginal cervical length was 26–35 mm
  —Every 4 weeks, if initial transvaginal cervical length was greater than 35 mm
- Fetal fibronectin test (at greater than 22 weeks of gestation, if symptoms)
- Digital cervical examination—cervical score preferred
- Office uterine activity monitoring

If transvaginal cervical length is less than 15 mm at 24 weeks of gestation or less, consider cerclage or strict bedrest

If transvaginal cervical length is 15–25 mm or positive fetal fibronectin test result or cervical score 0 or less:
- Prescribe discontinued work and activity
- Prescribe home bedrest
- Prescribe abstinence from sexual intercourse
- Consider home uterine activity monitoring

If transvaginal cervical length is 26–35 mm and cervical score is +1:
- Prescribe reduction of strenuous work
- Prescribe added rest
- Prescribe no travel

If transvaginal cervical length is greater than 35 mm, fetal fibronectin test result is negative, and cervical score greater than +1, reassurance will suffice

26–35 weeks of gestation
- Routine visits every 2 weeks, if all risk assessment results are negative
- Visits every 1 week, if any of the following risk assessment results is positive
  —Transvaginal cervical length of 25 mm or less
  —Positive fetal fibronectin test result
  —Cervical score of +1 or less

Ongoing preterm birth risk assessment:
- Weekly digital examination (for cervical score)
- Evaluation of symptomatic patients with
  —Transvaginal cervical length measurement
  —Fetal fibronectin test
  —Urine culture
  —Office uterine activity monitoring
- Cervical–vaginal wet prep and cultures, if symptomatic discharge

If transvaginal cervical length is 25 mm or less, or transvaginal cervical length is 26–35 mm with positive fetal fibronectin test result, or cervical score is 0 or less, or other maternal or fetal conditions, consider the following interventions:
- Antenatal corticosteroids
- Home bedrest
- Uterine activity monitoring
- Tocolytic therapy, if contractions
- Increased surveillance

Figure 11. Possible algorithm for integrating various preterm birth risk assessments and potential preterm birth prevention interventions into the antepartum management of twin gestations.

tions is more likely to be earlier in onset and more severe (15). Placental abruption as a complication of hypertension also is more common in twins, occurring with a threefold to eightfold increased frequency.

Intrauterine Growth Restriction and Discordant Growth

Up to one third of twin gestations are affected by intrauterine growth restriction (IUGR) by 36 weeks of gestation. Although twin and triplet growth curves exist, singleton fetal weight standards commonly are used to assess fetal growth in multiple gestations and are clinically acceptable. Before 30–32 weeks of gestation, growth in twins is similar to that of singletons. The fetal abdominal circumference begins to lag in the third trimester in some multifetal gestations, suggesting growth impairment rather than constitutional differences between these and singleton gestations.

Competition of multiple fetuses for limited maternal nutritional reserves as well as abnormalities of placentation are the two major contributors to twin IUGR. Vascular abnormalities in monochorionic placenta, suboptimal placental implantation, cord abnormalities, such as marginal or velamentous insertion, or a single umbilical artery are all more common in twin gestations. Serial ultrasonography is ideal for evaluating fetal growth in multiple pregnancies, and many obstetricians perform ultrasound examinations on a monthly basis in the third trimester. This interval is not evidence based. Once IUGR is diagnosed, more frequent monitoring of interval fetal growth and amniotic fluid volumes is suggested. Antenatal fetal surveillance is indicated, and early delivery may be considered (8).

Discordant fetal growth (difference in estimated fetal weights of the twins divided by the larger twin's weight expressed as a percentage) also is a risk factor for adverse outcomes. Much of the discrepancy in fetal weight is because of constitutional and genetic dissimilarities, but more severe degrees of discordance may result from twin–twin transfusion syndrome, anomalies, genetic syndromes, or placental factors leading to IUGR in one twin. The threshold at which discordant growth becomes a threat is controversial. Most centers will have a concern for discordance, with estimated weight differences between 20% and 30% (1). Intrauterine growth restriction is likely more predictive of serious fetal or neonatal morbidity than birth weight discordance (16, 17).

Fetal Death

In patients with twin gestations scanned in the first trimester, the reported rates of singleton demise ("vanishing twin") range from 13% to 78%. It is estimated that more than one in eight spontaneous pregnancies begin as twins, and for every liveborn twin pair there are 10–12 other twin pregnancies that result in a singleton birth (1).

During the second and third trimesters, death of one fetus complicates approximately 2–5% of twin pregnancies and up to 17% of triplet pregnancies. This estimate increases threefold to fourfold for monochorionic versus dichorionic twins (18) and also is more common when a structural malformation is present (19). Intrauterine fetal death of one twin in the second and third trimesters can adversely affect the surviving fetus or fetuses in two ways: 1) risk for multicystic encephalomalacia and multiorgan damage in monochorionic pregnancies and 2) preterm labor and delivery in both dichorionic and monochorionic twins.

In the period immediately after fetal death, the surviving twin in monochorionic gestations can develop an acute inter-twin transfusion to a degree that may cause fetal injury. It is believed that blood from the surviving twin may acutely pass into the dead twin through ubiquitous placental anastomoses (a capacitance effect). This results in hypotension and hypoperfusion in the surviving twin. This acute inter-twin transfusion can result in sublethal ischemic or hypoxic end organ injury and can lead to fetal death. Evidence for this "back-bleeding" theory comes from fetal heart rate tracings suggesting fetal anemia (sinusoidal pattern) in the survivor soon after the co-twin's demise and hematologic information obtained by percutaneous fetal blood sampling of the surviving twin that reveal marked anemia rather than clotting abnormalities (20). Of surviving twins, 5–25% have ischemic organ injury after death of a co-twin (generally after third-trimester loss), including neurologic defects (4, 21–24). Immediate delivery has not been shown to be effective in preventing multicystic encephalomalacia in the surviving twin (25). Consequently, immediate delivery of the surviving twin may have the unintended consequence of increasing the risk of prematurity without reducing the risk of hypoxic injury. If fetal testing is not reassuring, delivery should be performed. Even with reassuring results, complications may become apparent only on follow-up ultrasound imaging. Fetal magnetic resonance imaging results may be helpful, but the technique is still investigational.

It has been reported that multiple gestations with an intrauterine fetal death carry a 25% risk of disseminated intravascular coagulation if the fetal demise is retained for at least 4 weeks, but others have suggested that the risk with multiples is not as high as in a retained singleton demise. Only a few cases of maternal coagulopathy have been reported after single intrauterine fetal death in twins (4). Initial maternal testing under this circumstance includes a prothrombin time, partial thromboplastin time, fibrinogen level, and platelet count. If these values are within normal limits, further surveillance is not indicated. Women with normal results do not appear to be at increased risk for infection because of the retained dead fetus. Dystocia secondary to the demised fetus has been reported infrequently, but cesarean delivery seems to be more common with single intrauterine fetal death.

Neurodevelopmental Injury

In 1897, Sigmund Freud suggested that multiple birth was a greater cause of spastic diplegia than asphyxia (26). The risk of cerebral palsy is increased in multiple gestations even if delivered at term. Compared with singletons, twins are 4.6 times more likely to have cerebral palsy (7.32 versus 1.6 per 1,000 first-year survivors) (27). Moreover, triplets are 17.4-fold more likely to develop cerebral palsy (27.91 per 1,000 first-year survivors). A similar relationship is seen regarding lesser degrees of neurodevelopmental handicaps (Table 13). Low birth weight, firstborn birth order, and monochorionicity were more common in twins with cerebral palsy than in twins without the condition. The risk of neurologic injury is threefold to fivefold higher in monochorionic twins compared with dichorionic twins and higher among single survivors of a monochorionic pair (8, 28, 29). The prevalence of cerebral palsy ranges from 6.7 to 12.6 per 1,000 surviving twins. The risk of producing at least one child with cerebral palsy in twin, triplet, or quadruplet gestations has been reported as 15 per 1,000 twins, 80 per 1,000 triplets, and 429 per 1,000 quadruplets, respectively (30).

Problems Specific to Monochorionic Twins

The general obstetrician–gynecologist rarely encounters severe twin–twin transfusion syndrome, monoamnionicity, conjoined twins, or acardia. Consultation with an obstetrician–gynecologist with expertise in the management of high-risk pregnancies, such as a maternal–fetal medicine specialist, is advised (8).

Twin–Twin Transfusion Syndrome

Twin–twin transfusion syndrome accounts for approximately 15% of perinatal mortality in twins. It is characterized by placental arterial–venous shunts in monochorionic gestations that result in unbalanced blood flow across the shared placenta. Although all monochorionic twins share a portion of their vasculature, only 15–30% of them will develop clinical evidence of twin–twin transfusion syndrome. Though the syndrome can manifest at any gestational age, detection in the second trimester is associated with a poorer prognosis, including a loss rate for both twins approaching 100% if untreated.

The progression of the twin–twin transfusion syndrome is believed to follow a pattern (31):

Stage 1   Polyhydramnios–oligohydramnios, with the bladder visible in the donor twin.

Stage 2   The donor bladder is no longer visible.

Stage 3   Abnormal Doppler flow seen in the donor twin, with absent or reversed flow in the umbilical artery, reversed flow in the ductus venous, or pulsatile umbilical venous flow.

Stage 4   Hydrops in either twin (high output cardiac failure in the donor or congestive heart failure in the recipient).

Stage 5   Demise of one or both twins.

When the smaller fetus is enshrouded by the fetal membrane and restricted to the side of the uterine wall ("stuck twins"), it is at a very high risk for death unless in utero treatment or delivery occurs. Treatment options for twin–twin transfusion syndrome include serial large-volume amnioreduction, fetoscopic laser photocoagulation of communicating vessels, septostomy, and selective feticide.

The overall perinatal survival rate with large-volume amnioreduction has been reported as 60–65% (32). A randomized comparison of serial amnioreduction and fetoscopic laser occlusion found significantly more survival of at least one twin in the laser group (76% versus 56%) (33). Septostomy normalizes the amniotic fluid differences between the fetuses but carries the risk of cord entanglement and does not correct the underlying vascular abnormality. No difference in survival was seen in a study comparing amnioreduction with septostomy (34). Selective feticide using ultrasound-guided cord occlusion or radio frequency ablation also has been used, especially when there is evidence of a fetal anomaly, severe growth restriction or neurologic injury in the co-twin (35). Bipolar coagulation of the umbilical cord has been associated with a liveborn twin in 83% of cases and intact neurologic survival in 70% (36).

Monoamnionicity

Approximately 3% of monozygotic twin gestations are monoamniotic. Monoamniotic twins have a high rate of perinatal mortality (as high as 50%) caused by cord entanglement, congenital anomalies, cord accidents, and growth restriction. Recent studies indicate a perinatal mortality rate ranging from 10% to 21% (37, 38).

Table 13. Rates of Neurodevelopmental Handicap by Plurality per 1,000 Postneonatal Survivors*

	Singletons	Twins	Triplets or More
Moderate handicap	70.8	92.0	121.0
Severe handicap	19.8	33.7	57.1
Overall handicap	90.8	125.6	178.1

*Calculated using birth-specific rates obtained from Healthy children: investing in the future. Washington, DC: U.S. Government Office of Technology Assessment; 1988

Because of the unpredictability of acute cord compression, the optimal approach to monoamniotic twins remains unknown. In the largest reported series with good outcomes, the frequency of antenatal surveillance ranged from two to three times per week to daily testing once viability was achieved. Despite even high intensity surveillance, demise can still occur at any gestational age (37), and because of this some experts have suggested early delivery. Most reviews recommend delivery sometime between 32 weeks and 34 weeks of gestation after antenatal corticosteroid administration to enhance fetal lung maturity (1). Assessment of fetal lung maturity also can be considered in this situation. Cesarean delivery is recommended because of the near universal presence of umbilical cord entanglement.

TWIN REVERSED ARTERIAL PERFUSION SYNDROME

Twin reversed arterial perfusion syndrome results from artery-to-artery placental anastomoses in a monochorionic gestation. The normal "pump" fetus perfuses an abnormal recipient with blood flow in the recipient twin's umbilical artery being reversed. The result is an amorphous acardiac twin. A range of anomalies can be seen in the acardiac twin, including anencephaly, absent limbs, intestinal atresia, abdominal wall defects, and absent organs. The pump twin generally is morphologically normal, but in approximately 9% of cases the pump twin will have trisomy. Because of the increased cardiac workload, the pump twin can develop heart failure and fetal hydrops. The true incidence of twin reversed arterial perfusion syndrome is unknown because many cases result in early pregnancy loss, but it is estimated to occur in 1% of monozygotic twins and approximately 1 in 35,000 pregnancies overall. Approximately 75% of cases are monochorionic diamniotic and 25% are monochorionic monoamniotic.

Polyhydramnios and congestive heart failure in the pump twin are associated with a poor prognosis. The risk of this occurring increases with a proportionately larger acardiac twin (39). In the absence of poor prognostic indicators (congestive heart failure, polyhydramnios, or a twin weight ratio of greater than 70%), expectant management with serial ultrasonography is suggested. Amnioreduction can treat associated polyhydramnios. Management with the administration of indomethacin (for polyhydramnios, preterm labor, or both) and digoxin (to facilitate cardiac contractility) has been reported. Hysterotomy for removal of the acardiac twin is associated with both high maternal and perinatal morbidity. Ultrasound guided insertion of thrombogenic coils, injection of silk soaked in alcohol, injection of absolute alcohol, endoscopic ligation, and radioablation of the recipient's umbilical cord have been described (40). These methods usually are reserved for cases where the pump twin has already developed cardiac failure or is at high risk at a previable gestational age.

General Management of Multifetal Pregnancies

Initial education should include a discussion of prematurity, the leading cause of morbidity and mortality in multiple gestations. The short-term and long-term sequelae of preterm birth should be explained so that patients can appreciate the seriousness of the issue and the need for compliance with antepartum care. Other more frequent complications, such as IUGR, congenital anomalies, preeclampsia, gestational diabetes mellitus, and cesarean delivery should be discussed.

Maternal Nutrition

Maternal nutritional requirements are increased with twins because of the greater expansion of blood volume and uterine growth, establishment of glycogen and fat reserves, and the doubling of the fetal–placental mass. Depletion of maternal nutritional reserves has been associated with poor fetal growth and possibly earlier delivery.

Table 14 provides suggested body mass index (BMI)–specific individual dietary recommendations for twin gestations based on nonpregnant and singleton recommended dietary allowances published by the Food and Nutrition Board of the National Research Council and BMI-specific extrapolations for twins (41). Increased protein intake is essential for normal fetal and placental growth. Inadequate protein can be the result of inadequate protein intake (vegan diet or poverty), intake of poor quality protein, or an inadequate caloric intake that results in dietary protein being diverted to meet acute energy needs. The Institute of Medicine has recommended a maternal weight gain of 16–20 kg (35–45 lb) for term twin pregnancies. Body mass index-specific weight gain recommendations also have been developed for twins (Figure 12) (42). Early gestation and midgestation maternal weight gain has the greatest ultimate impact on twin birth weight, and this effect is most pronounced in underweight women. Even with catch-up weight gain after 24 weeks of gestation, there is still a strong association between poor early pregnancy weight gain and adverse outcomes, including poor fetal growth (43).

Women with twins have lower hemoglobin levels in the first and second trimester, higher rates of iron-deficiency anemia, and more iron-deficiency anemia in their infants 6 months of age or younger. The frequency of maternal anemia is related to overall nutritional status and justifies an emphasis on heme-iron rich dietary sources. Red meat, pork, poultry, fish, and eggs offer both a higher quality and quantity of protein as well as better iron absorption. Non–heme-iron sources, such as iron-fortified breads, leafy green vegetables, and nuts also are encouraged both for their iron and folate because a deficiency in these nutrients also can cause

Table 14. Body Mass Index*—Specific Nutritional Recommendations by Pregnancy Status

	Calories (kcal)	Protein (g)	Carbohydrates (g)	Fat (g)
Nonpregnant	2,200	110	220	98
Pregnant with a singleton	2,500	126	248	112
Pregnant with twins				
Underweight (BMI less than 18.5)	4,000	200	400	178
Normal weight (BMI of 18.5–24.9)	3,500	175	350	156
Overweight (BMI of 25–29.9)	3,250	163	325	144
Obese (BMI 30 and greater)	3,000	150	300	133

Abbreviation: BMI indicates body mass index.

*A body mass index is expressed as weight in kilograms divided by height in meters squared.

Data from Luke B, Brown MD, Misiunas R, Anderson E, Nugent C, van de Ven C, et al. Specialized prenatal care and maternal and infant outcomes in twin pregnancy. Am J Obstet Gynecol 2003;189:934–8.

maternal anemia. Some clinicians choose to routinely provide supplements of extra iron (60 mg/day of elemental iron) and folic acid (1 mg/day), whereas others prefer to emphasize dietary intake. Most clinicians also recommend a supplemental prenatal vitamin, or target specific nutrients lacking in the diets of women carrying twins (ie, calcium, magnesium, and zinc). In a study of 928 twin gestations, consultation with a registered dietician was associated with higher maternal weight gains and a significant reduction in the risk of having a very low birth weight infant (2%) compared with women who did not receive a nutritional consultation (12%) (44).

Prenatal Diagnosis of Genetic Disorders

Dichorionic twin gestations have twice the risk of aneuploidy because of the presence of two independently fertilized eggs. Monozygotic twins do not have a higher incidence of aneuploidy compared with singleton gestations at the same maternal age, but both fetuses would be affected. If maternal age is being considered as an indication for invasive genetic testing, a 33-year-old woman with dichorionic twins and a 31-year-old woman with trichorionic triplets will have the same risk for aneuploidy as a 35-year-old woman with a singleton gestation (1). Multiple gestations have higher levels of all the critical serum analytes, and a lower value in one fetus can potentially counteract a higher level in the other twin. During precounseling regarding screening for fetal aneuploidy or neural tube defects, women should consider the potential implications of identifying an abnormality in one fetus and a normal result in the other. Adjusted matenal serum alpha-fetoprotein levels can be used for neural tube defects screening in twins. However, maternal serum alpha-fetoprotein screening in high-order multiple gestations and serum screening for Down syndrome in multiples have not been validated. Currently, Down syndrome screening in multiple gesta-

tions using first trimester serum markers (β-hCG and pregnancy-associated plasma protein A levels) combined with nuchal translucency testing and maternal age remains investigational. In monochorionic twins, the results of nuchal translucency testing are averaged to calculate a single risk for both fetuses, whereas in dichorionic twins, the risk for each fetus is calculated independently. The combined test using first-trimester analyte levels and nuchal translucency measurement has a reported Down syndrome detection rate of 84% for monochorionic twins and 70% for dichorionic twins compared with detection rates of 85–90% for singletons at a 5% screen-positive rate (45). Second-trimester screening using the quadruple analyte screen also has a lower detection rate in twins compared with singleton gestations.

Amniocentesis is an appropriate option, and chorionic villus sampling of two or more fetuses also is suitable in experienced hands. The fetal loss rates appear to be similar. Monozygotic fetuses commonly are discordant for anatomic abnormalities; however, genetic discordance is exceedingly rare. When this occurs, the discordancy in karyotype usually involves the sex chromosomes and is probably the result of early mitotic nondisjunction followed by the twinning event (46).

Multifetal Pregnancy Reduction

The purpose of first-trimester multifetal pregnancy reduction is to improve perinatal outcomes by decreasing maternal complications secondary to high-order multiples and by decreasing adverse perinatal outcomes primarily associated with preterm delivery. Reducing high-order multiple gestations to twins reduces the risk of preterm labor and increases birth weight and gestational age at delivery. In selected cases, such as a history of a previous second-trimester loss, reduction from a twin gestation to a singleton gestation may be indicated.

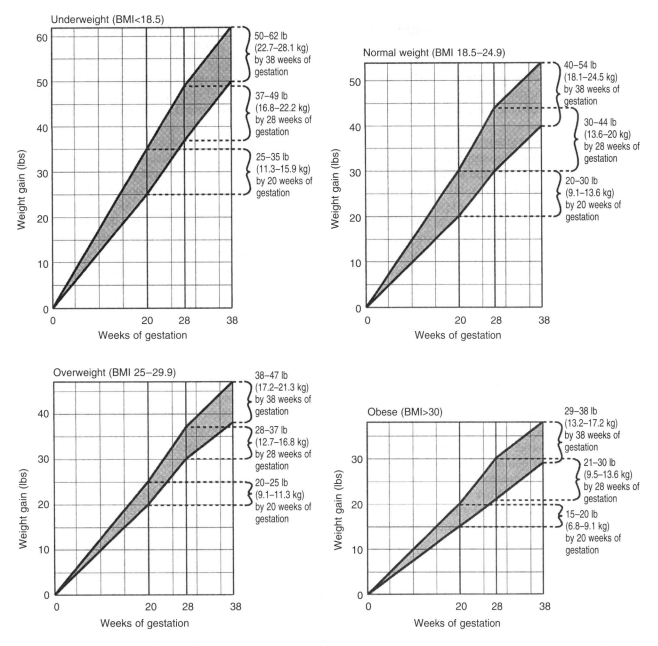

Figure 12. Body mass index-specific weight gain recommendations for women carrying a twin gestation. (Luke B, Hediger ML, Nugent C, Newman RB, Mauldin JG, Witter FR, et al. Body mass index–specific weight gains associated with optimal birth weights in twin pregnancies. J Reprod Medicine 2003;48:217-24.)

Nonetheless, multifetal pregnancy reduction is an ethical dilemma, and the starting number of fetuses needed to justify the procedure is controversial. Most of this controversy has related to whether or not multifetal reduction from triplets to twins results in better perinatal outcomes than expectant management. Although most women do not regret their decision, women undergoing multifetal pregnancy reduction do have feelings of loss, guilt, and sadness.

With accumulated experience, the loss rate associated with multifetal pregnancy reduction is approximately 6% (47). There is little maternal risk associated with the

procedure and there have been no reports of coagulation disorders developing afterwards.

Selective Reduction

Patients with twins discordant for severe anomalies or chromosomal abnormalities may choose selective reduction. Selective reduction procedures generally are performed later in gestation than multifetal reduction because anomalies often are undetected until the second trimester. Most selective reductions have been performed in twins, but also have been undertaken in high-order multiple gestations. In dichorionic pregnancies, ultrasound-guided intracardiac injection of potassium chloride is used. If selective fetal reduction is desired in a monochorionic pregnancy, complete ablation of the umbilical cord of the anomalous fetus is recommended to avoid damage to the remaining fetus.

A recent study reported favorable outcomes with selective reduction in 200 cases, including 164 cases of twins, 32 cases of triplets, and 4 cases of quadruplets. The unintended pregnancy loss rate was 4%. The average gestational age at delivery was 36 1/7 weeks of gestation and approximately 84% of these women gave birth after 32 weeks of gestation (48).

Preterm rupture of membranes complicates approximately 20% of these cases. Maternal coagulopathy has not been reported. Midtrimester maternal serum alpha-fetoprotein levels will be elevated following fetal reduction and should not be used as a screening test in these pregnancies.

Antepartum Surveillance

Routine antepartum surveillance of uncomplicated multifetal pregnancies has not been shown to be beneficial in prospective randomized trials, but is suggested for twin pregnancies complicated by growth abnormalities, abnormal fluid volume, fetal anomalies, monoamnionicity, or other pregnancy complications (1). Antenatal surveillance can include the nonstress test, or the standard or modified biophysical profile. Doppler imaging may be useful in evaluating fetal growth restriction or for the twin–twin transfusion syndrome (8).

Timing of Delivery

Current American College of Obstetricians and Gynecologists recommendations suggest that uncomplicated twins be delivered by 40 weeks of gestation (8). Recent studies suggest that multiple pregnancies may benefit from delivery before 40 weeks of gestation. The underlying theory is that early uteroplacental insufficiency in multiple pregnancies may place the fetuses at risk for compromise analogous to postterm status in a singleton gestation. Fetal mortality data from the United States between 1983 and 1988 reveals that the lowest risk of fetal death for twins occurred at birth weights of 2,500–2,800 g and at 36–37 weeks of gestation. The risk of fetal death increased at gestational ages beyond 37 weeks even if fetal growth remained appropriate. A similar population-based analysis from Japan showed that the risks of both fetal and early neonatal death (within 7 days of delivery) began to increase in twins delivered after 38 weeks of gestation. A population-based study from the state of Washington found that rates of respiratory distress syndrome and prolonged hospital stay (greater than 5 days) were slightly lower at 38 weeks of gestation compared with

37 weeks of gestation for twins, but neither improved by delivery at 39 weeks of gestation (49).

A more accurate impression for risk of intrauterine fetal death can be obtained with "the prospective risk of fetal death" (the number of fetal deaths at a particular gestational age divided by the number of fetuses in all ongoing pregnancies at that time). For twins, the prospective risk of fetal death at approximately 36–37 weeks of gestation appears to be equivalent to that of postterm singletons. However, delivering these pregnancies at such a gestational age could lead to complications secondary to prematurity. As a result, gestational age-specific prospective risk of fetal death must be considered in context with gestational age-specific neonatal death rates. Because the prospective risk of fetal death for twins exceeded the neonatal death rate at 39 weeks of gestation, the investigators in one study have recommended consideration of delivery of uncomplicated twins between 38 weeks and 39 weeks of gestation rather than at 40 weeks of gestation (50).

It appears to be a reasonable management option to offer elective delivery during the 38th week of gestation in well-dated, uncomplicated twin pregnancies (Figure 13). Prolonging the pregnancy to 39–40 weeks of gestational age is reasonable if all measures of fetal well-being are reassuring. In complicated twin gestations, neither maternal nor fetal status should be compromised in an effort to prolong pregnancy beyond 37–38 weeks of gestation (Figure 14). The severity of some maternal or fetal conditions will necessitate delivery at even earlier gestational ages, with enhancement of fetal lung maturity if time permits. Delivery based on such indications would not require confirmation of fetal lung maturity by amniocentesis.

Route of Delivery

The route of delivery in multiple gestations depends on fetal presentation in labor and health care provider's experience. If the presenting twin is nonvertex (20% of deliveries), cesarean delivery is suggested. A trial of labor and vaginal delivery is appropriate for vertex–vertex twins (40% of deliveries) regardless of gestational age or estimated fetal weight. However, 10–20% of second twins will change presentation after delivery of the first twin, and the obstetrician must be prepared for potential complications, such as fetal distress, cord prolapse, or placental separation. If the first twin is vertex and the second nonvertex (40% of deliveries), vaginal birth is preferred; however, cesarean delivery may be preferred if the second twin is substantially larger than the first (greater than 25% or 500 g larger after 34 weeks of gestation) or if the health care provider does not have adequate experience with vaginal breech deliveries (51). The option of external cephalic version for the second twin has been associated with a

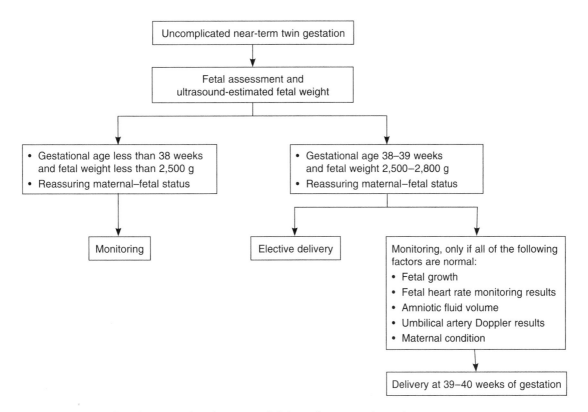

Figure 13. A potential algorithm regarding the timing of delivery for uncomplicated near-term twin gestations.

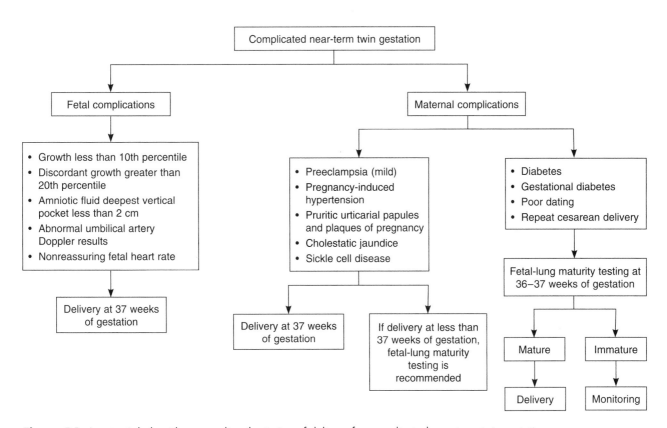

Figure 14. A potential algorithm regarding the timing of delivery for complicated near-term twin gestations.

lower likelihood of success and a higher rate of complications compared with planned breech extraction, and the risk of combined vaginal–cesarean delivery (52). Some obstetricians have had favorable experiences delivering triplets vaginally. Nonetheless, most health care providers deliver triplets and high-order multiple gestations by cesarean delivery because continuous fetal heart rate monitoring of triplets and high-order multiple gestations in labor is challenging, and there is a high likelihood of performing a breech extraction on a preterm and frequently very low birth weight infant.

References

1. Newman RB, Luke B, editors. Multifetal pregnancy : a handbook for care of the pregnant patient. Philadelphia (PA): Lippincott Williams & Wilkins; 2000.

2. Chow JS, Benson CB, Racowsky C, Doubilet PM, Ginsburg E. Frequency of a monochorionic pair in multiple gestations: relationship to mode of conception. J Ultrasound Med 2001;20:757–60; quiz 761.

3. Schachter M, Raziel A, Friedler S, Strassburger D, Bern O, Ron-El R. Monozygotic twinning after assisted reproductive techniques: a phenomenon independent of micromanipulation. Hum Reprod 2001;16:1264–9.

4. D'Alton ME, Simpson LL. Syndromes in twins. Semin Perinatol 1995;19:375–86.

5. Leduc L, Takser L, Rinfret D. Persistence of adverse obstetric and neonatal outcomes in monochorionic twins after exclusion of disorders unique to monochorionic placentation. Am J Obstet Gynecol 2005;193:1670–5.

6. Dube J, Dodds L, Armson BA. Does chorionicity or zygosity predict adverse perinatal outcomes in twins? Am J Obstet Gynecol 2002;186:579–83.

7. MacKay AP, Berg CJ, King JC, Duran C, Chang J. Pregnancy-related mortality among women with multifetal pregnancies. Obstet Gynecol 2006;107:563–8.

8. Multiple gestation: complicated twin, triplet, and high-order multifetal pregnancy. ACOG Practice Bulletin No. 56. American College of Obstetricians and Gynecologists. Obstet Gynecol 2004;104:869–83.

9. Newman RB, Godsey RK, Ellings JM, Campbell BA, Eller DP, Miller MC 3rd. Quantification of cervical change: relationship to preterm delivery in the multifetal gestation. Am J Obstet Gynecol 1991;165:264–9; discussion 269–71.

10. Neilson JP, Verkuyl DA, Crowther CA, Bannerman C. Preterm labor in twin pregnancies: prediction by cervical assessment. Obstet Gynecol 1988;72:719–23.

11. Goldenberg RL, Iams JD, Miodovnik M, Van Dorsten JP, Thurnau G, Bottoms S, et al. The preterm prediction study: risk factors in twin gestations. National Institute of Child Health and Human Development Maternal-Fetal Medicine Units Network. Am J Obstet Gynecol 1996;175:1047–53.

12. Imseis HM, Albert TA, Iams JD. Identifying twin gestations at low risk for preterm birth with a transvaginal ultrasonographic cervical measurement at 24 to 26 weeks' gestation. Am J Obstet Gynecol 1997;177:1149–55.

13. Edwards MS, Ellings JM, Newman RB, Menard MK. Predictive value of antepartum ultrasound examination for anomalies in twin gestations. Ultrasound Obstet Gynecol 1995;6:43–9.

14. Coonrod DV, Hickok DE, Zhu K, Easterling TR, Daling JR Risk factors for preeclampsia in twin pregnancies: a population-based cohort study. Obstet Gynecol 1995;85:645–50.

15. Krotz S, Fajardo J, Ghandi S, Patel A, Keith LG. Hypertensive disease in twin pregnancies: a review. Twin Res 2002;5:8–14.

16. Bronsteen R, Goyert G, Bottoms S. Classification of twins and neonatal morbidity. Obstet Gynecol 1989;74:98–101.

17. Fraser D, Picard R, Picard E, Leiberman JR. Birth weight discordance, intrauterine growth retardation and perinatal outcomes in twins. J Reprod Med 1994;39:504–8.

18. Kilby MD, Govind A, O'Brien PM. Outcome of twin pregnancies complicated by a single intrauterine death: a comparison with viable twin pregnancies. Obstet Gynecol 1994;84:107–9.

19. Malone FD, Craigo SD, Chelmow D, D'Alton ME. Outcome of twin gestations complicated by a single anomalous fetus. Obstet Gynecol 1996;88:1–5.

20. Okamura K, Murotsuki J, Tanigawara S, Uehara S, Yajima A. Funipuncture for evaluation of hematologic and coagulation indices in the surviving twin following co-twin's death. Obstet Gynecol 1994;83:975–8.

21. Fusi L, Gordon H. Twin pregnancy complicated by single intrauterine death. Problems and outcome with conservative management. Br J Obstet Gynaecol 1990;97:511–6.

22. Anderson RL, Golbus MS, Curry CJ, Callen PW, Hastrup WH. Central nervous system damage and other anomalies in surviving fetus following second trimester antenatal death of co-twin. Report of four cases and literature review. Prenat Diagn 1990;10:513–8.

23. Yoshida K, Matayoshi K. A study on prognosis of surviving cotwin. Acta Genet Med Gemellol (Roma) 1990;39:383–8.

24. Eglowstein MS, D'Alton ME. Single intrauterine demise in twin gestation. J Maternal-Fetal Invest 1993;2:272–5.

25. D'Alton ME, Newton ER, Cetrulo CL. Intrauterine fetal demise in multiple gestation. Acta Genet Med Gemellol (Roma) 1984;33:43–9.

26. Freud S. Infantile cerebral paralysis. Translated by Lester A Russin. Coral Gables (FL): Univ. of Miami Press; 1968.

27. Petterson B, Nelson KB, Watson L, Stanley F. Twins, triplets, and cerebral palsy in births in Western Australia in the 1980s. BMJ 1993;307:1239–43.

28. Adegbite AL, Castille S, Ward S, Bajoria R. Neuromorbidity in preterm twins in relation to chorionicity and discordant birth weight. Am J Obstet Gynecol 2004;190:156–63.

29. Lopriore E, Nagel HT, Vandenbussche FP, Walther FJ. Long-term neurodevelopmental outcome in twin-to-twin transfusion syndrome. Am J Obstet Gynecol 2003;189:1314–9.

30. Yokoyama Y, Shimizu T, Hayakawa K. Prevalence of cerebral palsy in twins, triplets and quadruplets. Int J Epidemiol 1995;24:943–8.

31. Quintero RA, Morales WJ, Allen MH, Bornick PW, Johnson PK, Kruger M. Staging of twin-twin transfusion syndrome. J Perinatol 1999;19:550-5.

32. Fisk N, Denbow M. Feto-fetal transfusion syndrome: amnioreduction as optimal treatment. In: Donnez J, Brosens L, editors. The uterus throughout the woman's life: 4th Congress of the European Society for Gynaecolgoical Endoscopy, Brussels, Belgium, December 6-9, 1995. European Society of Gynecologic Endoscopy. Congress. Bologna: Monduzzi Editore International Proceedings Division; 1996. p. 9-18.

33. Senat MV, Deprest J, Boulvain M, Paupe A, Winer N, Ville Y. Endoscopic laser surgery versus serial amnioreduction for severe twin-to-twin transfusion syndrome. N Engl J Med 2004;351:136-44.

34. Moise KJ Jr, Dorman K, Lamvu G, Saade GR, Fisk NM, Dickinson JE, et al. A randomized trial of amnioreduction versus septostomy in the treatment of twin-twin transfusion syndrome [published erratum appears in Am J Obstet Gynecol 2005;193:2183]. Am J Obstet Gynecol 2005;193: 701-7.

35. Robyr R, Yamamoto M, Ville Y. Selective feticide in complicated monochorionic twin pregnancies using ultrasound-guided bipolar cord coagulation. BJOG 2005;112:1344-8.

36. Shevell T, Malone FD, Weintraub J, Thaker HM, D'alton ME. Radiofrequency ablation in a monochorionic twin discordant for fetal anomalies. Am J Obstet Gynecol 2004;190:575-6.

37. Rodis JF, McIlveen PF, Egan JF, Borgida AF, Turner GW, Campbell WA. Monoamniotic twins: improved perinatal survival with accurate prenatal diagnosis and antenatal fetal surveillance. Am J Obstet Gynecol 1997;177:1046-9.

38. Allen VM, Windrim R, Barrett J, Ohlsson A. Management of monoamniotic twin pregnancies: a case series and systematic review of the literature. BJOG 2001;108:931-6.

39. Moore TR, Gale S, Benirschke K. Perinatal outcome of forty-nine pregnancies complicated by acardiac twinning. Am J Obstet Gynecol 1990;163:907-12.

40. Tsao K, Feldstein VA, Albanese CT, Sandberg PL, Lee H, Harrison MR, et al. Selective reduction of acardiac twin by radiofrequency ablation. Am J Obstet Gynecol 2002; 187:635-40.

41. Luke B, Brown MB, Misiunas R, Anderson E, Nugent C, van de Ven C, et al. Specialized prenatal care and maternal and infant outcomes in twin pregnancy. Am J Obstet Gynecol 2003;189:934-8.

42. Luke B, Hediger ML, Nugent C, Newman RB, Mauldin JG, Witter FR, et al. Body mass index--specific weight gains associated with optimal birth weights in twin pregnancies. J Reprod Med 2003;48:217-24.

43. Luke B, Min SJ, Gillespie B, Avni M, Witter FR, Newman RB, et al. The importance of early weight gain in the intrauterine growth and birth weight of twins. Am J Obstet Gynecol 1998;179:1155-61.

44. Luke B, Keith L, Keith D. Maternal nutrition in twin gestations: weight gain, cravings and aversions, and sources of nutrition advice. Acta Genet Med Gemellol (Roma) 1997; 46:157-66.

45. Wald NJ, Rish S. Prenatal screening for Down syndrome and neural tube defects in twin pregnancies. Prenat Diagn 2005;25:740-5.

46. Perlman EJ, Stetten G, Tuck-Muller CM, Farber RA, Neuman WL, Blakemore KJ, et al. Sexual discordance in monozygotic twins. Am J Med Genet 1990;37:551-7.

47. Stone J, Eddleman K, Lynch L, Berkowitz RL. A single center experience with 1000 consecutive cases of multifetal pregnancy reduction. Am J Obstet Gynecol 2002; 187:1163-7.

48. Eddleman KA, Stone JL, Lynch L, Berkowitz RL. Selective termination of anomalous fetuses in multifetal pregnancies: two hundred cases at a single center. Am J Obstet Gynecol 2002;187:1168-72.

49. Hartley RS, Emanuel I, Hitti J. Perinatal mortality and neonatal morbidity rates among twin pairs at different gestational ages: optimal delivery timing at 37 to 38 weeks' gestation. Am J Obstet Gynecol 2001;184:451-8.

50. Kahn B, Lumey LH, Zybert PA, Lorenz JM, Cleary-Goldman J, D'Alton ME, et al. Prospective risk of fetal death in singleton, twin, and triplet gestations: implications for practice. Obstet Gynecol 2003;102:685-92.

51. Cruikshank DP. Intrapartum management of twin gestations. Obstet Gynecol 2007;109:1167-76.

52. Chauhan SP, Roberts WE, McLaren RA, Roach H, Morrison JC, Martin JN Jr. Delivery of the nonvertex second twin: breech extraction versus external cephalic version. Am J Obstet Gynecol 1995;173:1015-20.

Intrauterine Growth Restriction

Radek Bukowski

A small for gestational age (SGA) fetus is one with biometric measurements or an estimated weight below a chosen threshold. The threshold usually is arbitrarily selected as 10th or 5th percentile –2 standard deviations, but its actual value also will depend on the gestational age of pregnancy and on the population from which it was derived. Although such norms are easy to obtain and apply clinically, one has to keep in mind that many such identified SGA fetuses will be constitutionally small and normal. Only a small proportion will be growth restricted. Intrauterine growth restriction (IUGR) refers, to impairment of fetal growth, preventing the fetus from achieving its individual growth potential. This group of fetuses is substantially more difficult to identify, and it also is the group that has a high risk of adverse outcome of pregnancy.

There is a substantial overlap between SGA and IUGR fetuses (Figure 15). Many IUGR fetuses are SGA. The contribution of IUGR fetuses among SGA pregnancies increases as cutoff-defining SGA decreases. For SGA status defined as birth weight below 10th percentile, 30–50% of SGA fetuses are thought to be IUGR. This proportion is estimated to increase with lower cutoffs for SGA. This seems to be further supported by increasing perinatal mortality with declining percentile of birth weight. However, a fetus with IUGR does not have to be SGA. Its growth might be severely impaired but still be above a chosen cutoff that defines SGA. Declining growth trajectory of an IUGR fetus may not cross percentile-defining SGA even until delivery.

The importance of the accurate identification of IUGR is high. Intrauterine growth restriction poses substantial risk to the fetus not only in utero but also after delivery, and its consequences seem to imprint themselves on the whole lifespan of the individual. Growth restricted fetuses are at increased risk of stillbirth (odds ratio [OR], 6.1; 95% confidence interval [CI], 5–7.5), neonatal death (OR, 4.1; 95% CI, 2.4–4.8), and neonatal

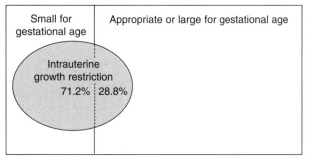

Figure 15. The overlap between small for gestational age fetuses and fetuses with intrauterine growth restriction.

encephalopathy (OR, 4.37; 95% CI, 1.4–13.4) as well as birth hypoxia, neonatal morbidity, cerebral palsy, impaired neurodevelopment, and cognitive function (IQ) and, possibly in adult life, type 2 diabetes mellitus, hypertension, and coronary artery disease. However, the association between IUGR and morbidity in adult life is confounded by common genetic and environmental milieu shared by mother and child. As a matter of fact, the IUGR status of the child was shown to be associated with mother's increased risk of coronary artery disease and stroke in later life (1). Thus, delivery of an IUGR infant may prognosticate future maternal health and longevity.

Evidence strongly indicates that at least a portion of IUGR originates in the first months of pregnancy as a result of chromosomal abnormalities and some congenital malformations. However, other studies demonstrate that IUGR fetuses without chromosomal or structural abnormalities are already smaller than their normally grown counterparts during the first trimester of pregnancy (2). This potentially could be a result of smaller amounts of placental proteins implicated in fetal growth that are produced in the first trimester in pregnancies that ultimately are growth restricted.

Clearly, IUGR is a culmination of multiple causes and pathways, originating in maternal, fetal, or placental abnormalities and resulting in impairment of fetal growth and not achieving its individual growth potential (Box 15). Serious implications of IUGR and poor accuracy and precision of traditionally used SGA definition for diagnosis of IUGR make diagnosis and management of IUGR extremely important but also very complex.

Diagnosis

The diagnosis of SGA and IUGR, as with other disorders, relies on the principles of Bayes theorem, which state that the chance of the disease increases with positive results of tests performed. The size of this increase in probability depends on how good the test is in detecting the disease. Physicians are intuitively proficient in combining these probabilities. Certainly it is not necessary for clinical purposes to conduct calculations of the probabilities before making a diagnosis and a clinical decision. However, it is useful to appreciate the effectiveness of the test used (ie, the magnitude of the change in probability of the disease when the test result is positive or negative). Bayes theorem uses for this purpose the likelihood ratio (LR) (ie, the sensitivity of the test divided by its reciprocal of specificity or false-positive rate). It is a very handy value because a

Selected Examples of Factors Associated With Intrauterine Growth Restriction

Maternal
- Smoking
- Alcohol
- Low prepregnancy weight
- Poor weight gain
- Malnutrition (less than 1,500 kcal/d)
- Age younger than 16 years or older than 35 years
- Diabetes mellitus
- Chronic renal disease
- Systemic lupus erythematosus
- Cyanotic heart disease
- Sickle cell anemia
- Antiphospholipid syndrome
- Chronic hypertension
- Preeclampsia
- Medications
  - Antiseizure agents
  - Corticosteroids
  - Folic acid antagonists (methotrexate)
- Low maternal socioeconomic status

Fetal
- Multiple gestation
- Anomalies
  - Chromosomal
  - Structural
- Infections
  - Viral: cytomegalovirus
  - Protozoal: toxoplasmosis
  - Spirochetal: syphilis
- Previous intrauterine growth restriction

Placental
- Abruption
- Previa
- Confined placental mosaicism

this increase in probability of the disease theoretically is a product of multiplication of all LRs of tests performed. Practically, however, the tests frequently are correlated and not independent; therefore, the final increase in probability of the disease is smaller than it would be expected from multiplying LRs of used tests. Also, repeating the same test over time (to demonstrate a trend) will provide additional information that, when translated into separate LRs, will further refine (increase or decrease) the probability of a disease. As a result, a trend has more predicting value than a single measurement.

Methods employed to diagnose SGA and IUGR evaluate either biometrical measurements of the fetus or biophysical parameters of fetal well-being. Biometrical measurements include abdominal palpation, fundal height measurement, and ultrasound biometry. Biophysical parameters include amniotic fluid volume estimates and uterine artery Doppler impedance measurements. Both types of tests crucially depend on an accurate estimate of gestational age. This dependence always has to be considered in interpreting the results of these tests, and, consequently, in clinical decision making.

Abdominal Palpation

Abdominal palpation is of a very limited value in detecting SGA and IUGR fetuses. Its sensitivity with regards to detection of a SGA fetus is only 44–50%. Palpation is, however, a part of the routine examination and its cost and effort required are minimal. When a small fetus is suspected during abdominal palpation further evaluation is indicated.

Ultrasound Biometry

Abdominal circumference and estimated fetal weight are the two most accurate ultrasound biometrical parameters for prediction of SGA fetuses at birth. The 10th percentile appears to be the best cutoff for both parameters in this respect. Published LR for abdominal circumference of less than 10th percentile range from 1.9 to 4.5, whereas the estimated fetal weight of less 10th percentile has a median LR of 2.8. Various formulas to calculate estimated fetal weight are used. Most demonstrate high validity and the tendency to underestimate the actual birth weight. Among them, the equation by Hadlock was reported to perform especially well in small fetuses. It appears that similarly to fundal height measurements, the performance of ultrasound biometry can be improved by performing serial examinations to demonstrate growth velocity and by individualization of the norms.

Postnatally, serial measurements are more accurate in identification of IUGR than abnormal ponderal index, subscapular skin fold thickness, or midarm circumference. Additionally, decreased fetal growth rate correlates

single number expresses validity of the test represented by its sensitivity and specificity. It also may help to estimate the posttest odds of the disease by simply multiplying the pretest odds of the disease, derived from the prevalence of the disease in the population, by the LR.

As a result, multiple tests employed to detect SGA or IUGR will diagnose those disorders with higher probability than each of the tests applied alone. The size of

with adverse pregnancy outcomes, including perinatal mortality. Decreases in abdominal circumference and estimated fetal weight values predict IUGR (defined by abnormal ponderal index after birth) with LRs of 2.1 and 3.9, respectively. Conversely, head circumference to abdominal circumference ratios, frequently found in standard ultrasound examination reports, perform worse than abdominal circumference or estimated fetal weight alone in predicting SGA fetus or IUGR.

Use of customized birth weight norms results in better prediction of adverse pregnancy outcomes than traditional population norms. This also appears to be true for antenatal ultrasound assessment of fetal growth using individualized norms. Such norms used prenatally result in better identification of SGA fetuses with LRs of 4–6.2. This is a result of both better sensitivity and a lower false-positive rate. The optimal cutoff for individualized norms appears to be 8th percentile for identification of SGA fetuses and adverse outcomes of pregnancy.

Individualized norms of fetal growth, or fetal growth potential, have been developed based on twenty pre-pregnancy and early-pregnancy physiologic determinants of birth weight. These novel norms have not yet been standardized but were shown to better identify normal and complicated pregnancy than either customized or ultrasound norms, and the number of variables used in their calculation can be adjusted as they become available during the course of pregnancy (3). Growth potential norms are a promising tool in the management of growth restriction, but they will have to be carefully validated in other populations before introduction into clinical practice.

A systematic review and meta-analysis published by the Cochrane Database of Systematic Reviews demonstrated that the use of routine ultrasound examinations after 24 weeks of gestation in a low-risk population is not associated with improvement of perinatal mortality. This might reflect a true lack of benefit, as well as a high false-positive rate, especially in low-risk pregnancies, of the norms used in those studies.

Biophysical Tests

Biophysical tests do not appear to be good predictors of SGA or IUGR. This is most likely because they measure fetal well-being rather than fetal growth. The two most likely parameters to be associated with the prediction of impaired fetal growth, amniotic fluid index and Doppler impedance measurements in umbilical and uterine arteries, demonstrate moderate predictive accuracy. Amniotic fluid index has an LR of 1.2 in predicting an abnormal ponderal index at birth. A meta-analysis of uterine artery Doppler imaging has shown its modest predictive accuracy of SGA fetuses at birth with an LR of 3.6 in the low-risk population and 2.7 in the high-risk population.

Three-Dimensional Ultrasonography

Three-dimensional ultrasonography can be used to estimate volumes of fetal body parts. Those volumetric measurements have been used to estimate fetal weight. However, the improvement in the estimate over traditional two-dimensional methods is, to date, marginal, with random error of 6–7% with three-dimensional ultrasonography and 7–8% with two-dimensional ultrasonography (4). If further improvement in technology will bring faster, more accurate estimates and possibly whole fetus volume estimates, three-dimensional ultrasonography may become the preferred method. Today three-dimensional ultrasonography remains a promising experimental methodology, awaiting its standardization and validation.

Management

A substantial proportion, up to 19%, of SGA fetuses has chromosomal abnormalities. Such pregnancies are frequently associated with structural malformations and have normal or increased amount of amniotic fluid and normal umbilical artery Doppler imaging impedance. In a large study of SGA pregnancies, ultrasound examination demonstrated structural malformations in 96% of chromosomally abnormal fetuses. From this study, the LR of a chromosomally abnormal fetus in the presence of structural malformation on ultrasound examination and SGA is approximately 9.1. Likelihood ratios for structural anomalies and markers of chromosomal abnormalities in the general population have been established. The finding of normal or increased amount of amniotic fluid in an SGA fetus increases the likelihood of chromosomal abnormalities almost three-fold (LR=2.7), whereas presence of end diastolic flow in the umbilical artery increases the likelihood by 60% (LR=1.6). Therefore, targeted ultrasound examination with evaluation of amniotic fluid volume and umbilical artery Doppler imaging impedance should constitute the initial step in evaluation of the SGA fetus.

Umbilical artery Doppler imaging impedance is well suited to be a pivotal test in the management of the SGA fetus. It is the only fetal surveillance method that, when used in a high-risk population, is associated with a trend towards improvement of perinatal mortality. Umbilical artery Doppler imaging is the only test able to predict neonatal morbidity in SGA fetuses. It is superior in this respect to fetal heart rate variability and biophysical profile. As intervention in fetuses with positive test results will lead to further testing and frequently preterm delivery, it is important that abnormal umbilical artery impedance has a low false-positive rate. Therefore, it is reassuring that absent end-diastolic flow is rare (only 2.7%) in SGA fetuses and has a low false-positive rate. The use of umbilical artery Doppler testing reduces false-positive results because it appears to decrease the rate of hospital admissions, labor inductions, and rates of cesarean deliveries for fetal distress. It also has few false-negative results. A persistently abnormal biophysical profile result is reported to be invariably associated with the absence of diastolic flow. Absent flow and reversed end-diastolic flow are associated with substantial risk of stillbirth (14% and 24%, respectively) and neonatal death (27% and 51%, respectively). However, the time interval from identification of abnormal umbilical artery impedance to onset of abnormalities of fetal heart rate or biophysical profile is variable, ranging from 2 days to 25 days. Therefore, after identification of the absent end-diastolic flow, the decision to perform delivery has to be based on other modes of fetal surveillance.

Fetal heart rate monitoring and biophysical profile are two of these methods most commonly applied, although fetal venous Doppler imaging also is promising. The benefit of umbilical artery impedance testing lies mainly in identification of a high-risk group of SGA fetuses that will require intensive surveillance. Fetuses with present end-diastolic flow can be safely managed on an outpatient basis. These patients also can be adequately monitored with testing performed every 2 weeks. Conversely, patients with absent or reversed end-diastolic flow of the umbilical artery (see Figure 7A in the section "Ultrasonography") require hospitalization and daily fetal monitoring. The recommendation for daily fetal surveillance is based on the reported very short time period within which fetal heart rate and biophysical profile results become abnormal in those patients.

The effects of both nonstress tests and biophysical profiles on reduction of perinatal mortality in a high-risk population have been evaluated by meta-analyses of interventional trials. Neither test, when used in the management, demonstrated a substantial improvement of perinatal mortality. There was actually a trend toward increased perinatal mortality in pregnancies monitored with nonstress testing, likely because of high false-positive rates. However, it is important to keep in mind that these analyses included far too few patients to determine if a clinically significant improvement in perinatal mortality exists. Because of a very low incidence of perinatal mortality, the meta-analysis of biophysical profile surveillance trials was powered sufficiently to detect only reduction in perinatal mortality in excess of

four times, whereas nonstress test meta-analysis was powered to detect only a larger effect. However, what transpires from these studies is a very low false-negative rate, a rarity of perinatal death among monitored pregnancies. The high false-positive rate of these tests is likely to be ameliorated by using them in conjunction with umbilical artery Doppler ultrasonography, which has a lower false-positive rate.

Most interventions aimed to treat IUGR do not demonstrate a substantial effect on perinatal outcome. Ultimately, delivery is the single intervention currently available. However, the question of timing of delivery remains unresolved. If we knew at what gestational age the incidence of stillbirth exceeds the incidence of neonatal death for fetuses with and without abnormal umbilical artery impedance, we could determine appropriate recommendations for timing of delivery. However, such data are not available and will be produced only by very large studies. Meanwhile, results of research of stillbirths demonstrates that most unexplained SGA stillbirths occur after 33 weeks of gestation. Many clinicians, therefore, deliver SGA pregnancies with absent or reversed end-diastolic flow in the umbilical artery at 34 weeks of gestation despite otherwise normal fetal surveillance. Small for gestational age fetuses with increased umbilical artery impedance frequently are delivered at 37 weeks of gestation.

References

1. Pell JP, Smith GC, Walsh D. Pregnancy complications and subsequent maternal cerebrovascular events: a retrospective cohort study of 119,668 births. Am J Epidemiol 2004;159:336–42.

2. Bukowski R, Smith GC, Malone FD, Ball RH, Nyberg DA, Comstock CH, et al. Fetal growth in early pregnancy and risk of delivering low birth weight infant: prospective cohort study. FASTER Research Consortium. BMJ 2007;334:836.

3. Bukowski R, Uchida T, Smith GC, Malone FD, Ball RH, Nyberg DA, et al. Individualized norms of optimal fetal growth: fetal growth potential. First and Second Trimester Evaluation of Risk (FASTER) Research Consortium. Obstet Gynecol 2008;111:1065–76.

4. Dudley NJ. A systematic review of the ultrasound estimation of fetal weight. Ultrasound Obstet Gynecol 2005;25:80–9.

Preterm Labor and Delivery

Maged Costantine and George Saade

Preterm birth, defined as delivery before 37 weeks 0 days of gestation, has increased by 20% since 1990 to approximately 12.8% of all births in 2006 (1). Much of this increase is a result of increases in rates of multiple gestations (driven by improvements in reproductive technologies) and of late preterm birth, defined as birth between 34 weeks of gestation and 37 weeks of gestation. Currently, twin births represent 3.2% of all births, but constitute 17% of all preterm births and 23% of all very preterm births (less than 32 weeks of gestation) (2). The rate of preterm birth is still highest among African Americans at 18.1%, compared with 12.8% in Hispanics and 11.8% in whites, with the increase affecting all three groups (1).

With an increase from 6.77% in 1990 to 9.15% in 2006, late preterm birth represents the fastest growing group of all preterm births (1) and makes up more than 70% of all preterm births (3). Late preterm infants still are at higher risk of neonatal complications than term infants. The infant mortality rate of late preterm infants is three times that of term infants (7.3 compared with 2.4 per 1,000 live births) (4). Moreover, these infants are at increased risks for temperature instability, hypoglycemia, respiratory distress, apnea, jaundice, and feeding difficulty. This has led the American College of Obstetricians and Gynecologists (the College) to recommend that late preterm delivery should occur only when an accepted maternal or fetal indication for delivery exists and should be documented in the patient's medical record (3).

Preterm birth is second only to congenital malformation as a cause of infant death (defined as death at less than 1 year of age) in the United States. In 2005, it accounted for 36.5% of all cases of infant death. Moreover, more than 65% of all cases of infant death occurred in preterm infants. In particular, very preterm infants (born at less than 32 weeks of gestation) account for only 2% of live birth rates but 55% of infant mortality rates. In addition, more than 60% of neonatal mortality (death occurring at less than 28 days) and morbidity in neonates without congenital anomalies were because of prematurity-related causes. Preterm-related infant mortality rates vary according to the race of the infant and mother. It is 3.4 times higher in non-Hispanic blacks compared with non-Hispanic whites. The percentage of total infant deaths that are preterm related is highest among infants of non-Hispanic black women (45.9%) compared with white women (32%) and Hispanic women (34%) (4, 5).

Data are now available from the most recent *Eunice Kennedy Shriver* National Institute of Child Health and Human Development Neonatal Research Network trial, a large prospective study of 4,633 infants weighing between 400 g and 1,500 g at birth, conducted at 14 tertiary centers across the United States between 1995 and 1996 (6). In this study, gestational age was determined by the best obstetric estimate, using last menstrual period, standard obstetric parameters, and ultrasound examination. All liveborn infants were included, including those not admitted to the neonatal intensive care unit. Because mortality was defined as death occurring before patient discharge, the reported rates do not include deaths during labor or deaths after 120 days of life; conversely, survival rates refer to those infants who lived to at least 120 days. Results of this study showed that a significant increase in survival of newborns occurs for each completed week from 21 weeks of gestation (0% survival) to 25 weeks of gestation (75% survival) (Figure 16) (7).

Pathophysiology

Preterm delivery in general is divided into two types: 1) indicated (maternal or fetal) or 2) spontaneous (with or without premature rupture of the membranes). Most spontaneous preterm deliveries occur as a result of one or more of four primary pathogenic processes. Each process has unique biochemical mediators, but all four processes share a common final biologic pathway that leads to cervical change and uterine contraction, with or without membrane rupture:

1. Activation of maternal–fetal hypothalamic–pituitary–adrenal axis caused by fetal or maternal stress—There is increasing epidemiologic, clinical, and experimental evidence that uteroplacental vascular abnormalities accompanied by intrauterine growth restriction are present in up to one third of preterm deliveries. Similarly, maternal psychosocial and physiologic indicators of stress have been increasingly linked to preterm delivery (8). The pathway responsible for stress-associated preterm delivery is likely to be similar to that for physiologic parturition.

2. Decidual–chorioamniotic or systemic inflammation—This inflammation may be the result of infectious or noninfectious processes. There are abundant epidemiologic, clinical, histologic, cell culture, and microbiologic data linking infection or inflammation with preterm delivery via the acti-

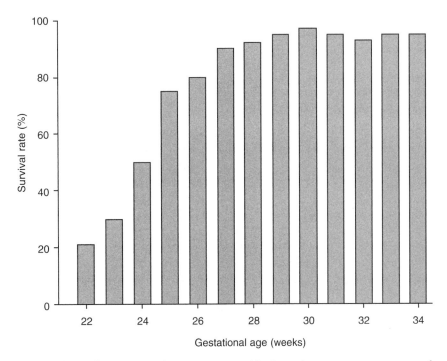

Figure 16. Survival until discharge by gestational age as estimated by best obstetric estimate among infants born in National Institute of Child Health and Human Development Neonatal Research Network Centers between January 1, 1995 and December 31, 1996. Data are expressed as percentage survived. (Data from Lemons JA, Bauer CR, Oh W, Korones SB, Papile LA, Stoll BJ, et al. Very low birth weight outcomes of the National Institute of Child Health and Human Development Neonatal Research Network, January 1995 through December 1996. NICHD Neonatal Research Network. Pediatrics 2001;107:E1.)

vation of cervical, decidual, and fetal membrane cytokine networks.

3. Decidual hemorrhage or uteroplacental ischemia— Decidual hemorrhage (*abruptio placentae*), regardless of whether it results in recurrent vaginal bleeding, has been strongly associated with a threefold to sevenfold increased risk of prematurity, particularly preceded by preterm rupture of membranes. The biochemical pathway by which such hemorrhage leads to preterm delivery appears to be mediated by thrombin generation. Thrombin binds to cellular receptors in the decidua to stimulate the production of various proteases (eg, plasminogen activators and matrix metalloproteases–collagenases) that ripen the cervix. Thrombin also may exert direct effects on the myometrium to stimulate contractions.

4. Pathologic uterine distention—Distention of the uterus activates the myometrium and increases the expression of fetal membrane cytokines.

Each of these four pathogenic mechanisms converges on a common pathway involving increased uterotonin and protease expression. More than one cascade may operate to produce preterm delivery in a given patient. The role of individual, genetically determined variations in inflammatory response is an active area of research that may explain the occurrence of preterm birth in some but not all women with common risk factors.

Risk Factors

It is important to identify women who are destined to give preterm birth. This would allow potentially risk-specific prevention or treatment practices (9). Currently, several risk factors are associated with an increased risk of preterm delivery (Box 16).

Scoring systems based on historical risk factors have low sensitivities in identifying women who will give birth preterm. Clinical symptoms and signs, such as uterine contractions, determined by self-perception or tocodynamometry, have low sensitivity and low positive predictive value, even in women with historical risk factors for preterm delivery (10).

Screening and Prevention

Identifying women who will give birth prematurely remains a challenge. A history of preterm birth, vaginal bleeding, and multifetal gestation are the strongest clinical predictors of preterm delivery; however, they lack sensitivity. Screening for bacterial vaginosis in low-risk women and treating them with antibiotics has not been shown to decrease the occurrence of preterm birth and, thus, is not recommended in asymptomatic patients (11, 12). Screening and treatment for bacterial vaginosis may be considered for women at high risk of preterm labor.

Second-trimester cervical length assessment by endovaginal ultrasonography and fetal fibronectin testing can

---

Box 16

Risk Factors for Preterm Birth

Demographic Factors

- Low socioeconomic and educational status
- Extremes of maternal ages (low and high)
- Single marital status
- Short interpregnancy interval (less than 6 months)
- Low prepregnancy body mass index
- Smoking
- Substance abuse (cocaine)
- Nutritional deficiencies

Obstetric Factors

- Previous preterm delivery (15–50% recurrence)
- Multiple gestations (twins, 40–50%; triplets and higher order, 75–95%)
- Vaginal bleeding (placental abruption or placenta previa)
- Hydramnios
- Uterine anomalies (septate uterus)
- History of cervical cone biopsy
- Intrauterine infection
- Infections: vaginal (bacterial vaginosis) and non-vaginal (pyelonephritis and pneumonia)
- Cervical shortening
- Excessive preterm uterine activity
- Maternal medical conditions (hypothyroidism, asthma, diabetes mellitus, hypertension, and depression)

---

identify women at increased risk of preterm delivery; however, they are not sufficiently sensitive, and their likelihood ratios are not in the clinically-useful range to be applied to routine prenatal care. However, they may be useful to evaluate women with clinical risk factors who, if test results are negative, may be spared ineffective traditional interventions, such as reduced physical activity. In symptomatic women presenting with preterm contractions, the usefulness of cervical length measurement and fetal fibronectin is limited to prevention of unnecessary interventions. However, the latter has not been shown to be better than clinical evaluation and judgment.

Cervical cerclage has been used in the treatment of women with history of incompetent cervix. It also has been proposed for prevention of preterm birth in women with a short cervix. Prophylactic cerclage reduced the rate of preterm birth (at less than 35 weeks of gestation) in women with both a history of preterm birth and a short cervix (less than 25 mm). However, cerclage has not been shown to be beneficial in women with a short

cervix (less than 15 mm) without history of prior preterm birth or in women with a history of preterm birth without a short cervix in the current pregnancy or in twin gestations. A recent study of the National Institutes of Health of women with a history of previous preterm birth showed that screening with transvaginal ultrasonography and cerclage for women with a cervical length less than 15 mm decreased the rate of preterm birth at less than 35 weeks of gestation (13–15).

Progesterone supplementation has been shown to reduce the risk of preterm birth in women at high risk (with a history of preterm birth or cervix of less than 15 mm); however, those at high risk secondary to twin or triplet gestations in current pregnancy did not benefit from progesterone therapy (16–20). Different progesterone formulations have been used with different routes of administration (Table 15). The American College of Obstetricians and Gynecologists currently recommends offering 17α-hydroxyprogesterone caproate to women with prior spontaneous preterm birth (21).

In addition, women planning to become pregnant should be counseled to stop smoking and to wait at least 1 year before attempting another pregnancy and their nutritional status should be assessed. Results from one recent study showed that preconceptional folic acid supplementation decreased the rate of preterm birth. Interconceptional antimicrobial treatment in women with prior preterm birth did not affect its frequency in the subsequent pregnancy (22).

Diagnosis

The symptoms and signs of preterm labor may include mild, menstrual-like cramps, constant low backache, uterine contractions that often are painless, and a recent increase in vaginal discharge or presence of a pink-stained discharge. Because these symptoms are subtle, they may not be recognized until the labor process and cervical dilation is in an advanced stage (greater than 4 cm). The diagnosis of true preterm labor early in its course is challenging, and providers often overdiagnose it. Often women who are treated after a diagnosis of preterm labor based on persistent contractions accompanied by cervical change are not actually in labor (up to 40%). Persistent contractions without additional evidence of labor are not sufficient to begin treatment. Ruptured membranes, bleeding, and clear evidence of cervical effacement (80% or more) or dilation (more than 2 cm) are the most reliable clinical signs. Studies have shown that waiting for evidence of cervical change does not affect the response to tocolysis. When measured in women with contractions whose cervical dilation is less than 3 cm, a negative fetal fibronectin test or a transvaginal ultrasound cervical length of 30 mm or more identify women who are not in labor, thus reducing the chance of false-positive diagnosis and overtreatment.

Table 15. Studies That Evaluated Progesterone Supplementation to Decrease Preterm Birth

Study	Patients Characteristics	Progesterone Supplementation	Results
da Fonseca*	High-risk (more than 90% with prior spontaneous singleton preterm birth)	Daily, 100 mg of progesterone, vaginally	Decreased risk of preterm birth at less than 34 weeks of gestation
Meis[†]	High-risk singleton or prior history of spontaneous singleton preterm birth	Weekly, 250 mg of 17 β-hydroxyprogesterone, intramuscularly	Decreased risk of preterm birth at less than 32 weeks of gestation, 35 weeks of gestation, and 37 weeks of gestation
Rouse[‡]	High-risk, twin	Weekly, 250 mg of 17 β-hydroxyprogesterone, intramuscularly	No benefit
O'Brien[§]	High-risk, prior spontaneous preterm birth	Daily, 90 mg of progesterone vaginal gel	No benefit
da Fonseca[ǁ]	Women in general population with short cervix (less than 15 mm)	Daily, 200 mg of micronized vaginal progesterone	Decreased risk of preterm birth at less than 34 weeks of gestation

*da Fonseca EB, Bittar RE, Carvalho MH, Zugaib M. Prophylactic administration of progesterone by vaginal suppository to reduce the incidence of spontaneous preterm birth in women at increased risk: a randomized placebo-controlled double-blind study. Am J Obstet Gynecol 2003;188:419–24.

[†]Meis PJ, Klebanoff M, Thom E, Dombrowski MP, Sibai B, Moawad AH, et al. Prevention of recurrent preterm delivery by 17 alpha-hydroxyprogesterone caproate. National Institute of Child Health and Human Development Maternal-Fetal Medicine Units Network [published erratum appears in N Engl J Med 2003;349:1299]. N Engl J Med 2003;348:2379–85.

[‡]Rouse DJ, Caritis SN, Peaceman AM, Sciscione A, Thom EA, Spong CY, et al. A trial of 17 alpha-hydroxyprogesterone caproate to prevent prematurity in twins. National Institute of Child Health and Human Development Maternal-Fetal Medicine Units Network. N Engl J Med 2007;357:454–61.

[§]O'Brien JM, Adair CD, Lewis DF, Hall DR, Defranco EA, Fusey S, et al. Progesterone vaginal gel for the reduction of recurrent preterm birth: primary results from a randomized, double-blind, placebo-controlled trial. Ultrasound Obstet Gynecol 2007;30:687–96.

[ǁ]Fonseca EB, Celik E, Parra M, Singh M, Nicolaides KH. Progesterone and the risk of preterm birth among women with a short cervix. Fetal Medicine Foundation Second Trimester Screening Group. N Engl J Med 2007;357:462–9.

Treatment

The initial evaluation of patients with suspected preterm labor should include assessment of uterine contractions and cervical status, performance of a sterile speculum examination to exclude ruptured membranes, determination of gestational age, and evaluation of maternal and fetal status. Ultrasonography for fetal evaluation is recommended because a number of structural fetal anomalies is associated with preterm labor. Before tocolysis is considered, a search should be made for treatable conditions associated with preterm labor, such as pyelonephritis, and an evaluation made to determine whether there are maternal or fetal contraindications to a specific tocolytic treatment. A urine culture often is obtained, and cultures for group B hemolytic streptococcus, *Chlamydia trachomatis*, and *Neisseria gonorrhoeae* are recommended. Amniocentesis may be performed to rule out intraamniotic infection, which is confirmed by the presence of microorganisms on a Gram stain, a positive culture, or a positive polymerase chain reaction test result for the presence of *Ureaplasma urealyticum*. In addition, fluid glucose level usually is low (less than 15 mg/dL) and white blood cells (especially neutrophils) are evident. The yield from amniocentesis is gestational-age dependent.

Chorioamnionitis is more common when preterm labor occurs at earlier gestational ages. Any patient presenting with preterm labor should initiate antibiotic therapy for group B streptococci prophylaxis unless a recent anovaginal culture result was negative.

After a diagnosis of preterm labor has been established, the clinician must weigh the risk–benefit ratio of tocolysis for each patient. Contraindications for tocolysis include chorioamnionitis and nonreassuring fetal or maternal status that require immediate delivery. The main objectives of using tocolytics are to allow transfer of the mother to a facility with a high level of neonatal care and to delay delivery for 48 hours in order to maximize the benefits of corticosteroids on improving neonatal survival and reducing neonatal morbidities. No tocolytic has been shown to decrease the rate of preterm birth, nor improve neonatal outcomes. It generally is advised not to combine tocolytic agents because of increased maternal side effects with no proven benefit. Before switching from one agent to another, it is prudent to reassess the clinical picture of the mother and to look for causes of preterm labor especially intraamniotic infection or abruption. Currently used tocolytics include magnesium sulfate, prostaglandin synthetase inhibitors, and calcium channel blockers.

Magnesium sulfate is a widely used tocolytic agent despite the absence of any proven efficacy. It works as a calcium competitive and inhibits myometrial contractility. Usually it is given as a loading dose of 4–6 g, intravenously, over 30 minutes followed by a continuous maintenance dose of 2–4 g/h. The usual effective maternal serum concentration is 6–8 mg/dL. The infusion rate is titrated to the clinical response, with careful maternal monitoring for toxicity. Magnesium sulfate is contraindicated in patients with myasthenia gravis (23, 24).

Prostaglandin synthetase inhibitors (eg, indomethacin) have been reported to be the most effective tocolytic agents. These agents may produce oligohydramnios and narrowing of the ductus arteriosus, but evidence shows that these effects are both rare and reversible if the drug is given before 32 weeks of gestation and when the duration of therapy is limited to 48–72 hours. Amniotic fluid volume and ductal flow assessment are not needed when these guidelines are followed. The advantages of indomethacin are its efficacy and relative safety. Unlike other agents, it rarely causes cardiovascular side effects. Gastric irritation is the most common maternal side effect but is usually mild. Asthma may occur in aspirin-sensitive women, and platelet function may be affected without leading to clinically excessive bleeding. Indomethacin should be avoided when either the mother or the fetus has a renal disorder as well as in mothers with active peptic ulcer disease or gastrointestinal bleeding. The initial dose is 50 mg orally or 100 mg rectally followed by 25 mg orally every 6 hours. It is a nonselective inhibitor of the enzyme COX and, thus, inhibits the production of prostaglandins involved in preterm labor.

Calcium channel-blocking drugs cause a decrease in intracellular free calcium and, hence, inhibition of myometrial contractility. Based on limited evidence, nifedipine is more effective than β-mimetics in increasing latency for 24 hours, 48 hours, and 1 week. The drug is given orally and has an onset of action in 20–30 minutes. Various regimens have been used with titration according to frequency of contractions. It should not be given sublingually because it may cause profound hypotension. Side effects, including hypotension and headache, are common and may be reduced with adequate pretreatment hydration. However, because pulmonary edema may occur with any tocolytic, including nifedipine, fluid balance should be carefully monitored. Calcium channel blockers are occasionally given to patients receiving magnesium sulfate. This combination should be used with caution. It is contraindicated in women with coronary artery disease or a history of stroke.

Beta-adrenergic drugs are less commonly used today. In the United States currently only oral and subcutaneous (intermittent and continuous therapy) agents are approved for use, but none of them have been shown effective. Their mechanism of action includes an increase in intracellular cyclic adenosine monophosphate leading to reduction in myometrial contractile activity. Study results have shown these drugs to be effective in delaying delivery by 48 hours; however, they are associated with frequent undesirable maternal side effects, such as hypotension, tachyarrhythmia, pulmonary edema, chest pain with or without myocardial injury, hyperglycemia, and hypokalemia. Fetal tachycardia also is very common. When beta-adrenergic drugs are used, maternal fluid balance should be carefully monitored (restriction of fluid administration to less than 2,500 mL per day and careful monitoring of urinary output) and any maternal symptom of chest pain should be thoroughly evaluated. Beta-adrenergic drugs are contraindicated in patients with cardiac disease and preexisting or gestational diabetes mellitus.

Oxytocin antagonists are the newest class of tocolytic drugs. Atosiban, the only drug available clinically, is not currently available in the United States. Its efficacy is comparable to β-mimetics, and this drug has a very favorable maternal safety profile (25).

Maintenance tocolytic therapy (with oral β-mimetic or calcium channel blocker) after successful arrest of preterm labor has not been proved to reduce the incidence of preterm delivery or recurrent preterm labor episodes or to improve neonatal outcomes. Other types of posthospitalization surveillance, such home uterine activity monitoring, also has no beneficial effects (26, 27).

Corticosteroid Therapy

A single course of antenatal corticosteroids is recommended for all pregnant women with intact membranes between 24–34 weeks of gestation (24–32 weeks of gestation for those with ruptured membranes) who are at risk of premature delivery within 7 days. Those at more than 34 weeks of gestation with documented pulmonary immaturity also should receive a course. The current recommended regimens are either betamethasone (two 12-mg doses given intramuscularly 24 hours apart) or dexamethasone (four 6-mg doses given intramuscularly 12 hours apart). Both cross the placenta and lack mineralocorticoid activity with only weak immunosuppressive activity. The American College of Obstetricians and Gynecologists does not recommend one agent instead of the other. Both agents have been shown to decrease the incidence of respiratory distress syndrome; however, only betamethasone has been shown to decrease mortality and the risk of cystic periventricular leukomalacia. Dexamethasone has been associated with fewer cases of intraventricular hemorrhage (28–31). No data exist on the efficacy of corticosteroid use before viability. Thus, corticosteroids are not recommended for this indication.

The current College recommendation is to limit antenatal corticosteroid administration to a single course and give rescue courses only to women enrolled in clinical trials, despite results from one study that showed decreased neonatal morbidities (especially respiratory) with repeated courses (28). Multiple studies showed that repeated courses of antenatal corticosteroids are associated with decreased birth weight and head circumference; however, long-term follow-up (2–3 years) showed no difference in physical or neurocognitive developmental outcomes except for a nonsignificant increase in the risk of cerebral palsy in infants exposed to repeat courses in one study (32). Maternal side effects from repeat courses include increase risk of infections and suppression of the hypothalamic–pituitary axis. These maternal and fetal side effects are unlikely if the corticosteroid course is repeated only once.

Resuscitation at the Threshold of Viability

Decision regarding intensive care to extremely premature infants has been traditionally based on gestational age at delivery, infant's weight, or both. However, recent data suggest that other factors play a role in predicting survival or long-term outcomes in infants receiving intensive care. In addition to gestational age, higher birth weight, exposure to antenatal corticosteroids, female gender, and singleton birth were associated with reduced risk of death, severe neurodevelopmental disabilities, or both (33).

All these parameters can assist obstetricians and neonatologists in counseling patients at risk for delivery at gestational ages at the threshold of viability. However, delivery room care of these so-called "micropreemies" is still the subject of ongoing concern and controversy. Most experts believe that informed parental preferences should be determined and followed concerning the degree of intervention to be undertaken. Although some informed parents will decide that resuscitation should not be initiated, a common course is to provide individualized care that involves ongoing judgment concerning extent and duration of resuscitation on the basis of clinical course and discussions with parents when possible. Many organizations, including the College and the American Academy of Pediatrics, provide guidelines that address management, outcomes, and ethical concerns (27, 34).

Magnesium Sulfate as a Neuroprotectant

A link between antenatal exposure to magnesium sulfate and a reduction in the risk of cerebral palsy was first suggested by a case–control analysis (35). Since then, a number of observational studies and clinical trials have been conducted to evaluate the utility of magnesium sulfate for neuroprotection. Four randomized trials were specifically designed to study the neuroprotection

effects of magnesium sulfate (36–39). Although the results from none of these trials demonstrated significant improvements in their primary outcome, in most of them significant benefit in some of their prespecified secondary outcomes was found. In the results from one of these studies, less "substantial gross motor dysfunction" (relative risk [RR], 0.51; 95% confidence interval [CI], 0.29–0.91) and "death or substantial motor gross motor dysfunction" (RR, 0.75; 95% CI, 0.59–0.96) was found with magnesium sulfate treatment compared with placebo (36). Results from another of these studies showed reductions in death or gross motor dysfunction (odds ratio [OR], 0.62; 95% CI, 0.41–0.93) and in death or motor or cognitive dysfunction (OR, 0.68; 95% CI, 0.47–0.99]) at a 2-year follow-up (37). Results from yet another of these studies demonstrated reduction in "moderate or severe cerebral palsy" (1.9% compared with 3.5% [RR 0.55; 95% CI, 0.32–0.95]) and overall cerebral palsy (4.2% compared with 7.3%, $P<0.004$) with magnesium sulfate treatment (39).

These trials in addition to available data from the follow-up study of the Magpie trial were pooled in a number of meta-analyses and systematic reviews (40–42). Although, the combined outcome of death or cerebral palsy was not significantly different when the five studies (MagNET, ACTOMgSO4, PREMAG, BEAM, and Magpie) were pooled, the benefit of antenatal magnesium sulfate became more evident when the analysis was limited to only the four trials specifically designed for fetal neuroprotection. The combined outcome of death or cerebral palsy was significantly reduced (RR, 0.86; 95% CI, 0.75–0.99) as well as that of death or moderate to severe cerebral palsy. Additionally, antenatal exposure to magnesium sulfate was found to decrease the risk of cerebral palsy (RR, 0.71; 95% CI, 0.55–0.91) and moderate to severe cerebral palsy (RR, 0.6; 95% CI, 0.43–0.84) without increasing the risk of perinatal or infant death (RR, 0.95; 95% CI, 0.8–1.13) or any other maternal or pediatric adverse events. Despite these findings, many questions remain unanswered especially magnesium sulfate dosing regimen, the ideal patient candidate, and concomitant use of tocolytics. It is important to note that the trial in the United States included patients who were not candidates for tocolysis (preterm premature rupture of membranes, advanced cervical dilatation, or indicated deliveries). Therefore, the findings of the trials should not be extrapolated to magnesium sulfate use as a tocolytic or to gestational ages beyond the upper limit included in the majority of the studies (32–34 weeks of gestation). If these criteria are followed, then only a minority of patients would be candidates for neuroprotection with magnesium sulfate. It is estimated that the number of patients needed to treat in order to prevent one case of cerebral palsy among infants who survive until age 18–24 months is 46 (95% CI, 26–187) in infants exposed to magnesium sulfate in utero before 30 weeks of gestation and 56 (95% CI, 34–164) in infants exposed to magnesium sulfate in utero before 32–34 weeks of gestation.

References

1. Martin JA, Hamilton BE, Sutton PD, Ventura SJ, Menacker F, Kimeyer S, et al. Births: final data for 2006. Natl Vital Stat Rep 2009;57(7):1–104.

2. Martin JA, Hamilton BE, Sutton PD, Ventura SJ, Menacker F, Kimeyer S, Munson ML. Births: Final data for 2005. Natl Vital Stat Rep 2007;56(6):1–104.

3. Late-preterm infants. ACOG Committee Opinion No. 404. American College of Obstetricians and Gynecologists. Obstet Gynecol 2008;111:1029–32.

4. Mathews TJ, MacDorman MF. Infant mortality statistics from the 2005 period linked birth/infant death data set. Natl Vital Stat Rep 2008;57(2):1–32.

5. Kung HC, Hoyert DL, Xu J, Murphy SL. Deaths: Final data for 2005. Natl Vital Stat Rep 2008;56(10):1–120. Available at: http://www.cdc.gov/nchs/data/nvsr/nvsr56/nvsr56_10.pdf. Retrieved September 11, 2009.

6. Lemons JA, Bauer CR, Oh W, Korones SB, Papile LA, Stoll BJ, et al. Very low birth weight outcomes of the National Institute of Child health and human development neonatal research network, January 1995 through December 1996. NICHD Neonatal Research Network. Pediatrics 2001;107:E1.

7. Perinatal care at the threshold of viability. ACOG Practice Bulletin No. 38. American College of Obstetricians and Gynecologists. Obstet Gynecol 2002;100:617–24.

8. Challis JR, Smith SK. Fetal endocrine signals and preterm labor. Biol Neonate 2001;79:163–7.

9. Goldenberg RL, Culhane JF, Iams JD, Romero R. Epidemiology and causes of preterm birth. Lancet 2008;371:75–84.

10. Iams JD, Newman RB, Thom EA, Goldenberg RL, Mueller-Heubach E, Moawad A, et al. Frequency of uterine contractions and the risk of spontaneous preterm delivery. National Institute of Child Health and Human Development Network of Maternal-Fetal Medicine Units [published erratum appears in N Engl J Med 2003;349:513]. N Engl J Med 2002;346:250–5.

11. Riggs MA, Klebanoff MA. Treatment of vaginal infections to prevent preterm birth: a meta-analysis. Clin Obstet Gynecol 2004;47:796,807; discussion 881–2.

12. McDonald HM, Brocklehurst P, Gordon A. Antibiotics for treating bacterial vaginosis in pregnancy. Cochrane Database of Systematic Reviews 2007, Issue 1. Art. No.: CD000262. DOI: 10.1002/14651858.CD000262.pub3; 10.1002/14651858.CD000262.pub3.

13. To MS, Alfirevic Z, Heath VC, Cicero S, Cacho AM, Williamson PR, et al. Cervical cerclage for prevention of preterm delivery in women with short cervix: randomised controlled trial. Fetal Medicine Foundation Second Trimester Screening Group. Lancet 2004;363:1849–53.

14. Berghella V, Odibo AO, To MS, Rust OA, Althuisius SM. Cerclage for short cervix on ultrasonography: meta-analysis of trials using individual patient-level data. Obstet Gynecol 2005;106:181–9.

15. Owen J, Hankins G, Iams JD, Berghella V, Sheffield JS, Perez-Delboy A, et al. Multicenter randomized trial of cerclage for preterm birth prevention in high-risk women with shortened midtrimester cervical length. Am J Obstet Gynecol 2009;201:375.e1–375.e8.

16. Fonseca EB, Celik E, Parra M, Singh M, Nicolaides KH. Progesterone and the risk of preterm birth among women with a short cervix. Fetal Medicine Foundation Second Trimester Screening Group. N Engl J Med 2007;357:462–9.

17. Meis PJ, Klebanoff M, Thom E, Dombrowski MP, Sibai B, Moawad AH, et al. Prevention of recurrent preterm delivery by 17 alpha-hydroxyprogesterone caproate. National Institute of Child Health and Human Development Maternal-Fetal Medicine Units Network [published erratum appears in N Engl J Med 2003;349:1299]. N Engl J Med 2003;348:2379–85.

18. Rouse DJ, Caritis SN, Peaceman AM, Sciscione A, Thom EA, Spong CY, et al. A trial of 17 alpha-hydroxyprogesterone caproate to prevent prematurity in twins. National Institute of Child Health and Human Development Maternal-Fetal Medicine Units Network. N Engl J Med 2007;357:454–61.

19. O'Brien JM, Adair CD, Lewis DF, Hall DR, Defranco EA, Fusey S, et al. Progesterone vaginal gel for the reduction of recurrent preterm birth: primary results from a randomized, double-blind, placebo-controlled trial. Ultrasound Obstet Gynecol 2007;30:687–96.

20. da Fonseca EB, Bittar RE, Carvalho MH, Zugaib M. Prophylactic administration of progesterone by vaginal suppository to reduce the incidence of spontaneous preterm birth in women at increased risk: a randomized placebo-controlled double-blind study. Am J Obstet Gynecol 2003;188:419–24.

21. Use of progesterone to reduce preterm birth. ACOG Committee Opinion No. 419. American College of Obstetricians and Gynecologists. Obstet Gynecol 2008;112:963–5.

22. Espinoza J, Erez O, Romero R. Preconceptional antibiotic treatment to prevent preterm birth in women with a previous preterm delivery. Am J Obstet Gynecol 2006;194:630–7.

23. Cox SM, Sherman ML, Leveno KJ. Randomized investigation of magnesium sulfate for prevention of preterm birth. Am J Obstet Gynecol 1990;163:767–72.

24. Crowther CA, Hiller JE, Doyle LW. Magnesium sulphate for preventing preterm birth in threatened preterm labour. The Cochrane Database of Systematic Reviews 2002, Issue 4. Art. No.: CD001060. DOI 10.1002/1465/858.CD001060.

25. Pryde PG, Janeczek S, Mittendorf R. Risk-benefit effects of tocolytic therapy. Expert Opin Drug Saf 2004;3:639–54.

26. Iams JD, Romero R, Culhane JF, Goldenberg RL. Primary, secondary, and tertiary interventions to reduce the morbidity and mortality of preterm birth. Lancet 2008;371:164–75.

27. Management of preterm labor. ACOG Practice Bulletin No. 43. American College of Obstetricians and Gynecologists. Obstet Gynecol 2003;101:1039–47.

28. Antenatal corticosteroid therapy for fetal maturation. ACOG Committee Opinion No. 402. American College of Obstetricians and Gynecologists. Obstet Gynecol 2008;11:805–7.

29. Ballard PL, Ballard RA. Scientific basis and therapeutic regimens for use of antenatal glucocorticoids. Am J Obstet Gynecol 1995;173:254–62.

30. Baud O, Foix-L'Helias L, Kaminski M, Audibert F, Jarreau PH, Papiernik E, et al. Antenatal glucocorticoid treatment and cystic periventricular leukomalacia in very premature infants. N Engl J Med 1999;341:1190–6.

31. Elimian A, Garry D, Figueroa R, Spitzer A, Wiencek V, Quirk JG. Antenatal betamethasone compared with dexamethasone (betacode trial): a randomized controlled trial. Obstet Gynecol 2007;110:26–30.

32. Wapner RJ, Sorokin Y, Mele L, Johnson F, Dudley DJ, Spong CY, et al. Long-term outcomes after repeat doses of antenatal corticosteroids. National Institute of Child Health and Human Development Maternal-Fetal Medicine Units Network. N Engl J Med 2007;357:1190–8.

33. Tyson JE, Parikh NA, Langer J, Green C, Higgins RD. Intensive care for extreme prematurity--moving beyond gestational age. National Institute of Child Health and Human Development Neonatal Research Network. N Engl J Med 2008;358:1672–81.

34. MacDonald H. Perinatal care at the threshold of viability. American Academy of Pediatrics. Committee on Fetus and Newborn. Pediatrics 2002;110:1024–7.

35. Nelson KB, Grether JK. Can magnesium sulfate reduce the risk of cerebral palsy in very low birthweight infants? Pediatrics 1995;95:263–9.

36. Mittendorf R, Dambrosia J, Pryde PG, Lee KS, Gianopoulos JG, Besinger RE, et al. Association between the use of antenatal magnesium sulfate in preterm labor and adverse health outcomes in infants. Am J Obstet Gynecol 2002;186:1111–8.

37. Crowther CA, Hiller JE, Doyle LW, Haslam RR. Effect of magnesium sulfate given for neuroprotection before preterm birth: a randomized controlled trial. Australasian Collaborative Trial of Magnesium Sulphate (ACTOMg SO4) Collaborative Group. JAMA 2003;290:2669–76.

38. Marret S, Marpeau L, Zupan-Simunek V, Eurin D, Leveque C, Hellot MF, et al. Magnesium sulphate given before very-preterm birth to protect infant brain: the randomised controlled PREMAG trial*. PREMAG trial group. BJOG 2007; 114:310–8.

39. Rouse DJ, Hirtz DG, Thom E, Varner MW, Spong CY, Mercer BM, et al. A randomized, controlled trial of magnesium sulfate for the prevention of cerebral palsy. Eunice Kennedy Shriver NICHD Maternal-Fetal Medicine Units Network. N Engl J Med 2008;359:895–905.

40. Doyle LW, Crowther CA, Middleton P, Marret S, Rouse D. Magnesium sulphate for women at risk of preterm birth for neuroprotection of the fetus. Cochrane Database of Systematic Reviews 2009, Issue 1. Art. No.: CD004661. DOI: 10.1002/14651858.CD004661.pub3; 10.1002/14651858. CD004661.pub3.

41. Conde-Agudelo A, Romero R. Antenatal magnesium sulfate for the prevention of cerebral palsy in preterm infants less than 34 weeks' gestation: a systematic review and metaanalysis. Am J Obstet Gynecol 2009;200:595–609.

42. Costantine MM, Weiner SJ. Effects of antenatal exposure to magnesium sulfate on neuroprotection and mortality in preterm infants: a meta-analysis. Eunice Kennedy Shriver National Institute of Child Health and Human Development Maternal-Fetal Medicine Units Network. Obstet Gynecol 2009;114:354–64.

Premature Rupture of Membranes

Brian M. Mercer

A hallmark of premature rupture of membranes (PROM) is early delivery; latency is inversely proportional to gestational age at membrane rupture. At term, 95% of expectantly managed pregnant women deliver within 28 hours of membrane rupture (1). Of all patients with membranes ruptured before 34 weeks of gestation, 93% will deliver in less than 1 week (2). Even with conservative management, 50–60% of women with preterm PROM remote from term will deliver within 1 week of membrane rupture. When PROM occurs near or before the limit of viability, up to one in four women remain pregnant for at least 1 month. Only a small proportion of women with membrane rupture will have spontaneous healing of the membranes (2.6–13%). The exception to this is when PROM occurs after amniocentesis, where resolution is common (3).

Risks

Maternal Risks

Chorioamnionitis is the most common maternal complication after PROM. The risk of infection decreases with increasing gestational age at membrane rupture and increases with increasing latency from membrane rupture to delivery. With PROM at term, 9% of pregnant women will develop intrauterine infection. The risk increases to 24% with membrane rupture longer than 24 hours. Intraamniotic infection complicates 13–60% of pregnancies, and endometritis occurs in approximately 2–13% of pregnancies after preterm PROM remote from term. Abruptio placentae may lead to PROM or may result secondarily, affecting 4–12% of these pregnancies. Retained placenta and postpartum hemorrhage necessitating uterine curettage, maternal sepsis, and death are uncommon but serious complications of expectantly managed PROM near or before the limit of viability.

Fetal and Neonatal Risks

At term, the fetus is at risk for umbilical cord compression from oligohydramnios and is susceptible to ascending infection, but the infant is anticipated to do well if intrapartum complications do not occur. The frequency and severity of neonatal complications after preterm PROM vary with the gestational age at which rupture and delivery occur and are potentially increased with perinatal infection, placental abruption, and umbilical cord compression.

Complications of preterm birth are the most significant risks to the infant born after preterm PROM, and respiratory distress syndrome is the most common serious complication after preterm delivery at any gestational age. Other serious acute morbidities, including necrotizing enterocolitis, intraventricular hemorrhage, and sepsis, are common with early preterm birth but relatively uncommon near term. Remote from term, serious perinatal morbidity that may lead to long-term sequelae or death is common. Current community-based survival and morbidity curves based on gestational age at delivery have been published (4). Although data specific to infants delivered after preterm PROM are not available, it has been found that perinatal sepsis is twofold more common after preterm PROM than after preterm birth caused by preterm labor with intact membranes.

Data linking perinatal infection to neurologic complications are accumulating. Because preterm PROM is associated with early delivery and with perinatal infection, it is a potential risk factor for long-term neurologic morbidity (5–7). However, no data suggest that immediate delivery of the candidate for conservative management after preterm PROM remote from term will prevent these sequelae.

Lethal pulmonary hypoplasia occurs when alveolar development is arrested when PROM occurs at the critical phase of development, generally before 20 weeks of gestation. Although lethal pulmonary hypoplasia rarely occurs with PROM after 24–26 weeks of gestation, presumably because alveolar development growth is adequate to support postnatal life, there remains the potential for nonlethal pulmonary hypoplasia, predisposing the infant to pulmonary complications related to poor pulmonary compliance and the need for high ventilatory pressures (eg, pneumothorax and pneumomediastinum). Restriction deformities can occur after oligohydramnios subsequent to PROM and are similar to those seen with Potter syndrome.

Diagnosis

The textbook description of using sterile techniques for examination, testing for pH of vaginal fluid, evaluating for ferning with a microscopic, obtaining of cervical cultures, and avoiding cervical digital examination all remain current. When a diagnostic dilemma occurs, injection of dilute sterile indigo carmine into a pocket of amniotic fluid under ultrasonographic guidance can include or refute the diagnosis. A number of markers, including placental alpha–microglobulin-1, insulin-like growth factor-binding protein-1, fetal fibronectin, alpha-fetoprotein, diamino-oxydase, total thyroxine and free thyroxine, prolactin, human chorionic gonadotropin, and interleukin-6, among others, have been found to be present in the vagina after PROM (8–10). These markers have not generally been evaluated for their accuracy when the diagnosis of PROM is unclear and they are unnecessary when the diagnosis is evident clinically. In a comparison of two rapid tests, placental alpha-microglobulin-1 was found to correctly identify lower concentrations of amniotic fluid than insulinlike growth factor-binding protein-1 in vitro (11). In results of a clinical study of women with suspected membrane rupture, an immunoassay was found for placental alpha-microglobulin-1 in cervicovaginal secretions to confirm PROM in 137 of 139 (98.6%) cases where the diagnosis was suspected and evident based on clinical examination or traditional nitrazine testing and ferning testing (8). However, the test result was positive in 24 cases where the diagnosis was not confirmed by initial traditional testing. Four of these had oligohydramnios, and eight had vaginal pooling (1), positive ferning (1), or a positive nitrazine test result alone (6). Eight of eleven remaining cases with no clinical evidence of membrane rupture but a positive placental alpha-microglobulin-1 result were later determined to have had membrane rupture on initial presentation. In a subsequent study a rapid test result for placental alpha-microglobulin-1 was positive in 30.9% of laboring women (25/81) and in 4.8% of nonlaboring women (6/125) without suspected membrane rupture, raising questions regarding the positive predictive value of this test when membrane rupture is not clinically apparent (12).

Management

At term, the patient with PROM is best served by expeditious delivery. Induction is associated with earlier delivery, without increasing the risk of intrauterine infection or cesarean delivery (1). Alternatively, conservative management of PROM at term increases the risk of chorioamnionitis and raises the potential for fetal compromise caused by umbilical cord compression while unmonitored.

The presence of advanced labor, intrauterine infection, significant uterine bleeding, or nonreassuring fetal test results are indications for delivery regardless of the gestational age. If feasible, maternal transfer to a facility with the resources to provide the care necessary for both the mother and premature neonate should be arranged early in the course of management to avoid emergent transfer once complications arise. When there is a suspicion of chorioamnionitis but the diagnosis remains unclear after clinical evaluation, a maternal white blood cell count above 18,000/mm³, or an amniocentesis sample revealing a glucose value of less than 16–20 mg/dL, or a positive Gram stain can be supportive of the diagnosis. Generally, amniotic fluid cultures will not be available until after a management decision needs to

be made in this regard. Intrapartum prophylaxis against group B streptococcus is recommended for women giving preterm birth and for those with PROM at term when the interval until delivery is expected to be 18 hours or more, unless recent anovaginal group B streptococcus cultures are negative (13).

Previable Premature Rupture of Membranes (Less Than 23 Weeks of Gestation)

With PROM occurring before the limit of viability, the most likely outcome is delivery of a previable or periviable infant near the limit of viability. The parents should be provided realistic information about the probability of delaying delivery for a substantial interval of time, including the limit of viability and the potential for extended latency thereafter. They also should be given the most current available information about the possibility for survival and the associated morbidities, both short term and long term, for a fetus delivered within that time frame. Initial observation for maternal infection, placental abruption, and labor is recommended, but there is no consensus regarding the advantages of continued inpatient management versus outpatient management before the limit of viability. The risks of infection, abruption, and cord complications need to be addressed in the initial monitoring and follow-up plan. If conservative management is chosen, a detailed ultrasound study of the fetus is indicated to look for anomalies. Pulmonary hypoplasia can be identified in many cases through serial ultrasound studies. Ultrasonographic measurement of lung growth either directly (lung length) or indirectly (eg, chest circumference, chest–abdomen circumference ratio, and chest circumference–femur length ratio), and Doppler imaging have a high positive predictive value for lethal pulmonary hypoplasia (14, 15). Experimental measures to reseal the membranes after previable PROM have been explored but cannot be recommended (16–19). When the patient elects not to pursue conservative management, the pregnancy can be terminated by dilatation and evacuation or induction of labor with oxytocin or with prostaglandins.

Preterm Premature Rupture of Membranes Remote From Term (23–31 Weeks of Gestation)

Advances in neonatal care have made possible the survival of very premature infants. However, the immediate and long-term morbidity of such early birth makes prolongation of pregnancy an important goal of conservative therapy after PROM remote from term. Initial therapy involves bed rest and continuous maternal and fetal monitoring for evidence of labor, abruption, chorioamnionitis, and umbilical cord complications. After the initial evaluation, daily evaluation of the fetal heart rate (FHR) pattern is advised because abnormalities are common (32–76%) as a result of cord compression and intrauterine infection. When FHR abnormalities are evident, continuous monitoring and reconsideration of delivery are advised. Fetal well-being can be assessed by nonstress test, biophysical profile, or both. Fetal heart rate patterns normally are less reactive remote from term, but low amniotic fluid volume may lower the biophysical profile score. Fetal heart rate monitoring offers the opportunity to concurrently evaluate for the presence of uterine contractions and the fetal response to these. Prolonged bed rest increases the maternal risk of thrombophlebitis (see the section "Deep Vein Thrombosis and Pulmonary Embolism") and its prevention should be considered when bed rest is prescribed (20).

The value of antibiotic therapy during conservative management of PROM at these gestational ages has been explored by numerous prospective studies, and together these have shown a positive effect in prolonging pregnancy and reducing perinatal infant morbidities. In one of the two largest studies, the *Eunice Kennedy Shriver* National Institute of Child Health and Human Development Maternal–Fetal Medicine Units network found that short-term (7 days) aggressive therapy with intravenous–oral ampicillin–amoxicillin and erythromycin improved latency and reduced gestational age-dependent morbidities (21). In results from another large multicenter trial, it was found that the use of a combination of ampicillin–clavulanic acid was not beneficial and could be harmful, increasing neonatal necrotizing enterocolitis, but the use of erythromycin alone prolonged pregnancy and reduced the incidence of the primary composite outcome of death or major cerebral abnormality or chronic neonatal lung disease (22). Follow-up of the infants described in this latter study revealed no increases or decreases in long-term morbidities for these infants at 7 years (23). Several studies have attempted to determine whether antibiotic therapy for less than 7 days is adequate after preterm PROM (24, 25). These studies are of inadequate size and power to demonstrate equivalent effectiveness against infant morbidity. Because of this, regimens such as that described by the *Eunice Kennedy Shriver* National Institute of Child Health and Human Development Maternal–Fetal Medicine Units network are recommended.

A single course of betamethasone (12 mg, intramuscularly, every 24 hours, two doses) or dexamethasone (6 mg, intramuscularly, every 12 hours, four doses) should be given during conservative management of PROM if this has not been previously administered. In the most recent meta-analysis, antenatal corticosteroid administration after preterm PROM substantially reduced the risks of respiratory distress syndrome (20% versus 35.4%), intraventricular hemorrhage (7.5% ver-

sus 15.9%), and necrotizing enterocolitis (0.8% versus 4.6%) without significantly increasing the risks of maternal infection (9.2% versus 5.1%) or neonatal infection (7.0% versus 6.6%) (26). Two randomized clinical trials have evaluated antenatal corticosteroid administration concurrent with antibiotic administration. In the results of one study less respiratory distress syndrome (18.4% versus 43.6%, $P=.03$) with no obvious increase in perinatal infection (3% versus 5%; P, not significant) was found with the use of antenatal corticosteroids after preterm PROM at 24–34 weeks of gestation (27). In the results of the second trial, although there was no significant reduction in respiratory distress syndrome with the use of antenatal corticosteroids, there was no increase in maternal or neonatal infectious morbidity with treatment. The women who remained pregnant after at least 24 hours of treatment had fewer perinatal deaths (1.3% versus 8.3%, $P=.05$) (28).

The use of tocolysis during conservative management of PROM remote from term has not been demonstrated to provide independent fetal benefit. It has been speculated that tocolysis may be useful in providing the opportunity to use antibiotic and corticosteroid therapy, but this effect is as yet unproved.

Preterm Premature Rupture of Membranes Near Term (32–36 Weeks of Gestation)

In general, delivery is recommended when preterm PROM occurs after 34 weeks 0 days of gestation because anticipated latency is brief, the risks of major neonatal morbidities is low, and because brief conservative management will not likely reduce these risks but does significantly increase the risk of maternal chorioamnionitis. At 32–33 weeks of gestation a test for fetal lung maturity can be assessed from the vaginal pool or an amniocentesis specimen. If the test result is positive, there is no apparent neonatal benefit for further conservative management, and delivery is indicated. Antenatal corticosteroids can be administered for those with pulmonary immaturity or, if fluid cannot be obtained, for testing.

Special Considerations
Cerclage Removal

Cervical cerclage is a known risk factor for PROM, which complicates approximately one in four pregnancies with a cerclage and approximately one half of pregnancies having emergent cerclage placement. No prospective studies exist on the management of women with preterm PROM and a cervical cerclage in situ. Results from retrospective studies have suggested that when cerclage is removed on admission the risk of adverse perinatal outcomes is not higher than after preterm PROM without a cerclage. Studies comparing pregnancies with cerclage retained or removed after preterm PROM have been small and have yielded conflicting results (29–31). In results from each study, insignificant trends toward increased maternal infection with retained cerclage have been found, and increased infant mortality and death from sepsis with retained cerclage, despite brief pregnancy prolongation, was found in the results of one of these studies. In results of one of these studies, comparing different practices at two institutions, significant pregnancy prolongation with cerclage retention was found. However, it is possible that this finding reflected population or practice differences rather than those related solely to cerclage retention. No controlled study results have indicated a significant reduction in infant morbidity with cerclage retention after preterm PROM. Given the potential risk without evident neonatal benefit, the general approach to management should include early cerclage removal after preterm PROM. The role for short-term cerclage retention while attempting to enhance fetal maturation with the use of antenatal corticosteroids in the periviable gestation has not been determined.

Antepartum Patient Discharge

In general, hospitalization for bed and pelvic rest is indicated after preterm PROM once the limit of viability has been reached. Because latency frequently is brief, intrauterine and fetal infection may occur, the fetus is at risk for umbilical cord compression, and labor or other complications can occur rapidly, ongoing surveillance of both mother and fetus is necessary. Results from one clinical trial have suggested that women who are stable can be discharged to reduce health care costs after initial observation. However, this trial lacked the necessary power to adequately evaluate the effect of discharge on these outcomes. Although the potential for a reduction in health care costs with antepartum patient discharge is enticing, it is important to establish that such management will not be associated with increased risks and costs related to perinatal morbidity. Any cost savings from antenatal discharge will be rapidly lost with a small increase in stays in the neonatal intensive care unit as a result of infectious or gestational age-dependent morbidity.

Prevention of Recurrent Preterm Premature Rupture of Membranes

In addition to general guidance directed against factors associated with an increased risk of spontaneous preterm birth (adequate nutrition, smoking cessation, and avoidance of heavy lifting and prolonged standing without breaks), research has identified antenatal 17 α-hydroxyprogesterone caproate therapy to be a specific intervention that can reduce the risk of recurrent spontaneous preterm birth caused by preterm labor or

PROM (32). In this multicenter trial, authors found 17 α-hydroxyprogesterone caproate treatment (250 mg, given intramuscularly each week through 36 weeks of gestation) reduced the risk of recurrent preterm birth (36.3% versus 54.9%; relative risk, 0.66; 95% confidence interval, 0.54–0.81) and spontaneous preterm birth (29.4% versus 45.1%; relative risk, 0.65; 95% confidence interval, 0.51–0.83), resulting in less frequent necrotizing enterocolitis, intraventricular hemorrhage, and need for supplemental oxygen. A study of the use of nightly vaginal progesterone suppositories (100 mg) also demonstrated less frequent preterm birth with treatment, whereas treatment with progesterone gel was not found to be effective in high-risk women (33, 34). Based on the available information, it is appropriate to offer weekly 17 α-hydroxyprogesterone caproate or daily progesterone vaginal suppositories to prevent recurrent preterm birth for women delivering preterm after PROM. Though vitamin C deficiency has been linked to preterm PROM, supplementation with this vitamin may actually increase the risk of this complication and is not recommended for this indication at present (35).

References

1. Hannah ME, Ohlsson A, Farine D, Hewson SA, Hodnett ED, Myhr TL, et al. Induction of labor compared with expectant management for prelabor rupture of the membranes at term. TERMPROM Study Group. N Engl J Med 1996; 334:1005–10.

2. Mercer BM, Arheart KL. Antimicrobial therapy in expectant management of preterm premature rupture of the membranes [published erratum appears in Lancet 1996;347:410]. Lancet 1995;346:1271–9.

3. Borgida AF, Mills AA, Feldman DM, Rodis JF, Egan JF. Outcome of pregnancies complicated by ruptured membranes after genetic amniocentesis. Am J Obstet Gynecol 2000;183:937–9.

4. Mercer BM. Preterm premature rupture of the membranes. Obstet Gynecol 2003;101:178–93.

5. Yoon BH, Jun JK, Romero R, Park KH, Gomez R, Choi JH, et al. Amniotic fluid inflammatory cytokines (interleukin-6, interleukin-1beta, and tumor necrosis factor-alpha), neonatal brain white matter lesions, and cerebral palsy. Am J Obstet Gynecol 1997;177:19–26.

6. Yoon BH, Romero R, Kim CJ, Koo JN, Choe G, Syn HC, et al. High expression of tumor necrosis factor-alpha and interleukin-6 in periventricular leukomalacia. Am J Obstet Gynecol 1997;177:406–11.

7. Yoon BH, Romero R, Yang SH, Jun JK, Kim IO, Choi JH, et al. Interleukin-6 concentrations in umbilical cord plasma are elevated in neonates with white matter lesions associated with periventricular leukomalacia. Am J Obstet Gynecol 1996;174:1433–40.

8. Lee SE, Park JS, Norwitz ER, Kim KW, Park HS, Jun JK. Measurement of placental alpha-microglobulin-1 in cervicovaginal discharge to diagnose rupture of membranes. Obstet Gynecol 2007;109:634–40.

9. Lockwood CJ, Wein R, Chien D, Ghidini A, Alvarez M, Berkowitz RL. Fetal membrane rupture is associated with the presence of insulin-like growth factor-binding protein-1 in vaginal secretions. Am J Obstet Gynecol 1994; 171:146–50.

10. Gaucherand P, Guibaud S, Awada A, Rudigoz RC. Comparative study of three amniotic fluid markers in premature rupture of membranes: fetal fibronectin, alpha-fetoprotein, diamino-oxydase. Acta Obstet Gynecol Scand 1995;74:118–21.

11. Chen FC, Dudenhausen JW. Comparison of two rapid strip tests based on IGFBP-1 and PAMG-1 for the detection of amniotic fluid. Am J Perinatol 2008;25:243–6.

12. Lee SM, Lee J, Seong HS, Lee SE, Park JS, Romero R, et al. The clinical significance of a positive Amnisure test in women with term labor with intact membranes. J Matern Fetal Neonatal Med 2009;22:305–10.

13. Prevention of early-onset group B streptococcal disease in newborns. ACOG Committee Opinion No. 279. American College of Obstetricians and Gynecologists. Obstet Gynecol 2002;100:1405–12.

14. Laudy JA, Tibboel D, Robben SG, de Krijger RR, de Ridder MA, Wladimiroff JW. Prenatal prediction of pulmonary hypoplasia: clinical, biometric, and Doppler velocity correlates. Pediatrics 2002;109:250–8.

15. Rizzo G, Capponi A, Angelini E, Mazzoleni A, Romanini C. Blood flow velocity waveforms from fetal peripheral pulmonary arteries in pregnancies with preterm premature rupture of the membranes: relationship with pulmonary hypoplasia. Ultrasound Obstet Gynecol 2000;15:98–103.

16. Sciscione AC, Manley JS, Pollock M, Maas B, Shlossman PA, Mulla W, et al. Intracervical fibrin sealants: a potential treatment for early preterm premature rupture of the membranes. Am J Obstet Gynecol 2001;184:368–73.

17. Quintero RA, Morales WJ, Bornick PW, Allen M, Garabelis N. Surgical treatment of spontaneous rupture of membranes: the amniograft--first experience. Am J Obstet Gynecol 2002;186:155–7.

18. O'Brien JM, Barton JR, Milligan DA. An aggressive interventional protocol for early midtrimester premature rupture of the membranes using gelatin sponge for cervical plugging. Am J Obstet Gynecol 2002;187:1143–6.

19. Devlieger R, Millar LK, Bryant-Greenwood G, Lewi L, Deprest JA. Fetal membrane healing after spontaneous and iatrogenic membrane rupture: a review of current evidence. Am J Obstet Gynecol 2006;195:1512–20.

20. Kovacevich GJ, Gaich SA, Lavin JP, Hopkins MP, Crane SS, Stewart J, et al. The prevalence of thromboembolic events among women with extended bed rest prescribed as part of the treatment for premature labor or preterm premature rupture of membranes. Am J Obstet Gynecol 2000; 182:1089–92.

21. Mercer BM, Miodovnik M, Thurnau GR, Goldenberg RL, Das AF, Ramsey RD, et al. Antibiotic therapy for reduction of infant morbidity after preterm premature rupture of the membranes. A randomized controlled trial. National Institute of Child Health and Human Development Maternal-Fetal Medicine Units Network. JAMA 1997;278:989–95.

22. Kenyon SL, Taylor DJ, Tarnow-Mordi W. Broad-spectrum antibiotics for preterm, prelabour rupture of fetal membranes: the ORACLE I randomised trial. ORACLE Collaborative Group [published erratum appears in Lancet 2001;358:156]. Lancet 2001;357:979–88.

23. Kenyon S, Pike K, Jones DR, Brocklehurst P, Marlow N, Salt A, et al. Childhood outcomes after prescription of antibiotics to pregnant women with preterm rupture of the membranes: 7-year follow-up of the ORACLE I trial. Lancet 2008;372:1310–8.

24. Lewis DF, Adair CD, Robichaux AG, Jaekle RK, Moore JA, Evans AT, et al. Antibiotic therapy in preterm premature rupture of membranes: Are seven days necessary? A preliminary, randomized clinical trial. Am J Obstet Gynecol 2003;188:1413–6; discussion 1416–7.

25. Segel SY, Miles AM, Clothier B, Parry S, Macones GA. Duration of antibiotic therapy after preterm premature rupture of fetal membranes. Am J Obstet Gynecol 2003;189:799–802.

26. Harding JE, Pang J, Knight DB, Liggins GC. Do antenatal corticosteroids help in the setting of preterm rupture of membranes? Am J Obstet Gynecol 2001;184:131–9.

27. Lewis DF, Brody K, Edwards MS, Brouillette RM, Burlison S, London SN. Preterm premature ruptured membranes: a randomized trial of steroids after treatment with antibiotics. Obstet Gynecol 1996;88:801–5.

28. Pattinson RC, Makin JD, Funk M, Delport SD, Macdonald AP, Norman K, et al. The use of dexamethasone in women with preterm premature rupture of membranes--a multicentre, double-blind, placebo-controlled, randomised trial. Dexiprom Study Group. S Afr Med J 1999;89:865–70.

29. Ludmir J, Bader T, Chen L, Lindenbaum C, Wong G. Poor perinatal outcome associated with retained cerclage in patients with premature rupture of membranes. Obstet Gynecol 1994;84:823–6.

30. Jenkins TM, Berghella V, Shlossman PA, McIntyre CJ, Maas BD, Pollock MA, et al. Timing of cerclage removal after preterm premature rupture of membranes: maternal and neonatal outcomes. Am J Obstet Gynecol 2000;183: 847–52.

31. McElrath TF, Norwitz ER, Lieberman ES, Heffner LJ. Perinatal outcome after preterm premature rupture of membranes with in situ cervical cerclage. Am J Obstet Gynecol 2002;187:1147–52.

32. Meis PJ, Klebanoff M, Thom E, Dombrowski MP, Sibai B, Moawad AH, et al. Prevention of recurrent preterm delivery by 17 alpha-hydroxyprogesterone caproate. National Institute of Child Health and Human Development Maternal-Fetal Medicine Units Network [published erratum appears in N Engl J Med 2003;349:1299]. N Engl J Med 2003;348:2379–85.

33. da Fonseca EB, Bittar RE, Carvalho MH, Zugaib M. Prophylactic administration of progesterone by vaginal suppository to reduce the incidence of spontaneous preterm birth in women at increased risk: a randomized placebo-controlled double-blind study. Am J Obstet Gynecol 2003;188:419–24.

34. O'Brien JM, Adair CD, Lewis DF, Hall DR, Defranco EA, Fusey S, et al. Progesterone vaginal gel for the reduction

of recurrent preterm birth: primary results from a randomized, double-blind, placebo-controlled trial. Ultrasound Obstet Gynecol 2007;30:687–96.

35. Spinnato JA 2nd, Freire S, Pinto e Silva JL, Rudge MV, Martins-Costa S, Koch MA, et al. Antioxidant supplement-

ation and premature rupture of the membranes: a planned secondary analysis. Am J Obstet Gynecol 2008;199:433. e1–433.e8.

Postterm Gestation

Susan M. Ramin

By definition, postterm pregnancy refers to a gestation that has extended to or beyond 42 weeks of gestation (ie, 294 days or estimated date of delivery plus 14 days). The incidence of postterm pregnancy is approximately 6%, and postterm pregnancy is associated with increased perinatal morbidity and mortality (1). Significant neonatal morbidity is related to oligohydramnios, meconium aspiration, macrosomia, and dysmaturity. Maternal complications include labor dystocia, cesarean delivery, perineal trauma, and postpartum hemorrhage.

The perinatal mortality rate (stillbirths plus early neonatal deaths) at greater than 42 weeks of gestation is twice that at term (4–7 deaths per 1,000 deliveries versus 2–3 deaths per 1,000 deliveries) and increases sixfold and higher at 43 weeks of gestation and beyond (2). Accurate pregnancy dating is critical. Although many cases of diagnosed postterm pregnancy are true prolongation of gestation beyond 294 days, the condition often is diagnosed in the setting of a poorly dated gestation.

Several risk factors are linked to postterm pregnancy. The most frequent cause of an apparently prolonged gestation is an error in dating. When postterm pregnancy truly exists, the cause usually is unknown. The most common identifiable risk factors for prolongation of pregnancy are primigravidity and prior postterm pregnancy. Other risk factors include male fetal gender, placental sulfatase deficiency, fetal anencephaly, and genetic predisposition.

Antenatal surveillance and induction of labor are two widely used strategies that theoretically may decrease the risk of an adverse fetal outcome; maternal risk factors for postterm pregnancy also should be considered (2). Despite the lack of evidence demonstrating a beneficial effect, antenatal fetal surveillance for postterm pregnancies has become a common practice on the basis of universal acceptance. It is reasonable to initiate antenatal surveillance of postterm pregnancies between 41 weeks (287 days or estimated delivery date plus 7 days) and 42 weeks (294 days or estimated delivery date plus 14 days) of gestation (2). Although no firm recommendations can be made based on the existing literature regarding the frequency of antenatal surveillance of postterm pregnancies, many practitioners use twice-weekly testing. Options for antenatal fetal surveillance include nonstress testing, biophysical profile or modified biophysical profile (nonstress test plus amniotic fluid volume estimation), contraction stress testing, and a combination of these modalities. No single form of antenatal fetal surveillance has been shown to be superior (3). Amniotic fluid volume assessment appears to be important. Regardless of the assessment modality, delivery should be effected in the presence of fetal compromise, oligohydramnios, or both. Amniotic fluid volume should be considered decreased if the amniotic fluid index is less than 5 cm or there is no vertical fluid pocket that is measurable and more than 2–3 cm in depth.

The data regarding sweeping of the membranes at term to reduce postterm pregnancy are conflicting; some study results indicate a benefit (4, 5), whereas others have found no difference in the incidence of postterm pregnancy (6). Results of a meta-analysis to assess the effects of membrane sweeping for inducing labor or preventing postterm pregnancy found that membrane sweeping was associated with a decreased frequency of pregnancy continuing beyond 41 weeks of gestation and 42 weeks of gestation (7).

Management of postterm pregnancy is controversial. Whether labor induction or expectant management results in an improved outcome is unclear because of insufficient data. In general, labor is induced in postterm pregnancies in which the cervix is favorable because of the low risk of failed induction and subsequent cesarean delivery. In postterm pregnancies with unfavorable cervices both expectant management with fetal surveillance and labor induction are associated with low complication rates and good perinatal outcomes (4–6). There does appear to be a slight advantage to labor induction using cervical-ripening preparations, when indicated, regardless of parity or method of induction.

In results of a meta-analysis of 19 trials of routine versus selective labor induction in postterm pregnancies, it was found that routine induction after 41 weeks of gestation was associated with a significantly lower rate of perinatal mortality (odds ratio, 0.2; 95% confidence interval, 0.06–0.7) and no increase in cesarean delivery rate (odds ratio, 1.02; 95% confidence interval, 0.75–1.38) (3). Routine induction of labor also had no effect on the instrumental delivery rate, use of analgesia, or incidence of fetal heart rate abnormality. The actual risk of stillbirth during the 41st week of gestation is estimated at 1.04–1.27 per 1,000 undelivered women, compared with 1.55–3.1 per 1,000 of those women at or beyond 42 weeks of gestation (8). These data suggest that routine labor induction at 41 weeks of gestation has fetal benefit without incurring the additional maternal risks of a higher rate of cesarean delivery (3, 9). Although this conclusion has not been universally accepted, if reliable dating establishes a gestational age of 41–42 weeks, induction of labor is an acceptable management strategy. Assessment of the cervix, pelvis, and fetal size and presentation should be done to determine if the patient is an eligible candidate for cervical ripening and induction of labor.

References

1. Martin JA, Hamilton BE, Sutton PD, Ventura SJ, Menacker F, Kimeyer S, et al. Births: final data for 2006. Natl Vital Stat Rep 2009;57(7):1–104.

2. Management of Postterm Pregnancy. ACOG Practice Bulletin No. 55. American College of Obstetricians and Gynecologists. Obstet Gynecol 2004;104:639–46.

3. Crowley P. Interventions for preventing or improving the outcome of delivery at or beyond term. Cochrane Database of Systematic Reviews 2006, Issue 4. Art. No.: CD000170. DOI: 10.1002/14651858.CD000170.pub2; 10.1002/14651858.CD000170.pub2.

4. Magann EF, Chauhan SP, Nevils BG, McNamara MF, Kinsella MJ, Morrison JC. Management of pregnancies beyond forty-one weeks' gestation with an unfavorable cervix. Am J Obstet Gynecol 1998;178:1279–87.

5. Magann EF, Chauhan SP, McNamara MF, Bass JD, Estes CM, Morrison JC. Membrane sweeping versus dinoprostone vaginal insert in the management of pregnancies beyond 41 weeks with an unfavorable cervix. J Perinatol 1999;19:88–91.

6. Wong SF, Hui SK, Choi H, Ho LC. Does sweeping of membranes beyond 40 weeks reduce the need for formal induction of labour? BJOG 2002;109:632–6.

7. Boulvain M, Stan CM, Irion O. Membrane sweeping for induction of labour. Cochrane Database of Systematic Reviews 2005, Issue 1. Art. No.: CD000451. DOI: 10.1002/14651858.CD000451.pub2; 10.1002/14651858.CD000451.pub2.

8. Menticoglou SM, Hall PF. Routine induction of labour at 41 weeks gestation: nonsensus consensus. BJOG 2002;109:485–91.

9. Rand L, Robinson JN, Economy KE, Norwitz ER. Post-term induction of labor revisited. Obstet Gynecol 2000;96:779–83.

Cardiac Disease

Steven L. Clark

Optimal care of a patient with cardiac disease in pregnancy is predicated on the health care providers' understanding of the physiologic changes of pregnancy, coupled with knowledge of the effects of pregnancy on the specific cardiac lesion. Care of patients with substantial cardiac disease often is best accomplished by a team approach, involving an obstetrician and specialists in maternal–fetal medicine, cardiology, and anesthesiology. A thorough history and physical examination at the initial prenatal visit, and careful follow-up of definitive or suspected cardiac disease uncovered at this time is essential in enabling such an approach.

The general categorizations of cardiac disease presented in Boxes 17 and 18 are useful first steps in considering general risk for pregnant cardiac patients, or those that are contemplating pregnancy (1). Patients in group I in Box 17 should, with appropriate care, have minimal risk of serious complications. In patients in group II in Box 17, the risk of adverse pregnancy outcome or significant illness is increased significantly despite optimal management. For most patients in group III in Box 17, there is an unacceptable risk of serious complications or death, even with optimal management. For such patients, avoiding or terminating pregnancy often is the treatment of choice. For specific patient counseling and planning of clinical care, a more detailed risk assessment system is useful. The most important risks apparently are the following factors (2):

- Prior congestive heart failure, stroke, or arrhythmia
- New York Heart Association functional class III or IV or clinical cyanosis
- Left ventricular outflow tract obstruction (mitral valve area less than 2 cm², aortic value area less than 1.5 cm², or peak flow gradient greater than 30 mm Hg)
- A baseline ejection fraction less than 40%

For each risk factor present, the patient is assigned a score of 1. In one large series, patients with a score of 0 had a 5% risk of major cardiac event during pregnancy, those with a score of 1 had a 27% risk of such an event, and those with a score of 2 or more had a 75% risk of a serious cardiac event (2). Most cardiac deaths will occur in patients in the latter category. Recent statistics and maternal mortality estimates suggest that with appropriate care in developed countries, maternal cardiac death

---

Box 17

Maternal Risk of Cardiac Disease Complications Associated with Pregnancy

Group I—Minimal Risk of Complications (Mortality Less Than 1%)

- Atrial septal defect*
- Ventricular septal defect*
- Patent ductus arteriosus*
- Pulmonic or tricuspid disease
- Corrected tetralogy of Fallot
- Bioprosthetic valve
- Mitral stenosis, New York Heart Association classes I and II
- Marfan syndrome with normal aorta

Group II—Moderate Risk of Complications (Mortality 5–15%)

- Mitral stenosis with atrial fibrillation†
- Artificial valve†
- Mitral stenosis, New York Heart Association classes III and IV
- Aortic stenosis
- Coarctation of aorta, uncomplicated
- Uncorrected tetralogy of Fallot
- Previous myocardial infarction

Group III—Major Risk of Complications or Death (Mortality Greater Than 25%)

- Pulmonary hypertension
- Coarctation of aorta, complicated
- Marfan syndrome with aortic involvement

*If unassociated with pulmonary hypertension

†If anticoagulation with heparin, rather than warfarin, is elected

Foley MR. Cardiac disease. In: Dildy GA 3d, Belfort MA, Svade GR, Phelan JP, Hankins GD, Clark SL, editors. Critical care obstetrics. 4th ed. Malden (MA): Wiley–Blackwell; 2004.

Box 18

New York Heart Association Classification of Cardiovascular Disease

- Class I—Patients who are not limited by cardiac disease in their physical activity. Ordinary physical activity does not precipitate the occurrence of symptoms, such as fatigue, palpitations, dyspnea, and angina.
- Class II—Patients in whom the cardiac disease causes a slight limitation in physical activity. These patients are comfortable at rest, but ordinary physical activity will precipitate symptoms.
- Class III—Patients in whom the cardiac disease results in a marked limitation of physical activity. They are comfortable at rest, but less than ordinary physical activity will precipitate symptoms.
- Class IV—Patients in whom the cardiac disease results in the inability to carry on physical activity without discomfort. Symptoms may be present even at rest, and discomfort is increased by any physical activity.

This box was published in Obstetric anesthesia, 2nd ed. Camann WR, Thornhill ML. Cardiovascular disease. Chestnut DH, editor. p. 776–808. Copyright Elsevier (1999).

---

generally is caused by pulmonary hypertension, endocarditis, ischemic cardiac disease, cardiomyopathy, and cardiac dysrhythmia (3–5).

Women with cardiac disease face four hemodynamic challenges during pregnancy, the first of which is the increased intravascular volume associated with pregnancy. This increase begins early and approaches 50% by the early third trimester. Thereafter, intravascular volume reaches a plateau. Patients with fixed cardiac output may be unable to tolerate such increases in intravascular volume, and pulmonary edema may result.

Second, patients experience a decline in systemic vascular resistance as pregnancy progresses. For some lesions, such as aortic stenosis, this decrease in cardiac afterload has the potential to improve cardiac function. However, the condition of patients with right-to-left shunts (such as ventricular–septal defect with Eisenmenger syndrome) may deteriorate because systemic vascular resistance decreases in the face of fixed and elevated pulmonary vascular resistance. This results in shunting of blood away from the lungs, desaturation, and clinical decompensation.

Third, the estrogen-induced hypercoagulability that is associated with pregnancy poses specific hazards for some patients with atrial fibrillation or mechanical cardiac valves. Such patients are prone to systemic thromboembolism, and this risk is increased during pregnancy. Both of these conditions may require full anticoagulation therapy. Unfortunately, pregnant women with mechanical cardiac devices retain a risk of embolism even with low molecular weight heparin therapy (6). For such patients, use of coumarin derivatives may be superior in preventing thromboembolism. Given the gravity of systemic (arterial) thromboembolism in pregnancy, therapy with warfarin may be considered despite the fetal risks incurred. With appropriate informed consent, options include the use of full anticoagulation therapy with low molecular weight heparin or low molecular weight heparin and aspirin for the duration of pregnancy or the substitution of warfarin during the middle trimester. The former approach eliminates any significant fetal risk but appears to incur an increased risk of maternal systemic thromboembolism; the latter will reduce but not eliminate fetal risk while decreasing maternal risk, at least during the middle trimester.

Finally, normal pregnancy is associated with marked fluctuations in cardiac output during labor, delivery, and the postpartum period. Patients with fixed cardiac output may be unable to tolerate such sudden shifts, and pulmonary edema may result.

With an appropriate understanding of these clinical issues, the obstetrician can be prepared, in consultation with maternal–fetal medicine, cardiology, and anesthesiology specialists, to develop a management scheme that minimizes the risk of complications. For example, with patients in whom increased preload may not be well tolerated, diuresis and heart rate control (in cases of mitral stenosis) may improve the chances for a successful pregnancy outcome. In a similar fashion, appropriate conduction anesthesia during labor, delivery, and even the immediate postpartum period may minimize cardiac output fluctuations and avoid pulmonary edema in patients whose cardiac lesions otherwise may not allow them to tolerate the fluid shifts associated with the delivery process.

Prophylaxis Against Subacute Bacterial Endocarditis

The most recent guidelines of the American Heart Association do not recommend endocarditis prophylaxis for any genitourinary procedures and recommend such prophylaxis only for select high-risk patients undergoing certain high-risk dental procedures (7). No class I or class II data exist to either support, or refute the application of these guidelines to vaginal or cesarean birth. Under these circumstances, a clinician would be within the standard of care to withhold prophylaxis from any woman undergoing delivery. A second appropriate option would be to restrict the use of such prophylaxis to patients with the highest risk, namely those with prosthetic heart valves, unrepaired cyanotic congenital heart disease, those with surgically constructed palliative shunts or conduits, and those within 6 months of repair of a congenital heart defect with prosthetic material and at any time for women with a repair that left a residual defect at or adjacent to the site of a prosthetic patch or device or women with cardiac valvulopathy after a cardiac transplant. The recommended treatment for patients without penicillin allergy is amoxicillin, 2 g, orally or ampicillin, 2 g, intravenously or intramuscularly, administered 30–60 minutes before delivery. Clindamycin use is the suggested alternative for patients who are allergic to penicillin (7).

Specific Maternal Conditions

Right-Sided Lesions

Right-sided structural cardiac lesions, when not associated with pulmonary hypertension, generally are tolerated well during pregnancy, labor, and delivery. Attention to appropriate fluid balance and the administration of oxygen are important management principles.

Left-Sided Lesions

Left-sided lesions are more complex than right-sided ones. In patients with mitral stenosis, control of heart rate with the use of β-blockers and, at times, judicious diuresis to avoid pulmonary edema are essential (1). Both of these treatments generally can be carried out without fear of adverse fetal effects. During labor and delivery in patients with severe mitral stenosis, pulmonary artery catheterization may sometimes be helpful in allowing the clinician to reduce preload through cautious diuresis while maintaining cardiac output. Patients undergoing delivery with pulmonary capillary wedge pressure levels exceeding 14–16 mm Hg or who have a mitral valve area of less than 2 cm^2 appear to have an increased likelihood of complications, including postpartum pulmonary edema (2, 8, 9).

In patients with aortic stenosis, particularly with an aortic valve area of less than 1.5 cm^2, the problem is somewhat different. In the presence of an intact mitral valve, pulmonary edema is uncommon. Rather, these patients are at risk of sudden hypotension, arrhythmia, and death should preload decrease. Thus, avoidance of hypovolemia or hypotension is essential. In addition, for patients with significant aortic stenosis, activity restriction during pregnancy is essential. Intrapartum fluid and blood component replacement should be geared to avoiding hypotension (1).

Patients with isolated mitral or aortic insufficiency generally tolerate labor and delivery without significant complication; again, careful attention to intake and output is essential. Most patients with significant cardiac disease will benefit from the intrapartum administration of oxygen and epidural anesthesia during labor.

Pulmonary Hypertension

Pulmonary hypertension, which remains one of the most dangerous complications of pregnancy, may be either primary or secondary to long-standing valvular lesions, such as mitral stenosis. Although patients with pulmonary hypertension may develop shortness of breath and cardiovascular decompensation during the antepartum period, the most critical time for these women is the peripartum and postpartum periods. During this time, any event that decreases cardiac preload, such as blood loss or, at times, conduction anesthesia, may dramatically and abruptly reduce pulmonary perfusion, resulting in desaturation and cardiovascular collapse. Thus, during labor in these patients, any decrease in cardiac preload must be scrupulously avoided and blood volume maintained, even at the risk of pulmonary edema. In severe cases, pulmonary artery catheterization may be of assistance in ensuring adequate cardiac output and intravascular volume. Such patients also may decompensate and develop intractable and ultimately fatal right heart failure in the postpartum period. Although the exact cause of this event is unknown, a rebound worsening of pulmonary hypertension associated with the loss of placental hormones is suspected. Many clinicians working with pregnant women have found the correlation between echocardiographic and invasive assessments of pulmonary artery pressures to be inconsistent, especially in mild–moderate cases. False-positive diagnoses of pulmonary hypertension may lead to inappropriate counseling and management. For this reason, many authorities would suggest a broader use of confirmatory right-heart catheterization for direct assessment of pulmonary artery pressures in pregnant women in whom pulmonary hypertension is suspected on echocardiography (10).

Ischemic Cardiac Disease

Ischemic cardiac disease carries a significant risk during pregnancy because of the increased oxygen demand on the heart (11). Thus, patients with a history of coronary artery cardiac disease should be counseled against pregnancy. If pregnancy is to be undertaken, bed rest often is essential to minimize myocardial oxygen demands as the fetus grows. The use of nitrates for angina is acceptable during pregnancy as well as the use of β-blocking agents. The prevalence of ischemic heart disease seems to be increasing possibly because more women are becoming pregnant at an older age.

Mitral Valve Prolapse

Mitral valve prolapse, a relatively common and generally benign syndrome, affects up to 17% of women of childbearing age. The diagnosis is suspected by auscultation of a systolic murmur and click and can be confirmed by echocardiography. Patients may develop troublesome palpitations, which are amenable to treatment with β-blocking agents.

Fetal Considerations

Patients with cyanotic heart disease or those with reduced cardiac output are at risk for intrauterine growth restriction and stillbirth. In such patients, delivery indicated for fetal rather than maternal deterioration is relatively common (12). Thus, serial ultrasonography to assess fetal growth and antepartum fetal heart rate assessment in the third trimester are important in any woman with cardiac disease complicated by maternal hypoxia or reduced cardiac output.

The risk of fetal cardiac defects is increased in women with congenital cardiac anomalies. This risk is on the order of 5% but may approach 10% or higher in women with congenital outflow tract obstruction. Thus, in any woman with congenital cardiac disease, fetal echocardiography is essential.

Peripartum Cardiomyopathy

Peripartum cardiomyopathy is defined as the development of cardiac failure with echocardiographic evidence of left ventricular dysfunction in the last month of pregnancy or within 5 months of delivery in the absence of both an identifiable cause of cardiac failure and recognizable cardiac disease before the final month of pregnancy (13). In practice, disregard of this definition often leads to overdiagnosis. Maternal mortality from peripartum cardiomyopathy approaches 20% (14). Treatment is nonspecific and may include inotropic support, diuresis, and afterload reduction in addition to delivery. In survivors, subclinical reductions in contractile reserve generally persist, increasing the maternal risk during future pregnancies (15, 16).

References

1. Foley MR. Cardiac disease. In: Dildy GA 3rd, Belfort MA, Saade GR, Phelan JP, Hankins GD, Clark SL, editors. Critical care obstetrics. 4th ed. Malden (MA): Blackwell Science; 2004. p. 252–74.

2. Siu SC, Sermer M, Colman JM, Alvarez AN, Mercier LA, Morton BC, et al. Prospective multicenter study of pregnancy outcomes in women with heart disease. Cardiac Disease in Pregnancy (CARPREG) Investigators. Circulation 2001;104:515–21.

3. Berg CJ, Atrash HK, Koonin LM, Tucker M. Pregnancy-related mortality in the United States, 1987-1990. Obstet Gynecol 1996;88:161–7.

4. de Swiet M. Maternal mortality: confidential enquiries into maternal deaths in the United Kingdom. Am J Obstet Gynecol 2000;182:760–6.

5. Clark SL, Belfort MA, Dildy GA, Herbst MA, Meyers JA, Hankins GD. Maternal death in the 21st century: causes, prevention, and relationship to cesarean delivery. Am J Obstet Gynecol 2008;199:36.e1–5; discussion 91–2.e7–11.

6. Curtis SL, Trinder J, Stuart AG. Acute thrombosis of a prosthetic mitral valve in pregnancy in spite of adjusted-dose low-molecular-weight heparin and aspirin. J Heart Valve Dis 2008;17:133–4.

7. Major changes in endocarditis prophylaxis for dental, GI and GU procedures [published erratum appears in Med Lett Drugs Ther 2007;49:104]. Med Lett Drugs Ther 2007;49:99–100.

8. Desai DK, Adanlawo M, Naidoo DP, Moodley J, Kleinschmidt I. Mitral stenosis in pregnancy: a four-year experience at King Edward VIII Hospital, Durban, South Africa. BJOG 2000;107:953–8.

9. Clark SL, Phelan JP, Greenspoon J, Aldahl D, Horenstein J. Labor and delivery in the presence of mitral stenosis: central hemodynamic observations. Am J Obstet Gynecol 1985;152:984–8.

10. Penning S, Robinson KD, Major CA, Garite TJ. A comparison of echocardiography and pulmonary artery catheterization for evaluation of pulmonary artery pressures in pregnant patients with suspected pulmonary hypertension. Am J Obstet Gynecol 2001;184:1568–70.

11. Roth A, Elkayam U. Acute myocardial infarction associated with pregnancy. Ann Intern Med 1996;125:751–62.

12. Patton DE, Lee W, Cotton DB, Miller J, Carpenter RJ Jr, Huhta J, et al. Cyanotic maternal heart disease in pregnancy. Obstet Gynecol Surv 1990;45:594–600.

13. Pearson GD, Veille JC, Rahimtoola S, Hsia J, Oakley CM, Hosenpud JD, et al. Peripartum cardiomyopathy: National Heart, Lung, and Blood Institute and Office of Rare Diseases (National Institutes of Health) workshop recommendations and review. JAMA 2000;283:1183–8.

14. Witlin AG, Mabie WC, Sibai BM. Peripartum cardiomyopathy: an ominous diagnosis. Am J Obstet Gynecol 1997; 176:182–8.

15. Lampert MB, Weinert L, Hibbard J, Korcarz C, Lindheimer M, Lang RM. Contractile reserve in patients with peripartum cardiomyopathy and recovered left ventricular function. Am J Obstet Gynecol 1997;176:189–95.

16. Chapa JB, Heiberger HB, Weinert L, Decara J, Lang RM, Hibbard JU. Prognostic value of echocardiography in peripartum cardiomyopathy. Obstet Gynecol 2005;105:1303–8.

Chronic Hypertension

Larry C. Gilstrap III

Chronic hypertension is preexisting hypertension or hypertension present before the 20th week of pregnancy. *Hypertension* is defined as a systolic blood pressure of 140 mm Hg or more, a diastolic blood pressure of 90 mm Hg or more, or both. Chronic hypertension is classified as mild (140 mm Hg/90 mm Hg or greater) or severe (180 mm Hg/110 mm Hg or greater) (1, 2). Preeclampsia superimposed on chronic hypertension is discussed in the section "Preeclampsia and Gestational Hypertension." Chronic hypertension appearing for the first time during pregnancy, especially after 20 weeks of gestation, can be difficult (if not impossible) to distinguish from preeclampsia or gestational hypertension. In some cases, the diagnosis cannot be confirmed until 12 weeks postpartum when there is persistent hypertension (1, 2).

Effects in Pregnancy

Chronic hypertension complicates up to 5% of all pregnancies and is associated with substantial adverse outcomes, including superimposed preeclampsia, preterm birth, fetal growth restriction, stillbirth, placental abruption, cesarean delivery, and perinatal morbidity and mortality (1). For example, the risks of adverse outcomes are far greater in the presence of superimposed preeclampsia, which occurs in approximately 25% or more of women with preexisting hypertension (3). Chronic hypertension is related to an increase in both preterm and term small for gestational age births (4). The cesarean delivery rate also is increased.

The women who have had chronic hypertension for several years are more likely to have cardiac hypertrophy, ischemic heart disease, renal dysfunction, and retinopathy. Evaluation before or during early pregnancy may include electrocardiography, an ophthalmologic examination, serum creatinine measurement, blood urea nitrogen analysis, 24-hour urine collection for total protein and creatinine clearance analysis, and other tests based on clinical suspicion (eg, echocardiography or renal ultrasonography). Most women will have primary essential hypertension. Secondary etiologies of hypertension (eg, pheochromocytoma, Cushing disease, and renal artery stenosis) should be considered as clinically appropriate and specific laboratory testing directed toward these causes as needed (1).

Treatment

The only compelling reason to treat women with chronic hypertension is to prevent catastrophic maternal cardiovascular complications. Thus, there appears to be little, if any, benefit to treat pregnant women with mild to moderate hypertension unless they have other complications, such as preexisting renal or cardiovascular disease (1). In two meta-analyses of antihypertensive therapy versus no therapy, not only was there no fetal benefit of therapy but also the incidence of fetal growth restriction was increased (5, 6). In a more recent third meta-analysis involving 46 trials and over 4,000 women, the authors concluded that the benefit of antihypertensive drug therapy for mild to moderate hypertension during pregnancy remained unclear (7).

It is recommended, however, that women with severe chronic hypertension be treated, although, as mentioned previously, the benefit to the fetus of such therapy is less than clear (1, 8, 9). Probably the two most commonly used antihypertensive agents to treat pregnant women are methyldopa and labetalol. Various antihypertensives, including alternatives to standard treatment are mentioned in Table 16. The angiotensin-converting enzyme (ACE) inhibitors and angiotensin II receptor blockers should be avoided during pregnancy because of

Table 16. Antihypertensive Therapy for Pregnant Women With Chronic Hypertension

Agent*	Dosage	Comments
Central sympatholytic agent: methyldopa	Oral: 250 mg at bedtime, increasing to twice daily or every 6 hours (maximum dose: 500 mg every 6 hours) IV: 250–500 mg every 6 hours	Drowsiness, dry mouth, nasal congestion, rebound hypertension, sedation, lethargy, dizziness, nausea, diarrhea, depression, sodium and water retention, and drug-induced hepatitis; excreted by kidneys, half-life is 1.8 hours.
Diuretic (thiazide): hydrochlorothiazide	Oral: 12.5 mg daily, increasing to 25 mg daily	Decreased levels of potassium sodium, magnesium, and zinc; increased levels of uric acid, glucose, calcium, and cholesterol and blood urea nitrogen to creatine ratio.
Diuretic (loop): furosemide	Oral: 20–40 mg daily, increasing to 160 mg twice daily IV: 40–80 mg (4 mg/min)	Monitor for fluid and increasing electrolyte imbalances. Increased glucose and uric acid levels; decreased potassium and magnesium levels. Patients allergic to sulfon amides may be allergic to furosemide. Dizziness, headache, gastrointestinal irritation, and hypotension may occur.
β-Adrenergic blocker: atenolol	Oral: 25 mg, increasing to 100 mg daily	Bradycardia, fatigue, nausea and vomiting, dizziness, and depression. May increase cholesterol level and rebound hypertension. Not for use in patients with diabetes mellitus, hyperthyroidism, or intermittent claudication. Associated with fetal growth restriction.
α-Adrenergic blocker and β-adrenergic blocker: labetalol	Oral: 100 mg, two or three times daily for a maximum dose of 1,200 mg daily IV: 20 mg over 10 min (maximum dose: 2 mg/min infusion)	Gastrointestinal distress, fluid retention, dry mouth, and orthostatic hypotension; half-life is 5.8 hours, excreted by kidneys (55–60%) and in feces 30%).
Calcium channel blocker: felodipine	Oral: 5–10 mg daily, increasing to 10 mg twice daily	99% bound to plasma proteins. Hepatic metabolism and reflex increase in heart rate; selective effects on vascular smooth muscle are much greater than those on cardiac muscle. Peripheral edema, and headache.
Calcium channel blocker: nifedipine	30–90 mg daily as a sustained release tablet, increasing to a maximum dose of 120 mg daily at 7–14 day intervals	

Abbreviation: IV indicates intravenous.

*All medications are U.S. Food and Drug Administration pregnancy category C, except hydrochlorothiazide (category D). Angiotensin-converting enzyme inhibitors are contraindicated in pregnancy because of the risk of fetal effects starting in the second trimester. Pregnancy interruption is not advised when exposure has occurred in the early first trimester.

the potential for both teratogenic effects and subsequent fetal and neonatal effects from their use (1, 2). Use of beta-blockers may be associated with fetal growth restriction (1, 10). The treatment of superimposed preeclampsia in women with chronic hypertension is the same as that for preeclampsia (see the section "Preeclampsia and Gestational Hypertension").

References

1. Chronic hypertension in pregnancy. ACOG Practice Bulletin No. 29. American College of Obstetricians and Gynecologists. Obstet Gynecol 2001;98:177–85.

2. Report of the National High Blood Pressure Education Program Working Group on High Blood Pressure in Pregnancy. Am J Obstet Gynecol 2000;183:S1–S22.

3. Sibai BM, Lindheimer M, Hauth J, Caritis S, VanDorsten P, Klebanoff M, et al. Risk factors for preeclampsia, abruptio placentae, and adverse neonatal outcomes among women with chronic hypertension. National Institute of Child Health and Human Development Network of Maternal-Fetal Medicine Units. N Engl J Med 1998;339:667–71.

4. Catov JM, Nohr EA, Olsen J, Ness RB. Chronic hypertension related to risk for preterm and term small for gestational age births. Obstet Gynecol 2008;112:290–6.

5. von Dadelszen P, Ornstein MP, Bull SB, Logan AG, Koren G, Magee LA. Fall in mean arterial pressure and fetal growth restriction in pregnancy hypertension: a meta-analysis. Lancet 2000;355:87–92.

6. Magee LA, Ornstein MP, von Dadelszen P. Fortnightly review: management of hypertension in pregnancy. BMJ 1999;318:1332–6.

7. Abalos E, Duley L, Steyn DW, Henderson-Smart DJ. Antihypertensive drug therapy for mild to moderate hypertension during pregnancy. Cochrane Database of Systematic Reviews 2007, Issue 1. Art. No.: CD002252. DOI: 10.1002/14651858.CD002252.pub2; 10.1002/14651858.CD002252.pub2.

8. Sibai BM. Chronic hypertension in pregnancy. Obstet Gynecol 2002;100:369–77.

9. Roberts JM, Pearson GD, Cutler JA, Lindheimer MD. Summary of the NHLBI Working Group on Research on Hypertension During Pregnancy. National Heart Lung and Blood Institute. Hypertens Pregnancy 2003;22:109–27.

10. Bayliss H, Churchill D, Beevers M, Beevers DG. Antihypertensive drugs in pregnancy and fetal growth: evidence for "pharmacological programming" in the first trimester? Hypertens Pregnancy 2002;21:161–74.

Obesity

Judette M. Louis and Patrick M. Catalano

The prevalence of obesity has increased substantially over the recent years and has reached epidemic proportions in industrialized nations (1). The body mass index (BMI), calculated as weight in kilograms divided by height in meters squared, is used to define obesity. Body mass index provides a reliable estimate of body fat and its associated health risk. Individuals are categorized based on the value of their BMI (Table 17). Individuals with a BMI of 25–29.9 are overweight and those with a BMI of 30 or greater are considered obese (2). Overweight and obese individuals are at increased risk of many diseases and health conditions:

- Hypertension
- Dyslipidemia
- Type 2 diabetes mellitus
- Coronary heart disease
- Cerebrovascular disease
- Gallbladder disease
- Osteoarthritis
- Sleep apnea and respiratory problems
- Some types of cancer (endometrial, breast, and colon)

The Centers for Disease Control and Prevention estimates that 66% of U.S. adults are overweight and 30% meet the criteria for obesity. The overall prevalence is substantially greater among ethnic minority groups. The prevalence of obesity increases with age. With the recent trend of a delay in childbearing, more reproductive-aged women are obese. The practicing obstetrician–gynecologist faces numerous challenges in the pregnancy management of these patients. Comorbid conditions, limited information about certain diseases, and technical difficulties challenge the traditional paradigm for management.

In this section we will discuss the comorbid conditions associated with obesity, how obesity affects routine pregnancy management, and pertinent areas for intervention and patient counseling.

Comorbid Conditions

Hypertension

Hypertensive disease in pregnancy is a leading cause of maternal morbidity and mortality. It is associated with adverse pregnancy outcome including indicated preterm delivery, placental abruption, intrauterine fetal demise, intrauterine growth restriction, and perinatal mortality. Obesity is a risk factor for both chronic hypertension and pregnancy-related hypertensive diseases, such as preeclampsia. Results from population-based studies indicate that even after excluding cases with diabetes mellitus or chronic hypertension, obese women had a twofold to threefold increased risk compared with women of normal weight of developing preeclampsia.

Table 17. Body Mass Index Category Classification

Weight category	Body Mass Index*
Underweight	Less than 18.5
Normal weight	18.5–24.9
Overweight	25–29.9
Obesity	30 and greater

*A body mass index is expressed as weight in kilograms divided by height in meters squared.

Data from Rasmussen KM, Yaktine AL, editors. Weight gain during pregnancy: reexamining the guidelines. Institute of Medicine. Washington, DC: National Academies Press; 2009.

The odds increase with increasing obesity severity (3). The cause of this association is unclear but one postulated mechanism is the relationship between insulin resistance, hyperinsulinemia, and endothelial dysfunction, which is known to play a role in preeclampsia.

Gestational and Preexisting Diabetes Mellitus

Although type 1 diabetes mellitus can be observed in obese women, obesity during pregnancy usually is complicated by type 2 diabetes mellitus and gestational diabetes mellitus. Type 2 diabetes mellitus results from increased insulin resistance and inadequate beta cell response. The increased insulin resistance of normal pregnancy also is a factor in the development of gestational diabetes mellitus. Gestational diabetes mellitus is characterized by an increased insulin resistance and inadequate response to insulin. Obesity is a significant risk factor for increased insulin resistance, and the risk increases with the severity of obesity. This pattern also is observed for the risk of gestational diabetes mellitus. In an analysis of data from a large prospective trial, the odds of developing gestational diabetes mellitus were 2.6 in obese women and 4 for morbidly obese women compared with women of normal weight (4). The fetal risks associated with diabetes mellitus in pregnancy have been well described. They include an increased risk of miscarriage and congenital anomalies, predominately cardiac and neural tube defects (5).

Obese women should be considered candidates for early testing for gestational diabetes mellitus or undiagnosed type 2 diabetes mellitus. This testing can be completed with their initial evaluation rather than waiting until the late second trimester. Other patients at increased risk for gestational diabetes mellitus are women with previous gestational diabetes mellitus, history of fetal macrosomia, or a maternal family history of type 2 diabetes mellitus. It is important to recommend a 75-g 2-hour oral glucose tolerance test at the 6-week postpartum visit for women with gestational diabetes mellitus. There is an increased risk of type 2 diabetes mellitus in women with gestational diabetes mellitus, particularly if they are obese.

Obstructive Sleep Apnea

Obstructive sleep apnea is a disorder characterized by the cessation of air movement and breathing during sleep (6). The prevalence has increased over recent years. This is in part attributed to better recognition and diagnosis by physicians. However, the significant increase in the prevalence of obesity also has played a role. The recognized risk factors for this condition include obesity, increased age, and obesity-related comorbid conditions, such as chronic hypertension and diabetes mellitus (6). The increasing prevalence of obesity and the delay of childbearing age translate into a potential increase in the number of women with the condition complicating pregnancy. In the general population, obstructive sleep apnea is associated with increased daytime sleepiness, decreased effectiveness at work, and increased motor vehicle accidents. Long-term complications include cardiovascular disease and mortality (6).

Obstructive sleep apnea in pregnancy is not well studied. Most published studies have been limited to case reports. Recently, results from a small prospective observational study indicated that women with obstructive sleep apnea had neonates that were on average smaller and more likely to require a neonatal intensive care than those of women who did not have obstructive sleep apnea (7). This is consistent with the published case reports that have implicated obstructive sleep apnea as a contributing factor to preeclampsia and fetal growth restriction. Insulin resistance is more prevalent in people with sleep apnea than in those who do not have obstructive sleep apnea even after controlling for obesity. The role that this may play in pregnancy-related complications has yet to be determined. It is hypothesized that insulin resistance and its role in endothelial dysfunction may contribute substantially to the association of preeclampsia and fetal growth restriction in women with sleep apnea.

There are no standard recommendations for the treatment of an individual with obstructive sleep apnea during pregnancy. The treatment recommendations are an extrapolation from the general population. Women who have obstructive sleep apnea and are attempting pregnancy should be aware that weight loss before pregnancy improves many cases of obstructive sleep apnea and also would decrease pregnancy risks. This may be the most prudent intervention. Management of obstructive sleep apnea during the antepartum period should include evaluation by a pulmonary medicine specialist and readjustment of their continuous positive airway pressure or bilevel positive airway pressure machine to optimize treatment. Results from small studies indicate an improvement of apnea and hypopnea postpartum, perhaps suggesting that pregnancy and the associated weight gain may worsen obstructive sleep apnea (6).

Although there are no published data regarding intrapartum risk to obese patients, obesity may contribute to a decreased success rate of regional anesthesia. Antenatal consultation with an anesthesiologist may help optimize their intrapartum care. If general anesthesia is necessitated, studies in the general population indicate that the presence of obstructive sleep apnea further increases anesthesia related morbidity (8). Therefore, the following considerations may optimize care in the woman with obstructive sleep apnea:

- Early consultation with an anesthesiologist and a sleep disorder specialist
- Potential early placement of regional anesthesia

- Early evaluation of the airway in preparation for a potential emergency
- Adherence to an aspiration prevention protocol

For additional information on sleep apnea, see the section "Sleep Disorders" in *Precis: Primary and Preventive Care*, Fourth edition.

Bariatric Surgery

Increasingly, obstetricians will encounter patients desiring pregnancy who have undergone bariatric surgery, usually either gastric restriction (eg, gastric banding) or gastric bypass procedures. These procedures generally are indicated when a patient's BMI exceeds 40 or her BMI is greater than 35 and she has coexistent serious medical problems (eg, obstructive sleep apnea) that would resolve or improve with weight loss. Although bariatric surgery can be highly beneficial and even lifesaving, it may increase the risk of iron deficiency and megaloblastic anemias (B_{12} and folate deficiencies) and, by decreasing preconceptional folate absorption, may increase the risk of neural tube defects. Women with malabsorption and dumping syndromes are at the highest risk of having nutrient deficiencies and inadequate caloric intake, and may experience metabolic abnormalities, such as ketosis caused by starvation that produces rapid weight loss. Whenever possible, pregnancy should be postponed until weight loss is complete and the patient's weight has stabilized (at least 12–24 months [9]); this requires active contraception because women who were formally infertile because of obesity often become fertile as their weight normalizes. Iron, folate, and vitamin D and vitamin B_{12} supplementation should be provided, and consultation with a nutritionist may help assure adequate protein and calorie intake. Serial ultrasound scans to monitor fetal growth may be indicated.

A meta-analysis of matched cohort studies showed lower maternal complication rates in patients who underwent bariatric surgery than in obese women who did not undergo bariatric surgery (10). In results of one such study, maternal complication rates were lower in women who underwent laparoscopic adjustable gastric band surgery than in obese women who did not undergo this surgery, including the rates of gestational diabetes mellitus (0% versus 22.1%, $P<.05$, respectively) and preeclampsia (0% versus 3.1%, $P<.05$, respectively.) Among results of 13 bariatric cohort studies, neonatal outcomes were similar or better in women who underwent surgery compared with obese women who did not undergo surgery (7.1% versus 7.7% for premature delivery, $P<.05$; 7.7% versus 10.6% for low birth weight, $P<.05$; and 7.7% versus 14.6% for macrosomia, $P<.05$).

Surgical complications in pregnancy after bariatric surgery are uncommon. The data are limited to case reports. Of the 20 reported cases, the most common maternal complication was bowel obstruction. Other reported complications included gastric ulcer perforation, intragastric band migration, and gastrointestinal migration (10). It is important to note that all these patients had symptoms, of nonspecific abdominal pain and many of the patients had a delay before intervention. Although there is likely a reporting bias, the lessons from these cases stress the importance of thorough evaluation of the pregnant patient who has had a gastric bypass. The American College of Obstetricians and Gynecologists (the College) recommends a high index of suspicion for gastrointestinal complications when pregnant women who have had such surgery present with abdominal symptoms (9). In summary, for women who have undergone bariatric surgery, the College has issued the following recommendations:

- Women should delay pregnancy for 12–24 months.
- Women with a lap band should be monitored by their obstetrician and surgeon, but removal or adjustment is not necessary and may result in excessive weight gain.
- All women should have adequate supplementation with folate, calcium, vitamin D, and vitamin B_{12}.

Nonalcoholic Fatty Liver Disease

Nonalcoholic fatty liver disease is a term used to categorize a spectrum of diseases that are marked by fatty infiltration of the liver. It ranges in severity from mild to severe and has been described as one of the most common causes of incidentally detected liver enzyme elevation (11). The mild form is simple steatosis; the moderate is nonalcoholic steatohepatitis, which is fatty infiltration with inflammation; and the most severe form is cirrhosis that can progress to liver failure or hepatocellular carcinoma. Although described in the 1980s, there remains limited information about the treatment of this condition. It is a condition associated with obesity but risk is not completely predicted by BMI. It is more closely related to insulin resistance, with type 2 diabetes mellitus and hyperlipidemia being two additional major risk factors (11).

There is limited information about nonalcoholic fatty liver disease and pregnancy. The area for concern for the obstetrician is that one third of these women will have elevated liver transaminase levels. If the abnormal levels are not diagnosed before pregnancy, they can pose difficulty when the abnormal transaminase levels cloud the diagnosis of preeclampsia. Additionally, although nonalcoholic fatty liver disease is a subclinical disease in its early stages, progression to nonalcoholic steatohepatitis may be associated with right upper quadrant pain. In the evaluation of obese women with abdominal pain, steatohepatitis should be considered. The association with insulin resistance places these women at high risk of gestational diabetes mellitus or preexisting diabetes mellitus. Early testing with liver function tests for detection should be considered.

Antepartum Management

Office Evaluation

In order to appropriately manage pregnancy in overweight and obese women, the clinician must first identify the individual. A medical history should include elucidation of obesity related conditions. Height and weight measurements and calculation of the BMI should be included in the physical examination.

Technical challenges may exist in the office setting for obese patients. Various adaptations of the office environment may facilitate their care. These include wide examination tables that are preferably bolted to the floor to avoid tipping, extra-large examination gowns, and large speculums. The appropriate blood pressure cuff size should be used by the guidelines of the American Heart Association. If a patient has an arm circumference greater than 41 cm, a thigh cuff should be used to avoid overestimation of blood pressure. Other supplies that may be helpful are long phlebotomy needles and tourniquets as well as scales with adequate capacity for the obese patient and stadiometers for accurate height measurement.

Weight Gain During Pregnancy

Generally, there is an inverse relationship between pregravid BMI and weight gain during pregnancy. Women who are obese before pregnancy do not gain as much weight as women with normal weight, but they have greater postpartum weight retention (12). The weight gain is compounded over time by multiple pregnancies. This accumulation results in increased prepregnancy weight and the associated risks for each subsequent pregnancy. Increasing the weight by just 1–2 BMI units is associated with an increased risk of gestational diabetes mellitus, chronic diabetes mellitus, and hypertensive disorders (12). Additionally, they have an increased likelihood of worsening obesity throughout their adult life.

Given the increased prevalence in obesity and our improved understanding of pregnancy related weight gain, the recommendations for pregnancy weight gain were revised in May 2009. They take into account the prepregnancy BMI according to the Institute of Medicine guidelines. These guidelines suggest a weight gain of 11.5–16 kg (25–35 lb) for women of normal weight, 7–11.5 kg (15–25 lb) for overweight women, and 5–9 kg (11–20 lb) for obese women (2).

Obese women should be offered a consultation with a nutritionist to aid them in achieving their goal. In addition to a proper diet, the College recommends exercise during pregnancy, if there are no contraindications. The recommendation is for a cumulative 30 minutes of exercise at a moderate level most if not all days of the week (13). It is recommended for all women, especially those who are obese and severely obese. The use of diets in the attempt of weight loss during pregnancy is not recommended but it is a reasonable intervention postpartum when the woman has completed breastfeeding. Staying within the Institute of Medicine recommendations for weight gain will help avoid postpartum weight retention. Additional adjuncts would be the encouragement of breastfeeding and counseling (14).

Intrapartum Management

In addition to the comorbid conditions associated with pregnancy in obese women, there are other complications to consider during the intrapartum period. External fetal heart rate and uterine contraction monitoring may be difficult secondary to maternal obesity. If there is an inability to monitor adequately, precautions should be in place to determine how to best proceed when oxytocin augmentation or induction is being used. Without adequate monitoring, there is the risk of inadequate fetal assessment or uterine tachysystole. These challenges have led to the implementation of strategies to counter them. They may be the increased use of more sensitive external monitors that improve signal transduction in obese women. In an attempt to improve monitoring, there may be an increased use of early amniotomy and use of fetal scalp electrodes and intrauterine pressure catheters. This strategy is associated with an increase in the already high rates of puerperal infection.

Operative Considerations

After controlling for comorbid conditions, obese women are more likely to require induction of labor and more likely to require cesarean delivery (15). This puts them at increased risk for surgical morbidity and mortality. In the general population, cesarean deliveries are associated with an increased risk for hemorrhage, infectious morbidity, and future pregnancy complications. That risk is further increased by obesity. Furthermore, the rate of cesarean delivery related complications is significantly greater with increasing obesity (3). The highest risk is among women with morbid obesity. They have significantly increased rates of wound infection (odds ratio [OR], 4.79), venous thromboembolism (OR, 4.13), and anesthesia complications (OR, 2.01) (3).

Anesthesia considerations include the possibility that it may be difficult to place a regional anesthesia. Anatomic distortion leads to a higher rate of epidural failure in obese women compared with women of normal weight. In these same obese patients, intubation may be difficult because of neck circumference or a high Mallampati scores (8). Obese parturients also have an increased risk of failed intubation and are prone to rapid desaturation (8). Coordination of care with an anesthesiologist is necessary. When making the choice of which anesthesia technique to use, the physician must take into consideration maternal size, the number of prior cesarean deliveries, and the expected duration of the case. Where a difficult or prolonged case is anticipated, an epidural technique may be more beneficial than a spinal technique and may avoid the need to convert to general anesthesia. Early placement of labor epidurals also may help prevent the need for general anesthesia. However, there also is a higher rate of epidural failure among obese patients. Therefore, this strategy is not always effective. Early communication between the obstetrician, anesthesiologist, and key members of the labor and delivery team may be effective in devising a management plan for the patient.

Obesity is identified as one of the factors that contribute to the risk of preventable surgical errors. Studies have indicated obesity and emergent situations as another risk factor (17). This confers a significant danger for the obese obstetric patient. Potential interventions include a systematic count to decrease the risk of retained instruments. It becomes even more prudent in the presence of any complications or unexpected procedures because these situations further increase the risk of retained sponges or instruments. For patients in the highest class of obesity, other considerations include appropriate instrument size and having a table that can accommodate the patient's size (17).

Postpartum infectious morbidity risk has been shown to decrease by 25% with the administration of prophylactic antibiotics at the time of cesarean delivery (16). Although most hospitals have it as a standard procedure, it may prove even more efficacious for the obese pregnant patient. Additional interventions to decrease wound complications include suture closure of the subcutaneous tissue if there is a depth of 2 cm or greater (OR, 0.44; 95% confidence interval [CI], 0.26–0.74). Similar reductions were obtained by closure of the subcutaneous drain (16). Both of those strategies have not been beneficial in the normal weight patient but have demonstrated benefit in the obese patient with a subcutaneous fat thickness of 2 cm or greater. Additional postpartum risk in the form of venous thromboembolism also is increased in the obese patient. Although there are some data for the effectiveness of using sequential compression devices, prophylactic heparin, or both in the high-risk patients in the general population, there is inconsistent data to indicate that this is effective in obese pregnant women. Morbidly obese patients should be counseled about those risks.

Fetal Risks of Obesity

In addition to maternal morbidity, obesity confers both short-term and long-term risks for the fetus. Results of large population-based studies have indicated an increased risk of congenital heart defects (OR, 1.18; 95% CI, 1.09–1.27), omphalocele (OR, 3.3; 95% CI, 1–10.3), and neural tube defects (OR, 1.8; 95% CI, 1.1–3) among infants of obese women. Results of subsequent studies examining the etiology have indicated that this may be independent of the presence of diabetes mellitus and fortification of cereal with folic acid (15).

The higher rates of congenital malformations are compounded by the difficulty in ultrasound assessment in this group of women. In a large study of more than 11,000 women, obese women had a nonvisualization rate that was twice the rate of nonobese women (37.3% versus 18.7%). Therefore, there is an increased likelihood that a malformation will be missed. The difficulty of visualization is particularly noted for heart, umbilical cord, and spine, which are areas of reported increased malformation risk in obese women (18). Techniques to improve visualization include the use of transvaginal ultrasonography and more advanced equipment with optimal setting for tissue penetration. The limitations of ultrasonography should be conveyed to patients.

Although results of initial studies were controversial, results from recently published large studies indicate that obese women have lower rates of spontaneous preterm delivery. This may not hold true for indicated preterm birth. Obese women have more comorbid conditions and higher rates of hypertensive disease, which may increase the risk of necessitating delivery prematurely for maternal or fetal indications in a subset of this group (3).

Long-term fetal risks also have been described. The offspring of obese women have a twofold-increased risk of childhood obesity and early-onset metabolic syndrome. This risk appears to be independent of maternal diabetes mellitus or neonatal birth weight (15).

Maternal obesity is an established risk factor for excessive fetal growth. Excessive fetal growth can be described by two terms in the obstetric literature: 1) large for gestational age and 2) fetal macrosomia. *Large for gestational age* describes a fetus whose estimated weight has met or exceeded the 90th percentile on various growth curves, adjusting for gestational age, gender, and race. *Macrosomia* is more of an absolute term used to indicate a suspected fetal weight of 4,000 g or greater, regardless of gestational age. The predominant maternal risk is cesarean delivery secondary to labor abnormalities (19). The major risk for vaginal delivery is shoulder dystocia (see the section "Shoulder Dystocia").

Postpartum Management and Future Preconception Counseling

Weight loss interventions may be directed during the postpartum visit. After delivery, it is appropriate to refer these patients for weight management. However, this may pose a challenge for the health care provider because a substantial proportion of women do not show up for a postpartum visit. An appropriate approach is education, evaluation of the patient's readiness, and suggestions for interventions (14).

In order to minimize maternal and neonatal morbidity, obese women should be encouraged to lose weight before attempting a future pregnancy and aim to achieve a BMI in the normal range (14). The success of any weight loss program will be dependent on patient readiness.

Further preconception counseling should focus on the associated risks. Recommendations for obese women who are pregnant or planning a pregnancy include the following items:

- Preconception counseling for issues discussed in this chapter with an emphasis on preconception weight loss

- Provision of specific information concerning the maternal and fetal risks of obesity in pregnancy and nutrition counseling at the first prenatal visit

- Potential screening for gestational diabetes mellitus in the first trimester and repeated screening later in pregnancy, if results are initially negative

- Potential vitamin B_{12}, folate, iron, vitamin D, and calcium supplementation for women who have undergone bariatric surgery

- Possible use of graduated compression stockings and early mobilization during and after cesarean delivery

- Antenatal consultation with an anesthesiologist

- Continuation of nutrition counseling and exercise program after delivery and consultation with weight loss specialists before attempting another pregnancy

References

1. Katz DL, O'Connell M, Yeh MC, Nawaz H, Njike V, Anderson LM, et al. Public health strategies for preventing and controlling overweight and obesity in school and worksite settings: a report on recommendations of the Task Force on Community Preventive Services. Task Force on Community Preventive Services. MMWR Recomm Rep 2005;54:1–12.

2. Rasmussen KM, Yaktine AL, editors. Weight gain during pregnancy : reexamining the guidelines. Institute of medicine. Washington, DC: National Academies Press; 2009.

3. Ramachenderan J, Bradford J, McLean M. Maternal obesity and pregnancy complications: a review. Aust N Z J Obstet Gynaecol 2008;48:228–35.

4. Catalano PM. Management of obesity in pregnancy. Obstet Gynecol 2007;109:419–33.

5. Pregestational diabetes mellitus. ACOG Practice Bulletin No. 60. American College of Obstetricians and Gynecologists. Obstet Gynecol 2005;105:675–85.

6. Pien GW, Schwab RJ. Sleep disorders during pregnancy. Sleep 2004;27:1405–17.

7. Sahin FK, Koken G, Cosar E, Saylan F, Fidan F, Yilmazer M, et al. Obstructive sleep apnea in pregnancy and fetal outcome. Int J Gynaecol Obstet 2008;100:141–6.

8. Soens MA, Birnbach DJ, Ranasinghe JS, van Zundert A. Obstetric anesthesia for the obese and morbidly obese patient: an ounce of prevention is worth more than a pound of treatment. Acta Anaesthesiol Scand 2008;52:6–19.

9. Bariatric surgery and pregnancy. ACOG Practice Bulletin No. 105. American College of Obstetricians and Gynecologists. Obstet Gynecol 2009;113:1405–13.

10. Maggard MA, Yermilov I, Li Z, Maglione M, Newberry S, Suttorp M, et al. Pregnancy and fertility following bariatric surgery: a systematic review. JAMA 2008;300:2286–96.

11. Kim CH, Younossi ZM. Nonalcoholic fatty liver disease: a manifestation of the metabolic syndrome. Cleve Clin J Med 2008;75:721–8.

12. Cox JT, Phelan ST. Nutrition during pregnancy. Obstet Gynecol Clin North Am 2008;35:369–83, viii.

13. Exercise during pregnancy and the postpartum period. ACOG Committee Opinion No. 267. American College of Obstetricians and Gynecologists. Obstet Gynecol 2002;99:171–3.

14. Obesity in pregnancy. ACOG Committee Opinion No. 315. American College of Obstetricians and Gynecologists. Obstet Gynecol 2005;106:671–5.

15. Catalano PM, Ehrenberg HM. The short- and long-term implications of maternal obesity on the mother and her offspring. BJOG 2006;113:1126–33.

16. Berghella V, Baxter JK, Chauhan SP. Evidence-based surgery for cesarean delivery. Am J Obstet Gynecol 2005;193:1607–17.

17. Patient safety in the surgical environment. ACOG Committee Opinion No. 328. American College of Obstetricians and Gynecologists. Obstet Gynecol 2006;107:429–33.

18. Hendler I, Blackwell SC, Treadwell MC, Bujold E, Sokol RJ, Sorokin Y. Does advanced ultrasound equipment improve the adequacy of ultrasound visualization of fetal cardiac structures in the obese gravid woman? Am J Obstet Gynecol 2004;190:1616–9; discussion 1619–20.

19. Shoulder dystocia. ACOG Practice Bulletin No. 40. American College of Obstetricians and Gynecologists. Obstet Gynecol 2002;100:1045–50.

Deep Vein Thrombosis and Pulmonary Embolism

J. Gerald Quirk

Thromboembolism is a leading cause of maternal mortality and occurs 4–5 times more frequently in pregnancy and the puerperium compared with the nonpregnant state for reproductive-aged women (1). Deep vein thrombosis (DVT) complicates pregnancy and the puerperium in 1.72 per 1,000 women (2). It is diagnosed with equal frequency in each of the trimesters of pregnancy; in 45–60% of cases it is diagnosed in the puerperium (3).

Pregnancy-associated changes in hemostatic and fibrinolytic proteins promote thromboembolism. Pregnancy is associated with a 20–200% increase in levels of fibrinogen, prothrombin (factor II), and clotting factors VII, VIII, X, and XII (4). Levels of von Willebrand factor may increase up to 400% by term. Additionally, prothrombin and factor V levels remain unchanged and levels of factors XIII and XI decrease somewhat. These changes result in an overall increase in thrombin-generating potential. In contrast, levels of the endogenous anticoagulant protein S decrease substantially during pregnancy, reaching a nadir, whereas concentrations of the antifibrinolytic type 1 plasminogen activator inhibitor increase by up to threefold. These hemostatic alterations likely reduce the risk of antepartum, intrapartum, and postpartum hemorrhage, but their net effect is to promote clot formation, extension, and stability, thus contributing substantially to the 10-fold increase in pregnancy-associated vein thrombosis. The risk of vein thrombosis is increased further in pregnant women with antiphospholipid syndrome or inherited thrombophilias (5, 6).

Antiphospholipid Syndrome

Antiphospholipid syndrome is the most common acquired thrombophilia and accounts for 14% (2–20%) of vein thrombosis in pregnancy. The combination of venous thromboembolism, specific obstetric complications, and the presence of significant antiphospholipid antibodies defines antiphospholipid syndrome (5, 6). By definition, antiphospholipid antibody-related thrombosis can occur in any tissue or organ. Additionally, antiphospholipid syndrome is associated with thrombocytopenia and recurrent fetal loss.

The most commonly encountered forms of antiphospholipid syndrome antibodies are isolated lupus anticoagulant antibodies and anticardiolipin antibodies. For a diagnosis of antiphospholipid syndrome, the patient must meet one of two clinical criteria and at least one of two laboratory criteria (Box 19). None of the many other clinical manifestations of the disorder need be present. Although other antiphospholipid antibodies may be present, their clinical significance (other than those directed against anticardiolipin immunoglobulin G and immunoglobulin M) remains unclear.

Inherited Thrombophilias

The inherited forms of thrombophilia include a wide variety of relatively common genetic conditions that predispose women to DVT (Table 18). They also have been implicated in fetal loss, especially stillbirth and abruption.

Inherited thrombophilias increase the risk of thromboembolism in pregnancy eightfold. These episodes include not only typical lower-extremity DVT and pulmonary embolism but also unusual thrombotic manifestations, such as sagittal, mesenteric, and portal vein thromboses. Excluding hyperhomocysteinemia, only 8–14% of white women meets laboratory criteria for a thrombophilic disorder; however, these women account for 70% of cases of venous thromboses diagnosed in pregnancy (7, 8). A pregnant patient with an inherited thrombophilia of low thrombogenic potential (ie, heterozygotes for the factor V Leiden and prothrombin *G20210A* mutations, as well as protein C or protein S deficiencies, or rarely hyperhomocysteinemia unresponsive to folate and vitamin B_{12} therapy) and a history of thromboembolism should be treated with prophylactic unfractionated heparin or low molecular weight heparin during pregnancy and the postpartum period. However, patients with highly thrombogenic thrombophilias (ie, antithrombin deficiency or homozygotes or compound heterozygotes for the factor V Leiden or prothrombin *G20210A* mutations) appear to require the use of therapeutic heparin (see Prevention). For a detailed discussion of the inherited and acquired thrombophilias, see *Clinical Updates in Women's Health Care: Thrombosis, Thrombophilia, and Thromboembolism* (9).

Diagnosis

Deep Vein Thrombosis

The clinical diagnosis of DVT in pregnancy often is inaccurate and unreliable. The first step in assessing the patient is to estimate her risk. Of patients exhibiting the classic features of DVT (Box 20), more than one half do not have the condition. Any pregnant woman with signs and symptoms of DVT should undergo testing expeditiously and low molecular weight heparin or unfractionated heparin therapy should be initiated until the diagnosis has been excluded (3). Compression color Doppler ultrasonography of the femoral and popliteal

International Consensus Statement on Preliminary Criteria for the Classification of the Antiphospholipid Syndrome*

Clinical Criteria

- Vascular thrombosis—one or more clinical episodes of arterial, venous, or small-vessel thrombosis, occurring within any tissue or organ

Complications of Pregnancy

- One or more unexplained deaths of morphologically normal fetuses at or after the 10th week of gestation
- One or more premature births of morphologically normal neonates at or before the 34th week of gestation
- Three or more unexplained consecutive spontaneous abortions before the 10th week of gestation

Laboratory Criteria[†]

- Anticardiolipin antibodies (immunoglobulin G or immunoglobulin M) present at moderate or high levels in the blood on two or more occasions at least 6 weeks apart[‡]
- Lupus anticoagulant antibodies detected in the blood on two or more occasions at least 6 weeks apart, according to the guidelines of the International Society on Thrombosis and Hemostasis[§]

*A diagnosis of definite antiphospholipid syndrome requires the presence of at least one of the clinical criteria and at least one of the laboratory criteria. No limits are placed on the interval between the clinical event and the positive laboratory findings.

[†]The following antiphospholipid antibodies are currently not included in the laboratory criteria: anticardiolipin immunoglobulin A antibodies, anti-β_2-glycoprotein-I antibodies, and antiphospholipid antibodies directed against phospholipids other than cardiolipin (eg, phosphatidylserine and phosphatidylethanolamine) or against phospholipid-binding proteins other than cardiolipin-bound β_2-glycoprotein-I (eg, prothrombin, annexin V, protein C, or protein S).

[‡]The threshold used to distinguish moderate or high levels of anticardiolipin antibodies from low levels has not been standardized and may depend on the population under study. Many laboratories use 15 or 20 international phospholipid units as the threshold, separating low from moderate levels of anticardiolipin antibodies. Others define the threshold as 2 or 2.5 times the median level of anticardiolipin antibodies or as the 99th percentile of anticardiolipin levels within a normal population. Until an international consensus is reached, any of these three definitions seems reasonable.

[§]Guidelines are from Brandt JT, Triplett DA, Alving B, Scharrer I. Criteria for the diagnosis of lupus anticoagulants: an update. On behalf of the Subcommittee on Lupus Anticoagulant/Antiphospholipid Antibody of the Scientific and Standardisation Committee of the ISTH. Thromb Hemost 1995;74:1185–90.

Levine JS, Branch DW, Rauch J. The antiphospholipid syndrome. N Engl J Med 2002;346:752–63. Copyright 2002 Massachusetts Medical Society. All rights reserved.

veins and calf trifurcation has become the primary diagnostic modality to evaluate the pregnant patient thought to have DVT. This approach has been found to be highly sensitive (greater than 98%) and specific (greater than 96%) in detecting thromboses of the deep femoral and popliteal veins (10). If ultrasound findings are abnormal, venous thrombosis is diagnosed and treatment initiated. If ultrasound findings are equivocal or normal but there is a high index of suspicion (positive personal or immediate family history or clinical progression), magnetic resonance imaging (MRI) may be indicated. Some recommend assay for D-dimer as an intermediate test. Because D-dimer levels rise during normal pregnancy, assay for D-dimer should be used with other tests to establish the diagnosis of DVT. In results from a recent study, using a highly specific assay for D-dimer, a negative result was associated with a negative predictive value for DVT in the first and second trimesters of pregnancy (11). For femoropopliteal DVT, sensitivity and specificity of MRI approach 100%. Some experts have advocated use of D-dimer testing in low-risk patients as a "rule-out" test, given its high negative predictive value but low positive predictive value in pregnancy.

Pulmonary Embolism

The classic clinical triad of dyspnea, pleuritic chest pain, and hemoptysis occurs in only one quarter of patients with documented pulmonary embolism. Although patients may display hypoxia, 17% of patients will have normal Pa_{O_2} laboratory values. Echocardiographic findings in severe cases may include right ventricular dilation and hypokinesis, tricuspid regurgitation, and pulmonary artery dilation.

At this time, there is no clear consensus as to whether ventilation–perfusion scanning or spiral computerized tomography (CT) should be the first-line diagnostic modality. Each modality has a similar detection rate for acute pulmonary embolism, but each has its own advantages and disadvantages. Choice of approach often will depend on the experience of the local radiology team and the availability of the technology. The "high probability" ventilation–perfusion scan result is associated with acute pulmonary embolism 95% of the time, but only 41% of patients with acute pulmonary embolism have a high probability scan result (sensitivity of 41% and specificity of 97%) (12). Ventilation–perfusion scanning offers the advantage of exposing the breasts to less radiation compared with spiral CT. Spiral CT provides a definitive diagnosis more frequently than ventilation–perfusion scanning because it can detect nonembolic lesions. Spiral CT is of more limited value with subsegmental peripheral vessels and horizontal oriented vessels in the right middle lobe (12). A suggested paradigm for testing patients at high clinical risk of acute pulmonary embolism is illustrated in Figure 17.

Table 18. Inherited Thrombophilias

Disorder	Genetics	Screening Assays	Prevalence	Risk of Venous Thromboembolism
Factor V Leiden	AD	DNA	3–15%	3–8-fold (0.2%)
Prothrombin G20210A	AD	DNA	2–3%	3-fold (0.5%)
Antithrombin	AD	Activity assay	0.02%	25–50-fold (50%)
Protein C	AD	Activity assay	0.2–0.3%	10–15-fold (4%)
Protein S	AD	Activity assay; if decreased, assess total and free antigen levels	0.1–2.1%	2-fold (4%)
Hyperhomocysteinemia	AR	Fasting homocysteine level test with or without methylene tetrahydrofolate reductase mutation screening	11%	2.5-fold (levels greater than 18.5 micromol/L) and 3–4-fold (levels greater than 200 micromol/L) (0.25–0.35%)

Abbreviations: AD indicates autosomal dominant; AR, autosomal recessive.

Haemostasis and Thrombosis Task Force, British Committee for Standards in Haematology. Investigation and management of heritable thrombophilia. Brit J Haematol 2001;114:512–28. Adapted with permission from Wiley–Blackwell.

Box 20
Typically Cited Signs and Symptoms of Deep Vein Thrombosis and Differential Diagnosis

Typically Cited Signs and Symptoms

- Erythema
- Warmth
- Pain
- Edema
- Tenderness
- Positive Homans sign

Differential Diagnosis

- Cellulitis
- Ruptured or strained muscle or tendon
- Injury to the knee joint
- Ruptured popliteal cyst
- Cutaneous vasculitis
- Superficial thrombophlebitis
- Lymphedema

or family history of vein thrombosis, should be treated with full therapeutic anticoagulation during pregnancy and maintained on anticoagulation for at least 6 weeks postpartum and up to 3 months if they have a history of prior venous thromboembolism. In contrast, pregnant women with low-risk thrombophilias (ie, heterozygotes for the factor V Leiden and prothrombin G20210A mutations as well as protein C or protein S deficiencies or hyperhomocysteinemia unresponsive to folate and vitamin B$_{12}$ therapy) and no personal history of DVT have a low incidence of DVT in pregnancy (0.2–4%) and do not appear to require antepartum anticoagulation therapy (13). However, they should receive anticoagulation therapy postpartum if they require a cesarean delivery, because most fatal pulmonary emboli occur during this period, or if they have other major risk factors for thrombosis (eg, obesity, prior prolonged bed rest, or strong family history) (14). Although controversial, patients without an identifiable thrombophilia whose prior thrombosis occurred during pregnancy should probably be given low-dose heparin as antenatal prophylaxis.

Prevention

If there is a high degree of suspicion of DVT, treatment with heparin should be considered pending availability of diagnostic test results (Box 21). As noted previously, women with high-risk thrombophilias (ie, antithrombin deficiency and homozygosity and compound heterozygosity for the factor V Leiden and prothrombin G20210A mutations), regardless of personal

Treatment

The mainstays of therapy for DVT are anticoagulation, elevation of the extremity, and analgesia. For pulmonary embolism, therapy includes initiation of anticoagulation therapy and maintenance of adequate cardiac output and oxygenation. When DVT occurs during pregnancy or the puerperium or when a pregnant woman requires anticoagulation based on risk factors (eg, orthopedic

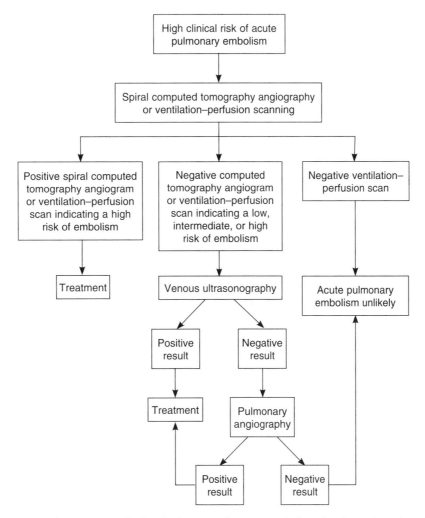

Figure 17. Testing paradigm for patients at high risk of acute pulmonary embolism. (Lockwood C. Thrombosis, thrombophilia, and thromboembolism. Clin Update Womens Health Care 2007; VI(4):1-95.)

surgery, immobilization, or mechanical heart valve) or medical history (prior DVT), heparin is the anticoagulant of choice for therapy. It can be administered as subcutaneous low molecular weight heparin, intravenous unfractionated heparin, or subcutaneous unfractionated heparin (14, 15). Heparin does not cross the placenta, appears to be safe for the fetus, and does not enter breast milk.

The maternal side effects of heparin therapy include hemorrhage, thrombocytopenia, and osteoporosis. Hemorrhage is more common with concomitant aspirin use or in the face of thrombocytopenia or liver disease and occurs less frequently when low molecular weight heparin preparations are used. Heparin-induced thrombocytopenia occurs in 3% of patients and has two forms: 1) early-onset, transient, heparin-induced platelet aggregation for which therapy need not be interrupted and 2) immunoglobulin G-mediated, heparin-induced, potentially severe, thrombotic thrombocytopenia occurring within 2 weeks of initiating therapy, which mandates cessation of therapy. Heparin-induced osteoporosis is far more common when doses of more than 15,000 units

per day are given for more than 6 months. These patients might benefit from dietary supplementation with 1,500 mg of calcium per day. Low molecular weight preparations are associated with lower risks of heparin-induced thrombocytopenia and osteoporosis.

The dose of unfractionated heparin required may vary secondary to differences in heparin-binding proteins in pregnancy. The activated partial thromboplastin time (aPTT), heparin level, or antifactor Xa level should be evaluated every 4 hours during the initial phase of therapy, and dosages should be adjusted as needed to maintain an aPTT between 1.5 times and 2.5 times control or antifactor Xa levels at 0.6–1 unit/mL. Intravenous therapeutic unfractionated heparin should be continued to be administered for at least 5 days or until clinical improvement is noted. Unfractionated heparin may then be administered subcutaneously every 8–12 hours to maintain the aPTT at 1.5–2 times control, 6 hours after the injection.

Women with a history of DVT remote from pregnancy and the puerperium that was associated with a nonrecurrent risk factor (eg, surgery or orthopedic immobilization) but who do not have acquired or inherited thrombophilias appear to be at very low risk of recurrence. Although anticoagulation during the antepartum period appears unnecessary in such patients, DVT prophylaxis should be used during the postpartum period.

Postpartum anticoagulation therapy should be continued for 6–12 weeks after DVT is diagnosed and for 4–6 months after pulmonary embolism or complex iliofemoral DVT is diagnosed. Oral anticoagulant therapy can be initiated postpartum by titrating the warfarin dose to maintain the patient's international normalized ratio at approximately 2. Because warfarin exerts a more rapid inhibitory effect on levels of protein C than on the procoagulant factors and given that protein S levels are suppressed during pregnancy, heparin should be maintained during the initial 4 days of warfarin therapy and until a therapeutic international normalized ratio is reached to avoid warfarin-induced skin necrosis and paradoxical thromboembolism.

Low Molecular Weight Heparin

Low molecular weight heparin has been shown to be a safe and effective alternative to traditional unfractionated heparin for both acute treatment and thromboprophylaxis of venous thromboembolism in pregnant patients (16–18). Like unfractionated heparin, low molecular weight heparin does not cross the placenta and has no teratogenic effects. However, compared with unfractionated heparin, low molecular weight heparin has a longer half-life and bioavailability, a more predictable dose–response relationship, and decreased risk of thrombocytopenia and hemorrhagic complications. Increased experience with the use of low molecular weight heparin during pregnancy suggests that it also can be used in pregnancy to treat patients with vein thrombosis, pulmonary embolism, or thrombophilic disorders. The dosage should be adjusted based on maternal weight. Because changes in maternal physiology unpredictably affect low molecular weight heparin levels, some experts recommend periodic (eg, monthly) evaluation of antifactor Xa levels during pregnancy in a woman on adjusted-dose therapeutic anticoagulation. Ideally, the dose should be sufficient to achieve a peak antifactor Xa level of 0.6–1.2 units/mL 4 hours after injection for those requiring therapeutic anticoagulation (19–21).

Regional anesthesia is contraindicated within 18–24 hours of administration of low molecular weight heparin. Epidural hematoma formation has been reported in patients receiving regional anesthesia while receiving low molecular weight heparin. To avoid this untoward event, therapy may be changed from low molecular weight heparin to unfractionated heparin at or near term. Alternatively, if the last dose of low molecular weight heparin was more than 24 hours before the administration of regional anesthesia, the risk of hematoma formation should be low. Consultation with an experienced anesthesiologist is indicated (22).

If vaginal or cesarean delivery occurs more than 12 hours from prophylaxis or 24 hours from therapeutic administration of doses of low molecular weight heparin, the patient should not experience anticoagulation-related problems with delivery (19). At this time, the synthetic heparin pentasaccharides (eg, fondaparinux) should be used only in special circumstances because they cross the placenta and there is a dearth of data supporting its safety in pregnancy.

Warfarin

The anticoagulant activity of warfarin is a result of its inhibition of vitamin K, which is a cofactor in the synthesis of functionally active factors VII, IX, X, and prothrombin (factor II). Warfarin is loosely bound to albumin and crosses the placenta. It carries a 33% risk of embryopathy (ie, nasal hypoplasia, stippled epiphysis, and central nervous system abnormalities) when exposure is between 7 weeks of gestation and 12 weeks of gestation. Fetal and placental bleeding also are serious complications of warfarin use throughout pregnancy. Vitamin K or fresh frozen plasma can be used to reverse the effect of warfarin. Warfarin use during pregnancy is normally contraindicated. However, pregnant women with mechanical heart valves may constitute a group that warrants warfarin use during the second trimester of pregnancy because current studies suggest an increase in thrombogenic complications using unfractionated heparin (23). Warfarin does not accumulate in breast milk or have an anticoagulant effect on the infant and is not contraindicated in women who breastfeeding.

Special Considerations

Retrievable Inferior Vena Caval Filter Placement

Indications for placement of an inferior vena caval filter are the same in the pregnant and nonpregnant patients and include the following conditions:

- Recurrent pulmonary embolism despite adequate anticoagulant therapy
- Pulmonary embolism or iliofemoral DVT in patients with contraindication to anticoagulation therapy (eg, active bleeding, hemorrhagic stroke, and recent surgery)
- Development of serious hemorrhagic sequelae with anticoagulant therapy

Thrombolytic Therapy

The most common complication of thrombolytic therapy for the treatment of pulmonary embolism is massive hemorrhage. Pregnancy poses special concerns about such therapy, given the risk of abruption and puerperal hemorrhage. The published experiences with thrombolytic therapy in pregnancy are observational studies and case reports.

Outcomes among 172 pregnant patients treated with thrombolytic therapy were reviewed, and it was reported that the maternal mortality rate was 1.2%, the fetal loss rate was 6%, and that the rate of maternal complications from hemorrhage was 8%. However, given the limited evidence of benefit of such therapy, its use in pregnant patients should be restricted to those rare settings in which the potential benefits of the therapy clearly outweigh the serious attendant risks (24).

Mechanical Heart Valves

Long-term anticoagulant therapy is indicated in most patients with mechanical heart valve prostheses. However, there is considerable controversy concerning optimal treatment methodologies. Compared with unfractionated heparin use throughout pregnancy, the use of warfarin in these women was associated with the greatest maternal protection (23). The risk of thrombosis in the heparin group and the warfarin group was 25% and 3.9%, respectively, whereas the risks of maternal mortality were 7% and 1.8%, respectively (25). Among the women in this study, the use of warfarin between 6 weeks of gestation and 12 weeks of gestation was associated with a doubling of the fetal loss rate to 30% and observation of stigmata of the fetal warfarin syndrome in 6% of cases. Thus, with appropriate informed consent, it may be an appropriate option to use full anticoagulation with unfractionated heparin in the first and third trimesters and to substitute warfarin during the middle trimester. However, although this approach may reduce fetal risk, this risk is not eliminated. Thus, therapeutic doses of heparin should be used in these patients seeking to maintain therapeutic anticoagulation during trough times. Subcutaneous low molecular weight heparin has been suggested as an alternative to protocols using warfarin and unfractionated heparin. Because platelet aggregation on the mechanical valve may contribute to valve thrombosis, low-dose aspirin also should be employed in these patients.

The manufacturer of enoxaparin specifically recommends against its use in this setting, based on a small number of reports to the U.S. Food and Drug Administration of valvular thrombosis in pregnant women treated with this agent (26). However, the 2008 American College of Chest Physicians guidelines referred to these reported cases of valvular thrombosis in pregnant patients receiving low molecular weight heparin for mechanical heart valve prostheses and concluded that virtually all such cases were associated with underdosage or inadequate monitoring and the group recommended enoxaparin therapy in such patients in lieu of warfarin (14). The starting dose should be 1 mg/kg, subcutaneously, every 12 hours, with subsequent monitoring of antifactor Xa peak levels 4 hours after injection and also trough levels before the next dose. Dose adjustments then should be made to maintain a trough level between 0.6 units/mL and 1.2 units/mL.

References

1. Heit JA, Kobbervig CE, James AH, Petterson TM, Bailey KR, Melton LJ 3rd. Trends in the incidence of venous thromboembolism during pregnancy or postpartum: a 30-year population-based study. Ann Intern Med 2005;143:697–706.

2. James AH, Jamison MG, Brancazio LR, Myers ER. Venous thromboembolism during pregnancy and the postpartum period: incidence, risk factors, and mortality. Am J Obstet Gynecol 2006;194:1311–5.

3. Marik PE, Plante LA. Venous thromboembolic disease and pregnancy. N Engl J Med 2008;359:2025–33.

4. Bremme KA. Haemostatic changes in pregnancy. Best Pract Res Clin Haematol 2003;16:153–68.

5. Girling JC, de Swiet M. Thromboembolism in pregnancy: an overview. Curr Opin Obstet Gynecol 1996;8:458–63.

6. Levine JS, Branch DW, Rauch J. The antiphospholipid syndrome. N Engl J Med 2002;346:752–63.

7. Investigation and management of heritable thrombophilia. Haemostasis and Thrombosis Task Force, British Committee for Standards in Haematology. Br J Haematol 2001;114:512–28.

8. Greer IA. The challenge of thrombophilia in maternal-fetal medicine. N Engl J Med 2000;342:424–5.

9. Lockwood C. Thrombosis, thrombophilia, and thromboembolism. Clin Update Womens Health Care 2007;VI(4): 1–95.

10. Douketis JD, Ginsberg JS. Diagnostic problems with venous thromboembolic disease in pregnancy. Haemostasis 1995; 25:58–71.

11. Chan WS, Chunilal S, Lee A, Crowther M, Rodger M, Ginsberg JS. A red blood cell agglutination D-dimer test to exclude deep venous thrombosis in pregnancy. Ann Intern Med 2007;147:165–70.

12. Tapson VF, Carroll BA, Davidson BL, Elliott CG, Fedullo PF, Hales CA, et al. The diagnostic approach to acute venous thromboembolism. Clinical practice guideline. American Thoracic Society. Am J Respir Crit Care Med 1999;160:1043–66.

13. Lockwood CJ. Inherited thrombophilias in pregnant patients: detection and treatment paradigm. Obstet Gynecol 2002;99:333–41.

14. Bates SM, Greer IA, Pabinger I, Sofaer S, Hirsh J. Venous thromboembolism, thrombophilia, antithrombotic therapy, and pregnancy: American College of Chest Physicians Evidence-Based Clinical Practice Guidelines (8th Edition). American College of Chest Physicians. Chest 2008;133:844S–86S.

15. Hirsh J, Bauer KA, Donati MB, Gould M, Samama MM, Weitz JI. Parenteral anticoagulants: American College of Chest Physicians Evidence-Based Clinical Practice Guidelines (8th Edition). American College of Chest Physicians. Chest 2008;133:141S–59S.

16. Greer IA, Nelson-Piercy C. Low-molecular-weight heparins for thromboprophylaxis and treatment of venous thromboembolism in pregnancy: a systematic review of safety and efficacy. Blood 2005;106:401–7.

17. Safety of Lovenox in pregnancy. ACOG Committee Opinion No. 276. American College of Obstetricians and Gynecologists. Obstet Gynecol 2002;100:845–6.

18. van Dongen CJ, van den Belt AG, Prins MH, Lensing AW. Fixed dose subcutaneous low molecular weight heparins versus adjusted dose unfractionated heparin for venous thromboembolism. Cochrane Database of Systematic Reviews 2004, Issue 4. Art. No.: CD001100. DOI: 10.1002/14651858.CD001100.pub2; 10.1002/14651858. CD001100.pub2.

19. American College of Obstetricians and Gynecologists. Thromboembolism in pregnancy. Practice Bulletin 19. Washington, DC: American College of Obstetricians and Gynecologists; 2000.

20. Nelson-Piercy C, Letsky EA, de Swiet M. Low-molecular-weight heparin for obstetric thromboprophylaxis: experience of sixty-nine pregnancies in sixty-one women at high risk. Am J Obstet Gynecol 1997;176:1062–8.

21. Ginsberg JS, Hirsh J. Use of antithrombotic agents during pregnancy. Chest 1998;114:524S–30S.

22. Horlocker TT, Wedel DJ, Benzon H, Brown DL, Enneking KF, Heit JA, et al. Regional Anesthesia in the Anticoagulated Patient: Defining the Risks. Reg Anesth Pain Med 2004;29:1–11.

23. Reimold SC, Rutherford JD. Clinical practice. Valvular heart disease in pregnancy. N Engl J Med 2003;349:52–9.

24. Ahearn GS, Hadjiliadis D, Govert JA, Tapson VF. Massive pulmonary embolism during pregnancy successfully treated with recombinant tissue plasminogen activator: a case report and review of treatment options. Arch Intern Med 2002; 162:1221–7.

25. Chan WS, Anand S, Ginsberg JS. Anticoagulation of pregnant women with mechanical heart valves: a systematic review of the literature. Arch Intern Med 2000;160:191–6.

26. U.S. Food and Drug Administration. Lovenox (enoxaparin sodium): safety information. Rockville (MD): FDA; 2002. Available at: http://www.fda.gov/Safety/MedWatch/Safety Information/SafetyAlertsforHumanMedicalProducts/ ucm154506.htm. Retrieved September 11, 2009.

Pulmonary Disorders

Luis D. Pacheco and Maged Costantine

Pregnant women undergo unique physiologic changes in pulmonary function that may predispose them to more severe sequelae from any given insult when compared with the same insult when not pregnant. Included are reductions in total lung volume that, by the third trimester, result in her tidal volume virtually overlapping her critical closing volume and a tendency to develop atelectasis even at base line, further exacerbated by disease states. This should translate into a need for closer observation of pregnant women.

Asthma

Asthma may complicate up to 4% of pregnancies, and its prevalence appears to be increasing. Pregnancies affected by asthma are at increased risk of preterm birth, preeclampsia, low birth weight, and perinatal mortality. Severe asthma is more likely to become worse during pregnancy. The course of asthma in an earlier pregnancy often predicts the course of asthma in a subsequent pregnancy.

Controlling asthma during pregnancy is important for the health and well-being of the mother and fetus. The Working Group on Asthma During Pregnancy of the National Institutes of Health has concluded that asthma should be treated as aggressively in pregnancy as in nonpregnant adults. That group identified four components of a management program for pregnant women with asthma (1):

1. Assessing and monitoring asthma monthly, with objective measures of lung function

2. Avoiding or controlling asthma triggers

3. Providing patient education

4. Using a stepwise approach to pharmacologic therapy

Environmental irritants, which may trigger asthma attacks, should be removed. These include cigarette smoke, dust mites, indoor mold, pollen, cockroaches, and animal dander.

Management of an asthma exacerbation requires assessment of its severity. Subjective assessments are notoriously inaccurate. Objective measures of lung function are necessary to assess the severity of disease and to tailor appropriate therapy for ongoing symptoms. The best measure is forced expiratory volume in the first second of expiration (FEV_1); however, the peak expiratory flow rate (PEFR) correlates with FEV_1 and can be measured with an inexpensive, hand-held flow meter. Home monitoring of the peak expiratory flow rate provides a daily assessment of lung function and response to ongoing therapy. Peak expiratory flow rate and FEV_1 do not change during a normal pregnancy. The patient with asthma should establish a personal best during an asymptomatic period. Adjustments of therapy and interventions are based on reductions from the patient's personal best benchmark.

First-trimester ultrasound confirmation of gestational age allows comparison for eventual fetal growth. Additional ultrasound examinations starting at 32 weeks of gestation may be warranted to evaluate fetal growth in patients with moderate to severe disease. In the third trimester, the need for fetal surveillance should be based on the severity of asthma.

Pharmacologic therapy for asthma should be individualized based on severity of disease (Table 19). Patients should not be undertreated because of pregnancy. Inhaled medications are preferred because they deliver the agent directly to the bronchial tree, thus decreasing the potential for systemic side effects. Inhaled short-acting β_2-agonists are the rescue therapy of choice for asthma during pregnancy. Inhaled albuterol is the first-choice, short-acting β_2-agonist for pregnant women, although other agents also may be appropriate. In general, patients should use up to two treatments of inhaled albuterol (two to six puffs) or nebulized albuterol at 20-minute intervals for most mild to moderate symptoms; higher doses can be used for severe symptom exacerbation. To avoid maternal and fetal hypoxia, patients should be counseled to start rescue therapy at home when they have an exacerbation of symptoms, such as coughing, chest tightness, dyspnea, wheezing, or a 20% decrease in the PEFR. With a good response (ie, symptoms reduce or resolve, and the PEFR reaches 80% of personal best) patients can continue normal activity. If a patient does not have a good response or if she notices a decrease in fetal activity, she should seek medical attention quickly.

For those with mild, intermittent asthma, no controller therapy is indicated. Use of inhaled corticosteroids is first-line controller therapy for persistent asthma during pregnancy. For patients with mild, persistent asthma, the use of low-dose inhaled corticosteroids is recommended (see Box 22). For patients with moderate persistent asthma or whose symptoms are not controlled with the use of low-dose inhaled corticosteroids, the use of medium-dose inhaled corticosteroids or low-dose inhaled corticosteroids and long-acting β_2-agonists are indicated. Budesonide is the preferred inhaled corticosteroid for use during pregnancy (2). However, there are no data indicating that the other inhaled corticosteroid preparations are unsafe during pregnancy. Therefore,

Table 19. Selected Medications for the Treatment of Asthma*

Name	Available Strengths	Usual Dosage	Side Effects
Short-Acting Inhaled β_2-Agonists			
Albuterol	Metered dose inhaler: 90 micrograms per puff	2–6 puffs every 4–6 hours as needed	Tachycardia, nervousness, tremor, headache, insomnia, and nausea
Pirbuterol	Autohaler: 200 micrograms per puff	2 puffs every 4–6 hours as needed	
Long-Acting Inhaled β_2-Agonists			
Formoterol	Aerolizer: 12 micrograms per inhalation	1 capsule twice daily	Headache, tremor, restlessness, and dizziness
Salmeterol	Diskus: 50 micrograms per inhalation	1 inhalation twice daily	
Inhaled Corticosteroids			
Beclomethasone	Metered dose inhaler: 40 micrograms or 80 micrograms per puff	40–240 micrograms twice daily or higher	Sore throat, dry mouth, hoarseness, and oral candidiasis
Budesonide	Turbuhaler: 200 micrograms per inhalation	200 micrograms daily to 600 micrograms twice daily or higher	
Flunisolide	Metered dose inhaler: 250 micrograms per puff	250–1,000 micrograms twice daily or higher	
Fluticasone	Metered dose inhaler: 44 micrograms, 110 micrograms, or 220 micrograms per puff	Metered dose inhaler: 44–330 micrograms, twice daily or higher	
	Rotadisk: 50 micrograms, 100 micrograms, or 250 micrograms per inhalation	Rotadisk: 50–500 micrograms, twice daily or higher	
Triamcinolone	Metered dose inhaler: 100 micrograms per puff	400–2,000 micrograms per day or higher divided into 2–4 doses	
Mast Cell Stabilizer			
Cromolyn	Metered dose inhaler: 1 mg per puff	2–4 puffs 3–4 times daily	Cough, sore throat, hoarseness, bad taste, and nausea
Leukotriene Modifiers			
Montelukast	10-mg tablet	10 mg nightly	Nausea, headache, and diarrhea
Zafirlukast	10-mg or 20-mg tablets	20 mg twice daily	
Methylxanthine			
Theophylline	Various regular and extended release tablets, capsules, and liquids	300–800 mg daily	Headache, tachycardia, insomnia, tremor, and restlessness

(continued)

the use of any inhaled corticosteroids may be continued in patients whose asthma was well controlled by these agents before pregnancy (2).

Use of long-acting β_2-agonists is the preferred add-on controller therapy for asthma during pregnancy. This therapy should be added when patients' symptoms are not controlled with the use of medium-dose inhaled corticosteroids. Alternative add-on therapies are theophylline or leukotriene receptor antagonists (montelukast and zafirlukast). However, the use of long-acting inhaled β_2-agonists is preferred because it has been shown to be a more effective add-on therapy in nonpregnant patients

Table 19. Selected Medications for the Treatment of Asthma* (continued)

Name	Available Strengths	Usual Dosage	Side Effects
		Combination Product	
Fluticasone–salmeterol	100 micrograms fluticasone–50 micrograms salmeterol, 250 micrograms fluticasone–50 micrograms salmeterol, or 500 micrograms fluticasone–50 micrograms salmeterol per inhalation	1 inhalation twice daily	Pharyngitis, oral candidiasis, and tremor

*Inhaled medications are available in the following devices: Autohaler® is breath-activated; Aerolizer® is used to inhale contents of a capsule, and patients must load the device before each use; Diskus® is used to inhale contents of a capsule, and doses are preloaded; metered dose inhaler is a traditional type of inhaler; Turbuhaler® is used to inhale a dry powder, and doses are preloaded. Albuterol, budesonide, and cromolyn also are available in nebulizer formulations.

Box 22

Step Therapy Medical Management of Asthma During Pregnancy

Mild Intermittent Asthma

• No daily medications; albuterol as needed

Mild Persistent Asthma

• Preferred—Low-dose inhaled corticosteroid

• Alternative—Cromolyn, leukotriene receptor antagonist, or theophylline (serum level 5–12 micrograms/mL)

Moderate Persistent Asthma

• Preferred—Low-dose inhaled corticosteroid and salmeterol or medium-dose inhaled corticosteroid or (if needed) medium-dose inhaled corticosteroid and salmeterol

• Alternative—Low-dose or (if needed) medium-dose inhaled corticosteroid and either leukotriene receptor antagonist or theophylline (serum level 5–12 micrograms/mL)

Severe Persistent Asthma

• Preferred—High-dose inhaled corticosteroid and salmeterol and (if needed) oral corticosteroid

• Alternative—High-dose inhaled corticosteroid and theophylline (serum level 5–12 micrograms/mL) and oral corticosteroid if needed

Asthma in pregnancy. ACOG Practice Bulletin No. 90. American College of Obstetricians and Gynecologists. Obstet Gynecol 2008;111:457–64.

---

than leukotriene receptor antagonists or theophylline. Long-acting inhaled β_2-agonists have fewer side effects than theophylline, which has a narrow therapeutic index and requires serum monitoring, and there are few data on the use of leukotriene receptor antagonists in humans during pregnancy. Because long-acting and short-acting inhaled β_2-agonists have similar pharmacology and toxicology, long-acting inhaled β_2-agonists are expected to have a safety profile similar to that of albuterol. Two long-acting inhaled β_2-agonists are available: salmeterol and formoterol. Limited observational data exist on their use during pregnancy. A step-wise approach to management is advised in order to achieve control. For patients whose symptoms are not well controlled (Table 20) with the use of medium-dose inhaled corticosteroids and long-acting inhaled β_2-agonists, treatment should be advanced to high-dose inhaled corticosteroids and long-acting inhaled β_2-agonists (salmeterol, one puff twice daily). Some patients with severe asthma may require regular oral corticosteroid use to achieve adequate asthma control. For patients whose symptoms are very poorly controlled, a course of oral corticosteroids may be necessary to attain control, along with a step up in therapy, as described previously.

Influenza

Because pregnant women are more susceptible to the serious complications associated with influenza infection, current recommendations are that all women who will be pregnant during the influenza season (October through the middle of May) should be vaccinated. The intramuscular, trivalent, inactivated vaccine may be applied during any trimester of pregnancy. The intranasal vaccine contains a live, attenuated virus and should not be used during pregnancy (3). Immunizing pregnant patients not only decreases symptomatic episodes in the mother but also provides passive immunization to the newborn, protecting infants against the disease up to the age of 6 months (4). The latter is important because the vaccine is not licensed for infants younger than 6 months.

Severe cases of influenza may warrant therapy with antivirals. Amantadine and rimantadine should no longer be used because of the high incidence of resistance. Alternatives include the neuraminidase inhibitors zana-

Table 20. Classification of Asthma Severity and Control in Pregnant Patients

Asthma Severity* (Control†)	Symptom Frequency	Nighttime Awakening	Interference With Normal Activity	FEV$_1$ or Peak Flow (Predicted Percentage of Personal Best)
Intermittent (well controlled)	2 days per week or less	Twice per month or less	None	More than 80%
Mild persistent (not well controlled)	More than 2 days per week, but not daily	More than twice per month	Minor limitation	More than 80%
Moderate persistent (not well controlled)	Daily symptoms	More than once per week	Some limitation	60–80%
Severe persistent (very poorly controlled)	Throughout the day or more	Four times per week	Extremely limited	Less than 60%

Abbreviation: FEV$_1$ indicates forced expiratory volume in the first second of expiration.

*Assess severity for patients who are not taking long-term control medications.

†Assess control in patients taking long-term control medications to determine whether step-up therapy, step-down therapy, or no change in therapy is indicated.

Asthma in pregnancy. ACOG Practice Bulletin No. 90. American College of Obstetricians and Gynecologists. Obstet Gynecol 2008; 111:457–64.

mivir and oseltamivir (5). The safety of these agents during pregnancy has not been established. They should be used in pregnancy only if the potential benefits outweigh the potential risks.

Avian influenza, H5N1 in humans mainly is the result of infection from contact with infected poultry or surfaces contaminated with secretions or excretions from infected birds. Transmission from one ill person to another is very unlikely. Treatment with neuraminidase inhibitors is indicated in infected pregnant patients.

In April 2009, the novel influenza A virus, H1N1, initiated a worldwide pandemia. Pregnant patients are at increased risk for developing severe disease if infected. Any pregnant patient with symptoms suggestive of H1N1 infection should undergo a rapid influenza diagnostic test. This point-of-care test provides results within 30 minutes or less. Importantly, treatment should not be delayed while awaiting test results. The sensitivity of this rapid diagnostic test is 10–70% (6). Confirmatory tests include reverse transcription–polymerase chain reaction test and viral culture. The optimal therapy is oseltamivir, 75 mg, twice daily for 5 days. Ideally, treatment should be started within 48 hours of onset of symptoms; however, pregnant patients should be started on oseltamivir even if more than 48 hours have elapsed. Pregnant women in close contact with suspected or confirmed cases should receive prophylaxis with oseltamivir, 75 mg, daily for 10 days. The antiviral therapy is not contraindicated during pregnancy or breastfeeding.

Pneumonia

Pulmonary disorders in pregnancy often require management of acute symptoms. Patients may require stabilization in a hospital setting to ensure adequate oxygenation. Over the last decade, an increase in the risk of infection with microorganisms like the *Pseudomonas* species, *Acinetobacter* species, methicillin-resistant *Staphylococcus aureus*, and drug resistant isolates of *Streptococcus pneumoniae*, have been noticed in the setting of community-acquired pneumonia.

Influenza A and influenza B viruses, respiratory syncytial virus, and parainfluenza virus can cause pneumonia. Influenza is by far the most frequent cause of community-acquired viral pneumonia, with annual outbreaks on a seasonal basis. These viruses usually are spread by aerosolized droplets produced from talking, sneezing, or coughing, which then quickly infect the epithelium of the respiratory tract. The incubation period typically is 1–3 days, and symptoms usually resolve spontaneously within 7–10 days. Roughly 1% of cases of influenza develop into pneumonia, with an associated mortality reported as high as 25–30%. Recent guidelines for the management of community-acquired pneumonia from the Infectious Diseases Society of America and the American Thoracic Society recommend therapy with a neuraminidase inhibitor (oseltamivir or zanamivir) in nonpregnant adults with influenza pneumonia (7). No data exists regarding the safety of use of these antivirals during pregnancy. Consequently, the benefit should outweigh any potential risks to the fetus if they are to be used during gestation.

The most common type of bacterial pneumonia is that caused by *Streptococcus pneumoniae* (pneumococcal pneumonia), followed in frequency by *Mycoplasma pneumoniae* and *Haemophilus influenzae*. The management of typical bacterial pneumonia should include both supportive measures for symptoms and pharmacologic agents directed at the responsible pathogen. Sputum Gram stain and culture may prove beneficial. An adequate specimen should contain more than 25 neutrophils and fewer than

10 epithelial cells. Because identifying the exact pathogen is the exception rather than the rule, initial antibiotic treatment usually is empirical. Most cases of pneumonia in adults are caused by pneumococci or mycoplasma, making macrolides an ideal first choice for treatment. Erythromycin, azithromycin, and clarithromycin are all acceptable alternatives. In patients with concomitant comorbidities such as heart, lung, liver, or renal disease, diabetes mellitus, or immunosuppressive states, the combination of treatment with a β-lactam plus a macrolide is recommended (eg, amoxicillin 1 g, three times per day plus a macrolide). Patients admitted to the hospital are better treated empirically with a parenteral β-lactam (eg, cefotaxime or ceftriaxone) plus a macrolide.

Sarcoidosis

The prognosis for patients with sarcoidosis is good. In almost 50% of patients, the condition resolves spontaneously; in the remaining 40–50% of patients, some permanent organ dysfunction persists. Corticosteroids are the hallmark of therapy. Their use generally is based on patient symptoms, chest X-ray findings, and pulmonary function testing. Unless there is severe preexisting disease, sarcoidosis seldom affects pregnancy adversely. Severe sarcoidosis in pregnancy warrants careful assessment and serial determinations of pulmonary function. Deterioration of lung function should prompt the use of prednisone 20–40 mg/day. Skin involvement may require the addition of hydroxychloroquine.

Cystic Fibrosis

When a pregnant woman has cystic fibrosis, outcomes for both the fetus and the mother are directly related to the degree of pulmonary disease at the time of conception. When the FEV_1 is less than 60% of predicted value, there is a substantially increased risk of preterm delivery, maternal pulmonary complications, and early death of the mother. In contrast, successful pregnancy outcomes can be expected when the prepregnancy FEV_1 is more than 80% predicted, and prepregnancy treatments, including pancreatic enzyme replacements, oral antibiotics, aerosolized bronchodilators, chest physiotherapy, and nutritional support, are continued. Other complications include poor maternal weight gain with requirement of parenteral nutrition and lower insulin secretion from the pancreas.

Pregnancy should be avoided in patients with cystic fibrosis with pulmonary hypertension and in those with a FEV_1 result less than 50% of predicted value (8). However, pregnancy by itself does not alter the natural evolution of the disease (9).

All patients with cystic fibrosis who are considering pregnancy should be encouraged to have preconception and genetic counseling. Once pregnancy is confirmed, serial pulmonary function testing should be performed on a regular basis. Frequent surveillance and early intervention are recommended for superimposed pulmonary infection, development of diabetes mellitus, and heart failure as a consequence of cor pulmonale. Diabetes mellitus screening should be performed early in pregnancy and again at 24–28 weeks of gestation. Meticulous attention should be paid to postural drainage and bronchodilator therapy to help maintain pulmonary function and prevent infection. Inhaled corticosteroids are not beneficial in patients with cystic fibrosis. Maternal nutrition status should be closely monitored. Cystic fibrosis exacerbations usually are treated with the use of antibiotics, short-acting β_2-agonists, inhaled hypertonic saline, and chest physiotherapy. Inhaled recombinant human deoxyribonuclease (dornase alfa) improves lung function by decreasing sputum viscosity.

Tuberculosis

In the United States, most cases of active tuberculosis during pregnancy occur as a result of reactivation or immunocompromise. Tuberculosis infection in pregnancy is associated with increased incidences of growth restriction, low birth weight, preterm delivery, and a sixfold increase in the perinatal mortality rate. Adverse outcomes are correlated with late diagnosis, incomplete treatment, and advanced pulmonary lesions.

Women seeking prenatal care should be screened if they are at high risk for acquiring tuberculosis (Box 23). The standard screening technique is the Mantoux tuberculin skin test, which consists of an intradermal administration of 5 units (0.1 mL) of purified protein derivative (PPD) tuberculin. Skin tests are interpreted 48–72 hours later. If the PPD tuberculin skin test result is negative, no further workup is warranted. If the result is positive, management is individualized as discussed below. However, a positive skin reaction should be interpreted according to the patient's risk factors (Table 21).

Chest radiography with abdominal shielding should be performed on all pregnant patients with positive PPD tuberculin skin test results to assess for pulmonary evidence of disease. Pregnant patients with positive PPD results should be treated during pregnancy with isoniazid (INH), if they have any of the following risk factors:

- Human immunodeficiency virus (HIV) infection
- Predisposing conditions, such as immunosuppressive therapy, diabetes mellitus, silicosis, hematologic malignancies, malnutrition, illicit drug use, end-stage renal disease, and previous gastrectomy
- Past tuberculosis without adequate therapy
- Chest X-ray result consistent with nonprogressive tuberculous disease
- New tuberculosis infection (PPD conversion in past 2 years)

Box 23

Risk Factors for *Mycobacterium Tuberculosis* Infection

1. Close contacts (ie, those sharing the same household or other enclosed environments) of persons known or suspected to have tuberculosis

2. Persons infected with human immunodeficiency virus (HIV)

3. Persons who inject drugs or other locally identified high-risk substance users (eg, crack cocaine users)

4. Persons who have medical risk factors known to increase the risk for disease if infection occurs

5. Residents and employees of high-risk congregate settings (eg, correctional institutions, nursing homes, mental institutions, other long-term residential facilities, and shelters for the homeless)

6. Healthcare providers who serve high-risk clients

7. Foreign-born persons, including children, recently arrived (within 5 years) from countries that have a high tuberculosis incidence or prevalence

8. Some medically underserved and low-income populations

9. High-risk racial or ethnic minority populations, as defined locally

10. Infants, children, and adolescents exposed to adults in high-risk categories

Data from Essential components of a tuberculosis prevention and control program. Recommendations of the Advisory Committee for Elimination of Tuberculosis. MMWR 1995;44(RR-11):1–34.

These factors put the patient at highest risk of progression to active disease (10).

The recommended regimen is INH, 300 mg daily, plus pyridoxine (10–50 mg/day) for 9 months. Especially in women with HIV and those recently infected, therapy should not be delayed, even during the first trimester of pregnancy. All other asymptomatic patients with a positive PPD result should receive their prophylaxis in the postpartum period for 9 months.

Patients with respiratory symptoms or those with findings on chest radiography suggestive of active disease should be evaluated for the presence of active infection with three morning sputum samples for acid-fast bacillus testing and culture. Because culture techniques take several weeks to yield results, therapy may be started if specimen test results are positive for acid-fast bacilli. Recently, polymerase chain reaction technology has been developed for the rapid diagnosis of tuberculosis. However, this technology has not replaced the traditional approach to diagnose tuberculosis.

Patients with positive acid-fast bacilli stain, *Mycobacterium tuberculosis* culture, or both, need to be treated immediately in the antepartum period with a three-drug regimen. If there is no suspicion of drug-resistant organism, INH with pyridoxine, rifampin, and ethambutol should be used for 9 months. Streptomycin is contraindicated (possible fetal ototoxicity). There is lack of information regarding the fetal effects of pyrazinamide use.

Isoniazid use generally is considered safe for the fetus in pregnancy, although it crosses the placenta readily. All pregnant women receiving INH also should receive pyridoxine (10–50 mg/day) to decrease the incidence of INH peripheral neuropathy and other central nervous system effects. Pregnant women taking INH should be monitored clinically for the development of hepatitis, and liver enzymes and bilirubin levels should be checked at baseline and throughout pregnancy and postpartum. Other risk factors that increase the risk of INH hepatitis include HIV infection, history of liver disease, and alcoholism. Isoniazid is present in small amounts in breast milk, and breastfeeding is not contraindicated. Infants breastfeeding whose mothers are taking INH should receive supplemental pyridoxine.

Although congenital infection can occur because of either hematogenous spread or fetal aspiration of the bacillus during delivery, most infections come from postpartum maternal contact. If the mother has active tuberculosis, the child should be separated from her until she is not contagious. Household contacts also should be screened and treated when necessary. If congenital tuberculosis is excluded, isoniazid should be given to the infant for 3–4 months after birth. Vaccination with bacillus Calmette–Guérin may be considered.

References

1. Management of asthma during pregnancy. Report of the Working Group on Asthma and Pregnancy. National Heart, Lung, and Blood Institute, National Asthma Education Program. Bethesda (MD): National Heart, Lung, and Blood Institute; 1993. Available at: http://www.nhlbi.nih.gov/health/prof/lung/asthma/astpreg.txt. Retrieved September 14, 2009.

2. Working Group report on managing asthma during pregnancy; recommendations for pharmacologic treatment: update 2004. National Heart, Lung, and Blood Institute, National Asthma Education Program, Working Group on Asthma and Pregnancy. Bethesda (MD): National Heart, Lung, and Blood Institute; 2005. Available at: http://www.nhlbi.nih.gov/health/prof/lung/asthma/astpreg/astpreg_full.pdf. Retrieved September 14, 2009.

3. Influenza vaccination and treatment during pregnancy. ACOG Committee Opinion No. 305. American College of Obstetricians and Gynecologists. Obstet Gynecol 2004; 104:1125–6.

4. Zaman K, Roy E, Arifeen SE, Rahman M, Raqib R, Wilson E, et al. Effectiveness of maternal influenza immunization in mothers and infants [published erratum appears in N Engl J Med 2009;360:648]. N Engl J Med 2008;359:1555–64.

Table 21. Guide to the Interpretation of Positive Purified Protein Derivative (Tuberculin) Skin Test Readings

Induration Diameter for the Test Result to be Positive	Risk Factors
5 mm or greater (high risk)	Recent close contact with persons who have active tuberculosis infection
	Human immunodeficiency virus (HIV) infection
	Fibrotic lesions of chest on radiography consistent with prior tuberculosis infection
	Prior organ transplantation and other causes of immunosuppression (eg, receipt of the equivalent of 15 mg/d or more of prednisone for 1 month or longer)
10 mm or greater (medium risk)	Injection drug use combined with negative or unknown HIV status
	Medical problems that increase the risk of tuberculosis activation (eg, silicosis, diabetes mellitus, chronic kidney disease, leukemia, lymphoma, carcinoma of the head or neck and lung, weight loss of 10% or greater of ideal body weight, gastrectomy, and jejunoileal bypass)
	Employment in high-risk facilities (eg, prisons, nursing homes, hospitals, and homeless shelters)
	Recent immigration (within the past 5 years) from countries of high tuberculosis prevalence
	Employment in a mycobacteriology laboratory
	Member of a medically underserved and low-income population
	Member of a high-risk racial or ethnic group
	Age younger than 4 years
	Exposure of children and adolescents to adults in high-risk categories
15 mm or greater (low risk)	Not meeting any of the previously listed criteria

5. Beigel JH. Influenza. Crit Care Med 2008;36:2660–6.

6. Hurt AC, Baas C, Deng YM, Roberts S, Kelso A, Barr IG. Performance of influenza rapid point-of-care tests in the detection of swine lineage A(H1N1) influenza viruses. Influenza Other Respi Viruses 2009;3:171–6.

7. Mandell LA, Wunderink RG, Anzueto A, Bartlett JG, Campbell GD, Dean NC, et al. Infectious Diseases Society of America/American Thoracic Society consensus guidelines on the management of community-acquired pneumonia in adults. Infectious Diseases Society of America; American Thoracic Society. Clin Infect Dis 2007;44(suppl 2):S27–72.

8. Cheng EY, Goss CH, McKone EF, Galic V, Debley CK, Tonelli MR, et al. Aggressive prenatal care results in successful fetal outcomes in CF women. J Cyst Fibros 2006; 5:85–91.

9. Goss CH, Rubenfeld GD, Otto K, Aitken ML. The effect of pregnancy on survival in women with cystic fibrosis. Chest 2003;124:1460–8.

10. Treatment of tuberculosis. American Thoracic Society; CDC; Infectious Diseases Society of America [published erratum appears in MMWR Recomm Rep 2005;53:1203]. MMWR Recomm Rep 2003;52:1–77.

Liver and Alimentary Tract Diseases

Thomas E. Nolan

Intrahepatic Cholestasis of Pregnancy

Intrahepatic cholestasis of pregnancy is the most common liver disorder unique to pregnancy. Patients usually present with pruritus during the third trimester of pregnancy. The normal course of the disorder is mild nocturnal pruritus of the palms and soles that gradually increases and migrates to the trunk with severe, unrelenting, generalized pruritus. The appearance of jaundice is highly variable and is not necessary for diagnosis. Intrahepatic cholestasis tends to recur in subsequent pregnancies and has a higher prevalence in the spring. The disease is common in women of Scandinavian and Chilean ancestry, but over the past 25 years its incidence has decreased in these populations. The disease is more common in close relatives of affected individuals with an autosomal-dominant, sex-limited inheritance (1). Its pathophysiology remains unknown, but seems to be related to increasing estrogen and progesterone levels associated with pregnancy, especially multiple gestations (2). Its histologic features are indistinguishable from those of other causes of cholestasis (centrilobular cholestasis, canaliculi-containing bile plugs, and bile pigment in hepatocytes).

The diagnosis of intrahepatic cholestasis of pregnancy is confirmed by demonstrating an increase in circulating bile acids (primarily cholic and chenodeoxycholic acids); however, this test often takes several weeks to yield results. Therefore, empiric therapy and additional testing are indicated. Levels of cholic acid are significantly higher than those of chenodeoxycholic acid, and thus determination of the former is more sensitive and specific for diagnosis (3). Fasting levels of bile acids 3–4 times the upper limit of normal are considered diagnostic. Ultrasonography of the gallbladder should be performed to rule out obstruction and stones. Mild to moderate increases in alanine aminotransferase and aspartate aminotransferase may be seen but are not diagnostic of the disease. There is no correlation between bile acids, liver function study results, and clinical symptoms. Total bilirubin levels usually are elevated less than 5 mg/dL. Impaired enterohepatic circulation of vitamin K may result in decreased production of vitamin K-dependent clotting factors (II, VII, IX, and X), leading to prolongation of prothrombin time in patients with severe and protracted intrahepatic cholestasis of pregnancy. Treatment with vitamin K at birth is recommended to prevent intracranial hemorrhage in the fetus and maternal hemorrhage postpartum (4).

Intrahepatic cholestasis of pregnancy is associated with an increased incidence of prematurity, fetal distress, and late fetal loss (at greater than 36 weeks of gestation). Fetal testing is of questionable value in predicting fetal demise (5). Because of late, sudden fetal loss, consideration of early delivery is recommended by some clinicians (6); others recommend induction of labor at 38 weeks of gestation (1). Deposits of bile salts in the placenta and increased levels of bile salt metabolites in amniotic fluid have been described, but how they adversely affect the fetus is unknown (7). Some clinicians have speculated that these deposits are related to an anoxic event. No clinical parameters have been correlated with fetal death in pregnant women with intrahepatic cholestasis of pregnancy.

Taking cornstarch baths or using antihistamines, such as diphenhydramine or hydroxyzine, may provide symptomatic relief in a few patients. Women with more severe symptoms require systemic therapy. Cholestyramine, phenobarbital, dexamethasone, S-adenosylmethionine, and epomediol have been used with varying success.

Ursodeoxycholic acid originally was introduced as an agent for the treatment of gallstones and is currently the medication of choice for cholestasis. It effectively reduces levels of cholic acids and bile acids while substantially decreasing pruritus. Additionally, research results suggest that fetal wastage is decreased in patients treated with ursodeoxycholic acid. In most cases, the pruritus resolves in the first 24–48 hours after delivery. Trials for all therapeutic interventions are small and inconsistent, and no consistent recommendations can be made (8).

Acute Fatty Liver of Pregnancy

Until recently, acute fatty liver of pregnancy was associated with a maternal mortality of nearly 90% of cases. Recent reports suggest that most patients survive with proper supportive care and early diagnosis and delivery. Acute fatty liver of pregnancy usually is first seen during the third trimester and is associated with first pregnancies, multiple gestations, and male fetuses. The signs and symptoms of preeclampsia may be found in approximately 20% of patients with acute fatty liver of pregnancy.

One possible etiology of acute fatty liver of pregnancy is an enzymatic defect in the fetus. Inherited as an autosomal recessive disorder, the fetus has a congenital deficiency of long-chain 3-hydroxyacyl coenzyme A dehydrogenases with a $1528G{\rightarrow}C$ mutation on one or both alleles (9). Because of this defect, there is an accumulation of straight-chain fatty acids that results in mitochondrial disruption and, eventually, severe liver dysfunction in the mother.

Pregnancy is associated with increased triglyceride breakdown, with the accumulated fatty acids causing a toxic reaction to hepatocytes (10). Results from one study suggests that 79% of the mothers of infants with this deficiency had either hemolysis, elevated liver enzymes, and low platelet count (HELLP) syndrome or acute fatty liver of pregnancy (11). Current recommendations are that metabolic screening for long-chain 3-hydroxyacyl coenzyme A dehydrogenase deficiency be performed on pregnant women affected with acute fatty liver of pregnancy or recurrent HELLP syndrome (12). Chorionic villus sampling or preimplantation genetic diagnosis to determine if the fetus is affected have been advocated for families where both partners are known carriers.

The clinical course of acute fatty liver of pregnancy begins with nonspecific constitutional symptoms and epigastric or abdominal pain, followed in approximately a week by jaundice and neurologic symptoms. Serum amylase, creatinine, bilirubin, uric acid, alanine aminotransferase, and aspartate aminotransferase levels are elevated. In contrast to viral hepatitis, liver transaminase levels are only moderately elevated, at 200–500 international units/L (13).

Coagulation abnormalities become evident as the disease progresses. These abnormalities include hypofibrinogenemia, increased fibrin degradation products, thrombocytopenia, and prolonged prothrombin and activated partial thromboplastin times. If the course of the disorder continues to progress, profound hypoglycemia can result from liver failure. Leukocytosis and anemia caused by microangiopathic destruction of red blood cells also are seen. Liver biopsy, with frozen section showing infiltration of hepatocytes with small droplets of fat (demonstrated with oil red O stain), remains the definitive diagnostic study, although this finding also may be present in preeclampsia. Electron microscopy examination reveals mitochondrial disruption. Computed tomography and magnetic resonance imaging have been helpful in establishing the diagnosis of acute fatty liver of pregnancy (Box 24).

Treatment of patients with acute fatty liver of pregnancy is immediate delivery. The route of delivery for women with the condition should depend on the clinical situation. Involvement of multiple organ systems is common. Special attention should be directed to combating infection with broad-spectrum antibiotics and treating coagulation dysfunction, usually with platelets, fresh frozen plasma, cryoprecipitate, and packed red cell transfusion. Use of H_2 receptor antagonists helps reduce the incidence of gastrointestinal bleeding. Although transaminase levels usually normalize promptly after delivery, other liver functions may remain abnormal for days to weeks. Multiple cases of successful liver transplantation have been reported, and transfer to a tertiary-care center with these services available should be considered.

Box 24

Differential Diagnoses for Acute Fatty Liver of Pregnancy

- Chemical hepatitis
- Cholangitis
- Hemolytic uremic syndrome
- Thrombotic thrombocytopenia purpura septicemia
- Budd–Chiari syndrome
- Pancreatitis
- Acute hepatitis
- Systematic lupus erythematosus
- Hemolysis, elevated liver enzymes, and low platelets syndrome
- Severe pregnancy-induced hypertension or eclampsia

Inflammatory Bowel Disease

Reports of pregnancy outcomes in patients with inflammatory bowel disease are conflicting. Important variables are the state of the disease at the beginning of gestation (ie, remission versus active disease) and its clinical course during gestation. Active disease is associated with a slight increase in spontaneous abortion and poor pregnancy outcome. These patients, particularly women with Crohn disease, should delay conception until their disease is in remission (14). Pregnancy is associated with a 15–30% chance of exacerbation of inflammatory bowel disease. Women with new onset disease during pregnancy are at increased risk for pregnancy loss. Patients with quiescent disease at conception usually do not have disease reactivation. Controversy exists as to whether flare-ups are more common in the postpartum period.

Treatment of inflammatory bowel disease is not altered greatly by pregnancy and includes the use of oral sulfasalazine, oral or rectal corticosteroids, and, occasionally, immunosuppression with systemic corticosteroids. Each of these medications may be continued during pregnancy. Infliximab, a new chimeric monoclonal antibody to tissue necrosis factor alpha given by infusion is being used in severe disease. Preliminary findings suggest that there have been no deleterious effects during pregnancy (15). Data on azathioprine in pregnancy vary widely because in most cases multiple other medications are used. In a database maintained by the National Transplantation Pregnancy Registry for renal transplants, there does not appear to be an increase in congenital anomalies related to azathioprine use (16). Surgery may be required to treat fistulae, bowel obstruction, hemorrhage, abscess formation, perforation, or malignancy or when medical management fails. Indications for surgery remain the same for the pregnant patient as for the nonpregnant patient. Occasionally, patients with active disease, severe dehydration, and perforations may require long periods of total parenteral nutrition.

Hyperemesis Gravidarum

Nausea and vomiting of pregnancy affect 70–85% of pregnant women (17). Hyperemesis gravidarum affects 0.5–2% of pregnancies, is the most common indication for hospital admission in the first part of pregnancy, and is second only to preterm labor as the most common reason for hospitalization during pregnancy (18). It appears to be an escalation of severity of nausea and vomiting of pregnancy. Commonly cited criteria for diagnosing hyperemesis gravidarum include persistent vomiting not related to other causes, a measure of acute starvation (usually large ketonuria), and some discrete measure of weight loss, most often at least 5% of prepregnancy weight.

Failure to treat early symptoms increases the likelihood of hospital admission for hyperemesis gravidarum. Recommendations for prevention and treatment are include in Box 25.

Nausea and vomiting of pregnancy occur before 9 weeks of gestation in virtually all affected women. If nausea and vomiting first occur after 9 weeks of gestation, other conditions, such as cholelithiasis, should be considered for the differential diagnosis.

Hepatitis

Hepatitis A Virus

The incidence of acute hepatitis A virus (HAV) during pregnancy is less than 1 in 1,000. Hepatitis A virus infection is acquired primarily by the fecal–oral route, either by person-to-person contact or ingestion of contaminated food or water. Most U.S. cases of HAV result from person-to-person transmission during community-wide outbreaks (19). Children have asymptomatic or unrecognized infections and therefore play an important role in HAV transmission by serving as a source of infection for others (20). Postexposure prophylaxis with immune globulin is indicated for household or other intimate contacts of a person with serologically (immunoglobulin [Ig] M anti-HAV) confirmed HAV and can be administered during pregnancy. Inactivated HAV vaccines are recommended for children older than 2 years in communities where HAV is endemic and among persons traveling to a developing country. Although not studied during pregnancy, the theoretical risk of this inactivated vaccine to the developing fetus is low, and the vaccine is not contraindicated in pregnancy. For this reason, the initiation of postexposure HAV vaccination should be considered in conjunction with immune globulin.

> **Box 25**
>
> ### Recommendations for Prevention and Treatment of Hyperemesis Gravidarum
>
> - Periconceptional multivitamin use may decrease the severity of nausea and vomiting of pregnancy.
> - Taking vitamin B_6 or vitamin B_6 plus doxylamine is safe and effective and should be considered first-line pharmacotherapy.
> - In patients with hyperemesis gravidarum who also have suppressed thyrotropin levels, treatment of hyperthyroidism should not be undertaken without evidence of intrinsic thyroid disease (including goiter or thyroid autoantibodies).
> - Treatment of nausea and vomiting of pregnancy with ginger has shown beneficial effects and can be considered as a nonpharmacologic option.
> - In refractory cases of nausea and vomiting of pregnancy, antihistamine H_1 receptor blockers, phenothiazines, and benzamides have been shown to be safe and efficacious in pregnancy.
> - Early treatment of nausea and vomiting of pregnancy is recommended to prevent progression to hyperemesis gravidarum.
> - Intravenous hydration should be used for the patient who cannot tolerate oral liquids for a prolonged period or if clinical signs of dehydration are present. Correction of ketosis and vitamin deficiency should be strongly considered. Dextrose and vitamins, especially thiamine, should be included in the therapy when prolonged vomiting is present.
> - Enteral or parenteral nutrition should be initiated for any patient who cannot maintain her weight because of vomiting.
> - Treatment of severe nausea and vomiting of pregnancy or hyperemesis gravidarum with methylprednisolone may be efficacious in refractory cases; however, the risk profile of methylprednisolone suggests it should be a treatment of last resort.

The usual clinical manifestations of HAV include fever, malaise, anorexia, nausea, abdominal discomfort, dark urine, and jaundice. Symptoms occur in more than 70% of infected adults. The diagnosis is confirmed by identifying IgM-specific antibody in the serum.

Serious complications of HAV infection are uncommon. A chronic carrier state does not exist, and perinatal transmission of the virus does not occur.

Hepatitis B Virus

Hepatitis B virus (HBV) infection is caused by a small DNA virus and accounts for 40% of all cases of hepatitis in the United States. Acute HBV infection occurs in 1–2 of 1,000 pregnancies, and chronic HBV infection occurs in 5–15 of 1,000 pregnancies.

Hepatitis B virus is transmitted efficiently by percutaneous or mucous membrane exposure to infectious body fluids. Sexual transmission among adults accounts for most HBV infections in the United States. In the 1990s, transmission among heterosexual partners accounted for 40% of infections, and transmission among men who have sex with men accounted for another 15% of infections. The most common risk factors include having multiple sex partners or a recent history of a sexually transmitted disease. Pregnant women who test negative for hepatitis B surface antigen (HbsAg), seek sexually transmitted disease treatment, and have not previously been vaccinated should receive HBV vaccine because pregnancy is not a contraindication to vaccination (21).

In adults, 50% of HBV infections are symptomatic, and about 1% of cases result in acute liver failure and death. In the acute stage of HBV infection, the diagnosis is confirmed by identification of HBsAg and IgM antibody to the core antigen. The presence of hepatitis B envelope antigen indicates an exceptionally high viral inoculum and active virus replication. No specific therapy is available for women with acute HBV infection. Risk of chronic infection is associated with age at infection: about 90% of infected infants, 60% of children older than 5 years, and 2–6% of adults become chronically infected. Chronic HBV infection is characterized by the persistence of HBsAg in the liver and serum. An estimated 1.25 million people are chronically infected with HBV. Among persons with chronic HBV infection, the risk of death from cirrhosis or hepatocellular carcinoma is 15–20%. Antiviral agents (ie, α-interferon or lamivudine) are available for treatment of women with chronic HBV.

Most cases (more than 90%) of perinatal transmission of HBV occur as a consequence of intrapartum exposure of the infant to maternal blood and genital tract secretions. The remaining cases result from hematogenous transplacental dissemination, breastfeeding, and close postnatal contact between the infant and the infected parent.

Immunoprophylaxis is the principal means of preventing HBV infection in adults and neonates. All pregnant women should be tested for HBsAg, and those who are seronegative should be vaccinated if they have a risk factor for HBV infection during pregnancy (eg, injection drug use, more than one sex partner in the previous 6 months, sex partner who tested positive for HBsAg, or evaluation or treatment for a sexually transmitted infection). Two recombinant vaccines are available. Before vaccination, individuals who have been exposed to HBV recently should initially receive passive immunization with hepatitis B IgG and simultaneously undergo the vaccination series. Hepatitis B IgG should be administered as soon as possible after exposure.

The Centers for Disease Control and Prevention recommends that all neonates be vaccinated for HBV (22). However, infants delivered to seropositive mothers also need to receive passive immunization with hepatitis B Ig.

Hepatitis C Virus

Hepatitis C virus (HCV) is the primary cause of the type of hepatitis previously known as non-A, non-B hepatitis. It is the most common chronic bloodborne infection in the United States; an estimated 3.2 million people are chronically infected. Persons with acute HCV infection are either asymptomatic or have a mild clinical illness. Pregnant women should be tested for anti-HCV only if they have risk factors for infection (eg, injection drug use or human immunodeficiency virus [HIV] infection) (23). Hepatitis C virus infection can be diagnosed by detecting either anti-HCV (enzyme immunoassay plus a supplemental antibody test—ie, recombinant immunoblot assay) or HCV RNA (by reverse transcription–polymerase chain reaction test). Chronic infection is common (75–85%), and 60–70% of infected persons have evidence of active liver disease (elevated transaminase levels). Although antibodies are produced, no protective antibody response has been identified after HCV infection. Antiviral therapy includes the use of pegylated interferon alone or in combination with oral ribavirin for a duration of 6–12 months (21).

Hepatitis C virus is most efficiently transmitted by direct percutaneous exposure to infected blood (eg, sharing needles). Although less efficient, perinatal and sexual exposures (1.5% prevalence in susceptible long-term spouses) can result in transmission. Perinatal transmission appears to be low (approximately 4%). This is more likely to occur in women with high titers of HCV RNA or who are coinfected with HIV (23). A problem with HCV infections in pregnancy is the variability in the level of viremia in pregnancy—a mother can have negative results at one stage and positive results at different times. There is a definite correlation with level of viremia (measured by quantitative polymerase chain reaction methods) and transmission. Infants born to mothers with HCV infection should be tested 2–4 months after birth at the earliest, and testing is most effective 12–18 months after birth. Therapy has been targeted to the pediatric group and not in pregnancy. Treatment of HCV infection with interferon monotherapy results in only 10–20% clearance of virus. Recent combined use of pegylated interferon and oral ribavirin has resulted in successful therapy in up to 50–80% of patients, depending on genotypes. Despite encouraging results in the nonpregnant patients, the use of antiviral agents to decrease viremia in pregnancy has not been studied. Because IgG does not protect against infection, postexposure prophylaxis for exposed women and immunoprophylaxis for the neonate are not available. There is no available vaccine against HCV infection.

Prevention and Screening

The HAV vaccine is available as both a single-antigen vaccine and as a combination vaccine (containing both HAV and HBV antigens). Both vaccines use inactivated HAV, and the HBV component is a recombinant protein nonviral antigen. There are two HAV vaccines available that are given in two doses, either 6–12 months apart or 6–18 months apart.

Two single antigen vaccines for HBV have been developed. Currently available vaccines are prepared from yeast cultures by using recombinant DNA technology. They are highly immunogenic and result in seroconversion in more than 95% of recipients.

There is one combination vaccine available for adults at risk of both HAV and HBV infection; it contains recombinant HBsAg and inactivated HAV. The dosage of the HAV component in the combination vaccine is lower than that in the single-antigen HAV vaccine, allowing it to be administered in a three-dose schedule (0 months, 1 month, and 6 months) instead of the two-dose schedule used for the single-antigen vaccine. An accelerated schedule (0 days, 7 days, and 21–30 days, followed by a booster dose at 12 months) is an option when a rapid immune response is needed for an occupational or behavioral imminent risk for HAV and HBV infection or for international travel (23, 24).

Screening in pregnancy is limited to surface antigen presence. If hepatitis B surface antibody is present in the absence of antibodies to HBcAg, it is a marker of vaccination. The presence of HBsAb and the antibodies hepatitis B core antigen are markers of natural immunity. Hepatitis B surface antibodies are rarely found concurrent with HBsAg. Time of infection and age of individuals are important when assessing for potential of chronic carrier status. Infants have a 90% risk of chronic infection, whereas young children only have a 25% risk. Chronic infections are associated with increased mortality from cirrhosis and liver cancer. To potentially decrease the transfer of HBV infections to the newborn, the use of lamivudine in the last month of pregnancy has been suggested. Lamivudine, given in doses of 100 mg daily beginning at 32 weeks of gestation, has been suggested to decrease the incidence of vertical transmission of HBV. Extensive data in this area is lacking, but the use of these drugs should be considered and literature experience consulted (25).

Patients with acute hepatitis in pregnancy who also have encephalopathy, coagulopathy, or severe debilitation should be hospitalized. Treatment should be symptomatic and address nutrition, fluid, and electrolyte imbalances and coagulopathy directed at specific deficiencies. Less ill individuals may be treated on an outpatient basis with decreased levels of activity and vaccination of household members and sexual partners.

References

1. Germain AM, Carvajal JA, Glasinovic JC, Kato CS, Williamson C. Intrahepatic cholestasis of pregnancy: an intriguing pregnancy-specific disorder. J Soc Gynecol Investig 2002;9:10–4.

2. Lammert F, Marschall HU, Glantz A, Matern S. Intrahepatic cholestasis of pregnancy: molecular pathogenesis, diagnosis and management. J Hepatol 2000;33:1012–21.

3. Walker IA, Nelson-Piercy C, Williamson C. Role of bile acid measurement in pregnancy. Ann Clin Biochem 2002;39:105–13.

4. Fagan EA. Intrahepatic cholestasis of pregnancy. Clin Liver Dis 1999;3:603–32.

5. Alsulyman OM, Ouzounian JG, Ames-Castro M, Goodwin TM. Intrahepatic cholestasis of pregnancy: perinatal outcome associated with expectant management. Am J Obstet Gynecol 1996;175:957–60.

6. Davies MH, da Silva RC, Jones SR, Weaver JB, Elias E. Fetal mortality associated with cholestasis of pregnancy and the potential benefit of therapy with ursodeoxycholic acid. Gut 1995;37:580–4.

7. Mullally BA, Hansen WF. Intrahepatic cholestasis of pregnancy: review of the literature. Obstet Gynecol Surv 2002;57:47–52.

8. Burrows R, Clavisi O, Burrows E. Interventions for treating cholestasis in pregnancy. Cochrane Database of Systematic Reviews 2001, Issue 4. Art. No.: CD000493. DOI: 10.1002/14651858.CD000493; 10.1002/14651858. CD000493.

9. Cappell MS. Hepatic disorders severely affected by pregnancy: medical and obstetric management. Med Clin North Am 2008;92:739,60, vii–viii.

10. Ibdah JA, Yang Z, Bennett MJ. Liver disease in pregnancy and fetal fatty acid oxidation defects. Mol Genet Metab 2000;71:182–9.

11. Ibdah JA, Bennett MJ, Rinaldo P, Zhao Y, Gibson B, Sims HF, et al. A fetal fatty-acid oxidation disorder as a cause of liver disease in pregnant women. N Engl J Med 1999;340:1723–31.

12. Strauss AW, Bennett MJ, Rinaldo P, Sims HF, O'Brien LK, Zhao Y, et al. Inherited long-chain 3-hydroxyacyl-CoA dehydrogenase deficiency and a fetal-maternal interaction cause maternal liver disease and other pregnancy complications. Semin Perinatol 1999;23:100–12.

13. Treem WR. Mitochondrial fatty acid oxidation and acute fatty liver of pregnancy. Semin Gastrointest Dis 2002;13:55–66.

14. Kane S. Inflammatory bowel disease in pregnancy. Gastroenterol Clin North Am 2003;32:323–40.

15. Katz JA, Antoni C, Keenan GF, Smith DE, Jacobs SJ, Lichtenstein GR. Outcome of pregnancy in women receiving infliximab for the treatment of Crohn's disease and rheumatoid arthritis. Am J Gastroenterol 2004;99:2385–92.

16. Polifka JE, Friedman JM. Teratogen update: azathioprine and 6-mercaptopurine. Teratology 2002;65:240–61.

17. Jewell D, Young G. Interventions for nausea and vomiting in early pregnancy. Cochrane Database of Systematic Reviews 2003, Issue 4. Art. No.: CD000145. DOI: 10.1002/14651858.CD000145; 10.1002/14651858.CD000145.

18. Gazmararian JA, Petersen R, Jamieson DJ, Schild L, Adams MM, Deshpande AD, et al. Hospitalizations during pregnancy among managed care enrollees. Obstet Gynecol 2002;100:94–100.

19. Fiore AE, Wasley A, Bell BP. Prevention of hepatitis A through active or passive immunization: recommedations of the Advisory Committee on Immunization Practices (ACIP). Advisory Committee on Immunization Practices. MMWR Recomm Rep 2006;55:1–23.

20. Staes CJ, Schlenker TL, Risk I, Cannon KG, Harris H, Pavia AT, et al. Sources of infection among persons with acute hepatitis A and no identified risk factors during a sustained community-wide outbreak. Pediatrics 2000;106:E54.

21. Workowski KA, Berman SM. Sexually transmitted diseases treatment guidelines, 2006. Centers for Disease Control and Prevention [published erratum appears in MMWR Morb Mortal Wkly Rep 2006;55:997]. MMWR Recomm Rep 2006;55:1–94.

22. Updated U.S. Public Health Service Guidelines for the Management of Occupational Exposures to HBV, HCV, and HIV and Recommendations for Postexposure Prophylaxis. U.S. Public Health Service. MMWR Recomm Rep 2001;50:1–52.

23. Viral hepatitis in pregnancy. ACOG Practice Bulletin No. 86. American College of Obstetricians and Gynecologists. Obstet Gynecol 2007;110:941–56.

24. Connor BA, Blatter MM, Beran J, Zou B, Trofa AF. Rapid and sustained immune response against hepatitis A and B achieved with combined vaccine using an accelerated administration schedule. J Travel Med 2007;14:9–15.

25. Gambarin-Gelwan M. Hepatitis B in pregnancy. Clin Liver Dis 2007;11:945,63,x.

Neurologic Diseases

Thomas C. Peng

Seizure Disorders

Seizure disorders affect between 0.5% and 2% of the population and are the most common neurologic problem in pregnancy. Approximately 75% of these disorders are idiopathic, generally classified as generalized tonic–clonic seizures, partial complex seizures that may or may not become generalized, and absence seizures (petit mal). Controversy exists about the effects of seizure disorders on pregnancy, the effects of pregnancy on seizure disorders, and the antiepileptic drugs used to treat these disorders.

Studies have shown that control of seizure disorders may deteriorate during pregnancy, and up to 25% of women with epilepsy will experience an increase in frequency (1). Factors that contribute to increased seizures include lower antiepileptic drug levels. If drug levels are monitored at regular intervals and dosages adjusted accordingly, seizure control can be maintained throughout pregnancy (2). Drug levels may fluctuate in pregnancy owing to a variety of factors. For example, gastrointestinal absorption is reduced and is often erratic as a result of progestational effects on bowel motility. Hepatic microsomal enzyme metabolism of many drugs increases during pregnancy. The large increase in glomerular filtration rate during pregnancy enhances the clearance of drugs that are eliminated by the kidneys. Monitoring free drug levels, which may increase in pregnancy because albumin levels are decreased, is recommended for the use of phenobarbital, phenytoin, carbamazepine, valproic acid, and primidone. Some experts recommend monthly monitoring of the use of lamotrigine because its clearance is markedly increased in pregnancy. Measuring the serum trough level of antiepileptic drugs has been recommended (3).

The underlying risk of fetal malformations is believed to be increased in women with untreated seizure disorders. Results from one study challenge this notion, documenting a rate of congenital anomalies that was similar among pregnant women with epilepsy but not exposed to antiepileptic drugs during the first trimester of pregnancy (0 of 98) and pregnant women without epilepsy and without exposure to antiepileptic drugs (9 of 508) (4). This study and others also demonstrated that compared with monotherapy, polytherapy with multiple antiepileptic drugs further increases the risk of fetal anomaly (4).

Although evidence that antiepileptic drugs are teratogenic is not conclusive, most studies suggest that the use of all antiepileptic drugs is associated with major congenital malformations at a twofold to threefold higher rate than in the general population (4, 5). Use of the older antiepileptic drugs has been associated with a variety of anomalies, including neural tube defects associated with the use of valproate; oral clefts and cardiac defects with the use of phenobarbital, carbamazepine, and valproate; and facial and digital dysmorphology with the use of phenytoin and carbamazepine. The teratogenic effects of the use of the newer antiepileptic drugs lamotrigine, gabapentin, topiramate, felbamate, oxcarbazepine, and levetiracetam are not yet defined. Preliminary reports of lamotrigine use by 200 pregnant women suggest that when used as monotherapy, the risk of major malformations may be as low as 2% (5). Gabapentin may be more commonly prescribed, with its low side-effect profile. It is well absorbed, neither protein bound nor metabolized, and is renally excreted.

Although the mechanisms of teratogenesis are unknown, two possibilities relate to the higher levels of free radical arene oxide metabolites and antifolate effects. Phenytoin, carbamazepine, and phenobarbital are metabolized to oxidative intermediates, which are inactivated by epoxide hydrolase. In pregnant women treated with antiepileptic drugs, fetuses with lower epoxide hydrolase activity as measured in amniotic fluid had an increased risk of congenital anomalies. The use of valproate, which is associated with fetal neural tube defects, inhibits epoxide hydrolase activity. This may explain in part the higher rates of major congenital anomalies in fetuses exposed to valproate in the first trimester when it is added to any other antiepileptic drugs in a polytherapy regimen and possibly when it is used as monotherapy. Therefore, avoidance of valproate as monotherapy and antiepileptic drug polytherapy in the first trimester should be considered to decrease the risk of major congenital malformations (6). Lower folic acid levels noted with antiepileptic drug treatment may contribute to the risk of anomalies. Folic acid supplementation of 1–4 mg per day is recommended, though the optimal dosage is unknown.

Preconception consultation with a neurologist is recommended to determine if patients treated with antiepileptic drugs can stop the use of antiepileptic drugs or, if they are receiving polytherapy, can reduce therapy to a single agent. In the second trimester, maternal biochemical testing such as maternal serum alpha-fetoprotein measurement, detailed fetal ultrasonography, and possibly amniocentesis to define risk of anomalies should be considered. A general recommendation to stop antiepileptic drug treatment is not appropriate if the risk of seizures is significant because the attendant complications (eg, status epilepticus and hazards of seizures with normal activity, including driving) can have serious effects on both the mother and fetus.

In the third trimester, oral vitamin K supplementation (10 mg or 20 mg daily) has been advocated by some experts because antiepileptic drugs are associated with a reduction in fetal vitamin K levels. Reduction in vitamin K–dependent coagulation factors may contribute to early hemorrhagic disease of the newborn. This recommendation remains controversial because study results have documented conflicting results as to whether maternal supplementation decreases the risk of early hemorrhagic disease. However, parenteral administration of vitamin K to the neonate is recommended at birth.

Myasthenia Gravis

Myasthenia gravis is an autoimmune neuromuscular disorder characterized pathologically by an immunologically mediated reduction of acetylcholine receptors at the neuromuscular junction in skeletal muscle. Clinically, patients note weakness and easy fatigue with repetitive skeletal muscle use. Respiratory muscles may become involved and respiratory difficulties may ensue (myasthenic crisis). Ptosis and diplopia are common presentations. The prevalence is 2–10 per 100,000 people, with women aged 20–30 years affected more often. Its occurrence in pregnancy, then, is not rare. Comanagement with a neurologist is a prudent course of action. In pregnancy, the course of myasthenia gravis is unpredictable, although recent studies confirm that in general, most patients experience either no change or improvement in symptoms (7). Relapse may manifest with worsening ptosis, dyspnea, respiratory difficulties, or other signs of skeletal muscle weakness.

Most patients who have myasthenia gravis are treated with an oral anticholinesterase drug such as pyridostigmine, a category C drug with no known adverse fetal effects. Other treatment options include thymectomy and the use of prednisone and other immunosuppressive drugs, such as azathioprine, cyclosporine, and, rarely, plasmapheresis. The need for the use of anticholinesterase drugs may increase during labor and delivery. Patients may experience respiratory difficulty or fatigue in the second stage of labor and may benefit from an assisted second stage. In this context, anticholinesterase drugs are best administered parenterally in the form of neostigmine because of poor oral absorption of pyridostigmine during labor. The conversion of an oral to intravenous dose is approximately 60 mg oral pyridostigmine to 0.5 mg intravenous neostigmine.

Consultation with an obstetric anesthesiologist before labor should be considered because of interactions between commonly used anesthetic agents and myasthenia. For example, patients with myasthenia can have prolonged weakness after nondepolarizing muscle relaxants and prolonged duration or increased toxicity from local ester anesthetics (eg, 2-chloroprocaine) metabolized by acetylcholinesterase. The use of these agents should be avoided in patients treated with anticholinesterase agents. For pain control, epidural analgesia should be considered to reduce respiratory requirements and fatigue. Narcotic analgesics (eg, meperidine) may be given, although patients with myasthenia gravis may be more sensitive than others to their respiratory depressant effects. The use of magnesium sulfate is contraindicated because of its effect on neuromuscular transmission. The use of aminoglycosides and several other drugs (eg, propranolol or barbiturates) have been noted to potentially exacerbate muscle weakness and should be used with caution (8).

Rarely, cholinergic crisis may occur as a result of overdosage of anticholinesterase drugs. It may be difficult to distinguish a cholinergic crisis and myasthenic crisis because both are characterized by muscle weakness. With cholinergic crisis, treatment with anticholinesterase drugs is discontinued and the use of atropine is recommended, whereas with myasthenic crisis, more intensive treatment is needed. Administration of a very short-acting anticholinesterase agent, such as edrophonium, may differentiate, with improvement in symptoms suggestive of inadequate anticholinesterase therapy and deterioration suggestive of too much therapy.

Transient neonatal myasthenia gravis is likely the result of transplacental passage of maternal antibodies directed against the acetylcholine receptor and may occur in up to 50% of newborns of women with myasthenia gravis (7). Its occurrence has not been associated with either severity of maternal disease or titer of maternal acetylcholine receptor antibodies. Clinical presentation usually occurs within the first week of life, with difficulties in sucking, swallowing, or respiration.

Multiple Sclerosis

Multiple sclerosis, the cause of which remains unknown, has no adverse effect on pregnancy, and pregnancy has no detrimental effect on multiple sclerosis. Clinically, symptoms include diplopia, transient blindness or eye pain (optic neuritis), weakness, spasticity, ataxia, tremor, dysarthria, and bladder dysfunction. No specific cure is available.

Treatment includes the use of medication (eg, corticosteroids) to diminish severity of an acute flare, the use of medications to address specific symptoms (eg, amitriptyline for neurogenic pain), and the use of newer agents to reduce the risk of recurrence. Currently, these newer agents include interferon β-1a and interferon β-1b and glatiramer. Experience with the use of these medications is insufficient to detail their risk to pregnancy or the fetus, but anecdotal reports suggest that the risk is small. During pregnancy, the rate of relapse decreases, with the greatest reduction in the third trimester. Conversely, relapse increases twofold in the first 3–6 months postpartum.

The course of disease is unpredictable, though certain factors, such as progressive disease from onset, motor and cerebellar signs, and an abnormal result on magnetic resonance imaging of the head, are associated with a poor prognosis, whereas complete recovery after the initial attack, dominant sensory symptoms, and absence of recurrence after 5 years are associated with a favorable prognosis.

Paraplegia and Quadriplegia

Patients with spinal cord injuries are able to become pregnant and give birth without major complications. In results of research, in general, pregnancy complications for patients with quadriplegia or paraplegia do not appear to increase except for urinary tract infections, pressure ulcers, and autonomic hyperreflexia. Urinary tract infections are more common in some patients because of an indwelling catheter. Cesarean deliveries also have been reported at a higher rate. Similar recommendations apply to patients who have spina bifida as to those with traumatic paralytic injuries, given comparable locations of the lesion.

Patients with traumatic spinal cord injury at T-5 vertebra spinal level or higher are at risk for autonomic hyperreflexia syndrome because central regulation of the sympathetic nervous system below the level of the lesion is lost. This syndrome is characterized by acute onset of headache, nasal congestion, upper thorax cutaneous vasodilation, flushing and blotching, hypertension, and reflex bradycardia. Blood pressures can reach malignant levels, leading to myocardial infarction and stroke. Any noxious stimuli to the nervous system below the level of the injury, such as labor, delivery, cervical examinations, and cystitis, have the potential to precipitate this syndrome. Before labor and delivery, consultation with an anesthesiologist is recommended. Epidural anesthesia has been advocated and appears to prevent the autonomic hyperreflexia syndrome in labor and delivery (9).

A concern in patients with quadriplegia or paraplegia (T-10 injury or higher) is the lack of sensation below the spinal cord injury and the inability to perceive uterine contractions. In the second and third trimesters, patients can be taught to palpate for uterine contractions or, if this is not possible, to use a home uterine contraction monitoring device. In the third trimester, examination of the cervix at each visit may be helpful. Cesarean delivery is reserved for obstetric indications. Vaginal delivery should be anticipated with a passive second stage of labor; the use of forceps or vacuum extraction may be necessary.

Cerebrovascular Disease

Cerebral infarction and transient ischemic attacks are rare in young women but are increased up to 13-fold in pregnancy and the postpartum period. An analysis from a large population data, the Nationwide Inpatient Sample, of approximately 9 million pregnancy related discharges between 2000 and 2001, noted discharge codes of stroke in 2,850 women, for an incidence of approximately 34 strokes per 100,000 discharges (10). The types of stroke identified included ischemic (27%), hemorrhagic (25%), cerebral venous thrombosis (2%), and pregnancy related (46%). Stroke occurred antepartum in 11%, around the time of delivery in 41% and postpartum in 48%. Risk may be highest in the postpartum period (11). Risk factors that have been identified as associated with an increased risk of stroke in pregnancy include advanced maternal age, African American race, migraine headaches, heart disease (eg, cardiomyopathy, atrial fibrillation, paradoxical embolus from venous thrombus, and endocarditis), sickle cell disease, hypertension, diabetes mellitus, substance use, smoking, anemia, and thrombocytopenia. Preeclampsia, gestational hypertension, and eclampsia are foremost among pregnancy-related complications that increase the risk of stroke (10). The etiology is unknown but is perhaps related to the hypercoagulable state of pregnancy. Atherosclerosis is responsible for less than 25% of cases during pregnancy. The diagnosis of cerebral infarction may be confirmed by magnetic resonance imaging and computed tomography. Evaluation should further include electrocardiography, echocardiography, thrombophilic assessment, prothrombin and partial thromboplastin time measurements, complete blood count, serum cholesterol and triglyceride measurements, and assessment of carotid arteries. It is unclear as to which thrombophilic factors increase the risk of stroke. Results of case–control studies of stroke in men and nonpregnant women found similar rates of thrombophilia (deficiency of protein C, protein S, antithrombin III, or factor V Leiden mutation or prothrombin *G20210A* mutation) in cases with stroke and controls without stroke (12). Evaluation for antiphospholipid antibodies and homocysteine level are reasonable because these factors that have been associated with an increased risk of stroke in some studies (13, 14) but not all (15). The recurrence risk of ischemic or occlusive cerebrovascular disease has been estimated in the 1–2% range for a subsequent pregnancy (16) whereas results from another study of 23 women indicated no recurrence (17). No consensus exists on therapy to reduce the risk of recurrent stroke. A published guideline offers the following recommendations (18):

1. For pregnant women with ischemic stroke or transient ischemic attack and high-risk thromboembolic conditions, such as known coagulopathy or mechanical heart valves, the following options may be considered: the use of adjusted-dose unfractionated heparin throughout pregnancy; the use of adjusted-dose low molecular weight heparin; or the use of unfractionated heparin or low molecular weight heparin until the 13th week of gestation, followed by the use of warfarin until the middle of the third trimester, when the use of unfractionated heparin or low molecular weight heparin is then reinstituted until delivery.

2. Pregnant women with lower-risk conditions may be considered for treatment with unfractionated heparin or low molecular weight heparin in the first trimester, followed by the use of low-dose aspirin for the remainder of pregnancy.

Vaginal delivery, unless obstetrically contraindicated, is preferable to cesarean delivery. Patients who present with severe acute headaches with or without other neurologic signs, such as mental status changes, seizures, cranial nerve abnormalities, and deficit in motor control of the extremities, are suspect for subarachnoid hemorrhage and intracranial venous thrombosis. Intracranial venous thrombosis is a rare complication, generally diagnosed with magnetic resonance angiography and computed tomography. Treatment is uncertain and prognosis in general is tenuous. Incidence of subarachnoid hemorrhage is 1–5 per 10,000 pregnancies, with a mortality rate of 30–40% (19). Hemorrhage typically occurs antepartum, in the latter half of pregnancy but also can occur postpartum. The two major etiologies of subarachnoid hemorrhage are cerebral vascular aneurysms and arteriovenous malformations, with indistinguishable clinical presentations. Initial evaluation generally depends on imaging such as computed tomography and magnetic resonance imaging. Cerebral angiography is useful in identifying the site of the lesion. After the initial hemorrhage, recurrent bleeding is a major morbidity that increases mortality with each subsequent bleed. Early neurosurgical intervention has been associated with better maternal and fetal outcomes. Some experts suggest that patients with a surgically corrected aneurysm can undergo labor and vaginal delivery. Delivery recommendations for uncorrected aneurysm or arteriovenous malformations are not well defined. Cesarean delivery has been recommended by some experts.

References

1. Liporace J, D'Abreu A. Epilepsy and women's health: family planning, bone health, menopause, and menstrual-related seizures. Mayo Clin Proc 2003;78:497–506.

2. Pennell PB. Antiepileptic drug pharmacokinetics during pregnancy and lactation. Neurology 2003;61:S35–42.

3. Schoenenberger RA, Tanasijevic MJ, Jha A, Bates DW. Appropriateness of antiepileptic drug level monitoring. JAMA 1995;274:1622–6.

4. Holmes LB, Harvey EA, Coull BA, Huntington KB, Khoshbin S, Hayes AM, et al. The teratogenicity of anticonvulsant drugs. N Engl J Med 2001;344:1132–8.

5. Pennell PB. The importance of monotherapy in pregnancy. Neurology 2003;60:S31–8.

6. Harden CL, Meador KJ, Pennell PB, Hauser WA, Gronseth GS, French JA, et al. Management issues for women with epilepsy-Focus on pregnancy (an evidence-based review): II. Teratogenesis and perinatal outcomes: Report of the Quality Standards Subcommittee and Therapeutics and Technology Subcommittee of the American Academy of Neurology and the American Epilepsy Society. American Academy of Neurology; American Epilepsy Society. Epilepsia 2009;50:1237–46.

7. Batocchi AP, Majolini L, Evoli A, Lino MM, Minisci C, Tonali P. Course and treatment of myasthenia gravis during pregnancy. Neurology 1999;52:447–52.

8. Porter TF, Branch DW. Autoimmune diseases. In: James DK, Steer PJ, Weiner CP, Gonik B, editors. High risk pregnancy:

managment options. 3rd ed. Philadelphia (PA): Saunders/Elsevier; 2006. p. 949–85.

9. Hambly PR, Martin B. Anaesthesia for chronic spinal cord lesions. Anaesthesia 1998;53:273–89.

10. James AH, Bushnell CD, Jamison MG, Myers ER. Incidence and risk factors for stroke in pregnancy and the puerperium. Obstet Gynecol 2005;106:509–16.

11. Kittner SJ, Stern BJ, Feeser BR, Hebel R, Nagey DA, Buchholz DW, et al. Pregnancy and the risk of stroke. N Engl J Med 1996;335:768–74.

12. Hankey GJ, Eikelboom JW, van Bockxmeer FM, Lofthouse E, Staples N, Baker RI. Inherited thrombophilia in ischemic stroke and its pathogenic subtypes. Stroke 2001;32:1793–9.

13. Finazzi G, Brancaccio V, Moia M, Ciaverella N, Mazzucconi MG, Schinco PC, et al. Natural history and risk factors for thrombosis in 360 patients with antiphospholipid antibodies: a four-year prospective study from the Italian Registry. Am J Med 1996;100:530–6.

14. Moller J, Nielsen GM, Tvedegaard KC, Andersen NT, Jorgensen PE. A meta-analysis of cerebrovascular disease and hyperhomocysteinaemia. Scand J Clin Lab Invest 2000; 60:491–9.

15. Rahemtullah A, Van Cott EM. Hypercoagulation testing in ischemic stroke. Arch Pathol Lab Med 2007;131:890–901.

16. Lamy C, Hamon JB, Coste J, Mas JL. Ischemic stroke in young women: risk of recurrence during subsequent pregnancies. French Study Group on Stroke in Pregnancy. Neurology 2000;55:269–74.

17. Coppage KH, Hinton AC, Moldenhauer J, Kovilam O, Barton JR, Sibai BM. Maternal and perinatal outcome in women with a history of stroke. Am J Obstet Gynecol 2004;190:1331–4.

18. Sacco RL, Adams R, Albers G, Alberts MJ, Benavente O, Furie K, et al. Guidelines for prevention of stroke in patients with ischemic stroke or transient ischemic attack: a statement for healthcare professionals from the American Heart Association/American Stroke Association Council on Stroke: co-sponsored by the Council on Cardiovascular Radiology and Intervention: the American Academy of Neurology affirms the value of this guideline. American Heart Association/American Stroke Association Council on Stroke; Council on Cardiovascular Radiology and Intervention; American Academy of Neurology. Circulation 2006;113:e409–49.

19. Fox MW, Harms RW, Davis DH. Selected neurologic complications of pregnancy. Mayo Clin Proc 1990;65:1595–618.

Diabetes Mellitus

Donald R. Coustan

Preexisting Diabetes Mellitus

Preexisting diabetes mellitus complicates approximately 0.1–0.3% of pregnancies in the United States. Perinatal mortality associated with diabetes mellitus has declined from approximately 65% before the discovery of insulin to well below 5% at present. The most significant remaining cause of perinatal death among women with diabetes mellitus is congenital malformation. The dramatic improvement in survival rates has resulted in part from general advances in perinatal care but particularly from the development of a team approach to the management of diabetes mellitus, which stresses maintaining excellent glycemic control during pregnancy.

Preconception Care

The incidence of congenital anomalies is fourfold higher among infants of women with diabetes mellitus than among the general population. Anomalies of the cardiac, renal, vertebral, and central nervous systems arise during the first 8 weeks of gestation, at a time when it is unusual for patients to seek prenatal care. Studies have demonstrated a strong correlation between elevated levels of glucose and ketone bodies (as well as other metabolic aberrations) in the embryonic and preembryonic

milieu and the likelihood of malformations. Furthermore, results from a number of case reviews have demonstrated a reduction in the rate of malformations when improved metabolic control is instituted before or during very early pregnancy. Therefore, the management and counseling of women with diabetes mellitus of reproductive age should begin before conception (1). In fact, every medical visit for a female of reproductive age with diabetes mellitus should be considered a preconception visit.

Ideally, metabolic control should be at optimal levels before conception. Many authorities suggest delaying conception until glycosylated hemoglobin levels have remained in the normal or near-normal range for at least 3 months. A thorough medical history, physical examination, and laboratory evaluation should be undertaken to determine the presence or absence of vascular disease and other potentially complicating factors. Appropriate contraceptive advice should be given so that women with diabetes mellitus can plan their pregnancies. Women with diabetes mellitus, like other women considering pregnancy, should be counseled to ingest at least 400 mg of folic acid daily before conception and in early pregnancy to lower the likelihood of neural tube defects in their offspring. Preconception care of women with diabetes mellitus is cost-effective in terms of preventing many of the complications of diabetes mellitus during pregnancy.

Self-Monitoring of Blood Glucose

Self-monitoring of blood glucose, along with intensive therapy, has made maintenance of near-normal glycemia a therapeutic reality for pregnant women with diabetes mellitus. Patients are instructed to monitor their ambient glucose levels frequently throughout the day by using reagent strips impregnated with glucose oxidase and a portable reflectance meter or similar system. Some diabetes mellitus care centers suggest fasting and preprandial measurements; others use fasting and 1-hour or 2-hour postprandial or peak postprandial testing. In results from a randomized trial of women with severe gestational diabetes mellitus, as well as two descriptive studies of pregnancies in women with preexisting diabetes mellitus, postprandial glucose measurements were more predictive than preprandial monitoring of certain adverse outcomes among infants of mothers with diabetes mellitus (2–4). Target glucose values are fasting levels of 60–90 mg/dL and 1-hour postprandial values below 130–140 mg/dL or 2-hour postprandial values below 120 mg/dL. All patients with type 1 diabetes mellitus and their families should be instructed in the use of glucagon to treat severe hypoglycemia.

Insulin, Oral Agents, and Diet Therapy

In most pregnant women with diabetes mellitus, the condition can be managed successfully with an insulin regimen consisting of multiple injections of mixtures of short-acting and intermediate-acting insulin timed to maintain blood glucose in the desired range. The second-generation oral agent glyburide was initially shown not to cross the placenta substantially at term in results from early in vitro and in vivo studies and has been demonstrated to be similarly effective to insulin in treating gestational diabetes mellitus in a single randomized trial, but little information is available regarding the use of oral antidiabetes agents in early to midpregnancy for treating preexisting diabetes mellitus (5, 6). However, a 2009 report from the National Institutes of Health-sponsored Obstetric–Fetal Pharmacology Research Unit Network, of a study using a particularly sensitive assay technique, demonstrated that umbilical cord glyburide levels averaged 70% of maternal levels at the time of delivery (7). This report raises concerns about the use of glyburide in pregnancy because this drug is an insulin secretogogue, and it would not be advantageous to increase fetal insulin secretion. Although none of the studies of the use of glyburide to date have reported adverse fetal effects, questions regarding the safety of use of this medication in pregnancy remain unanswered. Metformin is increasingly useful in treating insulin resistance syndrome, enhancing the likelihood of conception.

A number of case series have been published to describe its use at various times in pregnancy. Because this agent can cross the placenta, leading to fetal levels that exceed maternal levels and acts as an insulin sensitizer in addition to suppressing hepatic insulin production, it might be expected to enhance the effects of fetal hyperinsulinemia (8). Because of this theoretic possibility and a lack of well-controlled animal or human studies, women with diabetes mellitus who conceive while taking oral agents should be switched to insulin during pregnancy.

Diet is critical to successful regulation of maternal diabetes mellitus. Most diets include 30–35 kcal/kg of ideal body weight, with a high protein intake (90–125 g) and the addition of snacks between meals. The protein content may need to be reduced when diabetic nephropathy is present. Flexibility in the diet regimen is necessary to suit the patient's preferences and activity schedule.

Fetal Surveillance

Early ultrasound examination to confirm the gestational age of the fetus is suggested for women with diabetes mellitus. In an attempt to detect neural tube defects and other anomalies, various screening tests have been devised. Integrated screening, consisting of first-trimester serum and ultrasound evaluation of nuchal translucency combined with a determination of maternal serum alpha-fetoprotein levels and other serum markers measured at 16–20 weeks of gestation appears to be the most efficient approach. Women with diabetes mellitus also should be offered an ultrasound study at 18–20 weeks of gestation to detect fetal malformations. Because maternal serum alpha-fetoprotein values may be lower in pregnancies of women with diabetes mellitus, interpretations may need to be altered accordingly. Repeated ultrasound examinations at monthly intervals between 28 weeks of gestation and delivery are useful in establishing the pattern of fetal growth and changes in amniotic fluid volume.

Programs of fetal surveillance should be initiated in the third trimester, when the risk of fetal death appears to be greatest. The severity of the diabetes mellitus and the presence of other complicating factors (eg, nephropathy, hypertension, fetal growth disturbance, and poor or undocumented metabolic control) should determine the need for and frequency of fetal testing. Antenatal testing should be performed at least weekly and more often if complicating factors are present. The primary benefit of normal test results is reassurance for the physician and the patient that the pregnancy can continue, thus allowing further fetal maturation. For women with severe vascular disease, testing often is initiated at the time of potential extrauterine viability, whereas surveillance may be delayed until as late as 35 weeks of gestation when the diabetes mellitus is well controlled and the pregnancy is otherwise uncomplicated. The nonstress test, oxytocin challenge test, biophysical profile, and maternal assessment of fetal activity are all accepted methods of fetal evaluation.

Timing and Route of Delivery

Improved fetal surveillance and better metabolic management of diabetes mellitus have reduced the likelihood of unexplained fetal death in late pregnancy. As a result, scheduling elective preterm delivery for patients with diabetes mellitus is no longer routine, although the rate of elective intervention at 38 weeks of gestation or beyond continues to be higher than the rate for women without complications from diabetes mellitus. Before elective early delivery, amniocentesis should be performed to document fetal pulmonary maturity in patients with poor or undocumented metabolic control or those with fetuses at less than 39 weeks of gestation by accurate dating. Problems, such as hypertension, nephropathy, or altered fetal growth, may necessitate early delivery as soon as fetal maturity can be documented. Occasionally, evidence of fetal or maternal compromise may dictate delivery before fetal lung maturity.

Diabetes mellitus is not an indication for cesarean delivery, but its complications may be. For example, because of the increased likelihood of shoulder dystocia in the vaginal delivery of large infants of women with diabetes mellitus, recommendations have been made for elective cesarean delivery when fetal weight exceeds predetermined limits. Some authorities suggest a fetal weight threshold of 4,000 g; others recommend 4,500 g because the predictive accuracies of various methods of estimating fetal weight are less than optimal (9). A decision analytic model predicted that a policy of elective cesarean delivery for women with diabetes mellitus with fetal weight estimated by ultrasonography at above either 4,000 g or 4,500 g resulted in similar numbers of cesarean deliveries (443–489) and similar total costs (under $1,000,000) needed to prevent one permanent brachial plexus injury (10). These results were much more favorable than those generated using similar policies for pregnant women without diabetes mellitus.

Gestational Diabetes Mellitus

Gestational diabetes mellitus has been defined as glucose intolerance of varying severity diagnosed during pregnancy by glucose tolerance testing. Women with gestational diabetes mellitus should undergo a 75-g, 2-hour oral glucose tolerance test within 6–12 weeks after delivery to determine whether they have diabetes mellitus, prediabetes mellitus (impaired fasting glucose or impaired glucose tolerance), or normal glycemia (Table 22). Adherence currently is less than 60%, and clinicians should encourage postpartum testing (11). If the test shows impaired glucose tolerance or impaired fasting glucose, lifestyle interventions should be recom-

Table 22. Diagnostic Criteria for Diabetes Mellitus in the Nonpregnant State

Test	Diagnostic Levels		
	Diabetes Mellitus*	Prediabetes Mellitus	Normal
Fasting plasma glucose	126 mg/dL or greater	100–125 mg/dL	Less than 100 mg/dL
75 g, 2-hour OGTT	200 mg/dL or greater	140–199 mg/dL	Less than 140 mg/dL

Abbreviation: OGTT indicates oral glucose tolerance test.
*The values indicate provisional diagnosis of diabetes. The diagnosis must be confirmed by further testing. For detailed information, see Diagnosis and classification of diabetes mellitus. American Diabetes Association. Diabetes Care 2009;32(suppl 1):S62-7.

Diagnosis and classification of diabetes mellitus. American Diabetes Association. Diabetes Care 2009;32(suppl 1):S62-7.

mended and diabetes mellitus testing should be repeated annually. If the postpartum glucose tolerance test is normal, then glycemia should be reassessed at least every 3 years (12). Within 10–20 years after delivery, approximately one half of women who had gestational diabetes mellitus will develop type 2 diabetes mellitus. Among certain ethnic groups, women with gestational diabetes mellitus develop type 2 diabetes mellitus at an accelerated rate; up to 50% of Hispanic women will develop the disease within 5 years.

The clinical significance of gestational diabetes mellitus continues to be challenged. The risk of complications, such as fetal macrosomia, traumatic or operative delivery, neonatal hypoglycemia, and jaundice, are all increased in such pregnancies. Childhood and adult obesity, as well as diabetes mellitus, may be increased among offspring of mothers with gestational diabetes mellitus.

Screening and Diagnosis

In 2005, the Australian Carbohydrate Intolerance Study in Pregnant Women, a randomized trial, compared universal screening and treatment of gestational diabetes mellitus with testing and treatment only when considered to be clinically indicated (13). Universal screening and treatment were significantly beneficial. The American College of Obstetricians and Gynecologists and the American Diabetes Association recommendations for screening for gestational diabetes mellitus are similar (12, 14). Traditional risk factors (family history, previous macrosomic infant, poor obstetric history, and glycosuria) identify only 40–60% of cases of gestational diabetes mellitus. Certain factors, such as age younger than 25 years, normal body weight, no first-degree family history of diabetes mellitus, and not being a member of a high-risk ethnic group, place women at lower risk of gestational diabetes mellitus. Therefore, routine blood glucose screening may not be cost-effective in these women. Patients who manifest all of these characteristics may be candidates for selective screening based on obstetric risk factors.

A 50-g, 1-hour oral glucose challenge test has been suggested for screening for diabetes mellitus. This test usually is performed at 24–28 weeks of gestation, although performing the test earlier may be worthwhile when strong risk factors, such as a previous history of gestational diabetes mellitus, are present. A 3-hour oral glucose tolerance test should be performed when the screening test value exceeds a predetermined limit. When a threshold of 140 mg/dL is used for the 50-g, 1-hour challenge test, 14% of individuals will require a 3-hour glucose tolerance test. With a threshold of 130 mg/dL, an additional 10% of cases of gestational diabetes mellitus will be identified, but 23% of patients will be required to undergo the 3-hour diagnostic test.

Normal values for the glucose tolerance test differ from those used in nonpregnant women. Table 23 lists two conversions of the original O'Sullivan criteria. Any two values meeting or exceeding the threshold confirm the diagnosis of gestational diabetes mellitus. Results from a number of studies have demonstrated excess morbidity even when only the lower set of thresholds is exceeded. In 2007, the Fifth International Workshop Conference on Gestational Diabetes affirmed its previous recommendation that the lower of the two sets of thresholds be used. The Hyperglycemia and Adverse Pregnancy Outcomes study in 2008 demonstrated that the relation-

ship between maternal glucose levels and a number of important fetal outcomes is a continuum, implying that the choice of diagnostic criteria is relatively arbitrary (15). An international group currently is working to reach consensus on reasonable thresholds based on their predictive value for adverse pregnancy outcomes.

Treatment

The Australian Carbohydrate Intolerance Study in Pregnant Women, which demonstrated significant benefit from identifying and treating gestational diabetes mellitus, used dietary counseling, self-monitoring of blood glucose, and insulin as needed. This is a standard approach to treatment. Women with gestational diabetes mellitus should be counseled about appropriate diet. The use of oral hypoglycemic agents has been considered contraindicated in pregnancy because the earlier agents, whose mechanism of action is to stimulate pancreatic insulin production and release, cross the placenta. There was concern that they could stimulate the fetal pancreas, exacerbating the problem of fetal hyperinsulinemia. A randomized trial demonstrated no significant difference in neonatal outcome between women with severe gestational diabetes mellitus treated with glyburide, a second-generation sulfonylurea, and those treated with insulin (5). A previous study used isolated single cotyledons in vitro to demonstrate that very little glyburide was transferred across the human placenta (6). Such findings suggest that it might be acceptable to treat gestational diabetes mellitus with specific oral agents,

Table 23. Detection of Gestational Diabetes Mellitus

Test	Plasma Glucose Level (mg/dL)*
50-g, 1-hour screening	130 or 140
O'Sullivan criteria	
National Diabetes Data Group conversion: 100-g oral glucose tolerance test	
Fasting	105
1 hour	190
2 hours	165
3 hours	145
Carpenter conversion: 100-g oral glucose tolerance test	
Fasting	95
1 hour	180
2 hour	155
3 hour	140

*Result is upper limit of normal.

Data from Carpenter MW, Coustan DR. Criteria for screening tests for gestational diabetes. Am J Obstet Gynecol 1982;144:768–73 and Classification and diagnosis of diabetes mellitus and other categories of glucose intolerance. National Diabetes Data Group. Diabetes 1979;28:1039–57.

which would be more comfortable for patients than insulin injections (16). However, as noted earlier in the section in preexisting diabetes mellitus, results from recent studies have demonstrated that glyburide crosses the placenta and reaches the fetus in significant amounts. If it is prescribed for treatment of gestational diabetes mellitus, patients should be informed of the fact that fetal levels are 70% of maternal levels and that potential adverse consequences may be discovered at a later time.

A 2008 randomized trial compared metformin with insulin in treating gestational diabetes mellitus (17). Pregnancy outcomes were similar in the two groups, and there were no apparent adverse neonatal effects of metformin exposure. Predictably, subjects assigned to metformin stated that they would be more likely to choose the same therapy again. Forty-six percent of patients treated with metformin required supplemental insulin. The frequent need for supplemental insulin, coupled with the higher concentrations of metformin in fetal than maternal compartments, appear to have limited the adoption of this form of therapy for gestational diabetes mellitus (8).

The most important intervention in gestational diabetes mellitus is surveillance of maternal blood glucose levels during the third trimester. Circulating glucose should be monitored in the fasting state and postprandially. Most clinicians recommend daily self-monitoring of blood glucose, as described for women with preexisting diabetes mellitus, but the frequency of testing may be reduced for those patients whose circulating glucose levels are well controlled by diet.

The thresholds for initiating insulin therapy are somewhat arbitrary. The potential for perinatal mortality is probably increased, and insulin therapy should be instituted when the goals for metabolic control during pregnancy in women with preexisting diabetes mellitus are exceeded (fasting levels of 60–90 mg/dL and 1-hour postprandial values below 130–140 mg/dL or 2-hour postprandial values below 120 mg/dL). Even lower thresholds may be required to reduce the likelihood of macrosomia.

There are a number of insulin analogs currently available (18). The short-acting insulin analogs, lispro and aspart, each differ from human insulin by a single amino acid substitution, and both are more rapidly absorbed and have a shorter duration of action than regular human insulin. Available data suggest that neither of these analogs crosses the placenta to a meaningful extent, and both are commonly used in pregnancy. The use of long-acting insulin analogs, glargine and detemir, has been reported in small case series. Because the ability of these analogs to cross the placenta has not been well characterized, they are not as commonly used in pregnancy as the short-acting analogs.

For women with gestational diabetes mellitus who are receiving insulin or have hypertension, a history of stillbirth, or other risk factors, fetal evaluation should be instituted in a fashion similar to that described for women with preexisting diabetes mellitus. If glucose levels remain in the desired range throughout pregnancy and other complications are absent, the potential for perinatal mortality probably is not increased. Nevertheless, daily determinations of fetal movement may provide reassurance to the pregnant woman and the clinician and allow the pregnancy to proceed to term. Results from a randomized trial of induction of labor at 38 weeks of gestation versus expectant management revealed similar rates of cesarean delivery (19); however, the number of infants with macrosomia increased with expectant management. There was no statistically significant impact on shoulder dystocia. As with preexisting diabetes mellitus, ultrasound evaluation may be used to help identify macrosomia.

Postpartum, women with gestational diabetes mellitus should be offered a 75-g, 2-hour oral glucose tolerance test. Approximately 5% of these women will receive the diagnosis of type 2 diabetes mellitus, and 34–35% of these women will receive the diagnosis of impaired glucose (20). Women with impaired glucose may reduce progression and diagnosis of type 2 diabetes mellitus through lifestyle modifications (21).

References

1. Kitzmiller JL, Block JM, Brown FM, Catalano PM, Conway DL, Coustan DR, et al. Managing preexisting diabetes for pregnancy: summary of evidence and consensus recommendations for care. Diabetes Care 2008;31:1060–79.

2. Combs CA, Gunderson E, Kitzmiller JL, Gavin LA, Main EK. Relationship of fetal macrosomia to maternal postprandial glucose control during pregnancy. Diabetes Care 1992; 15:1251–7.

3. de Veciana M, Major CA, Morgan MA, Asrat T, Toohey JS, Lien JM, et al. Postprandial versus preprandial blood glucose monitoring in women with gestational diabetes mellitus requiring insulin therapy. N Engl J Med 1995; 333:1237–41.

4. Jovanovic-Peterson L, Peterson CM, Reed GF, Metzger BE, Mills JL, Knopp RH, et al. Maternal postprandial glucose levels and infant birth weight: the Diabetes in Early Pregnancy Study. The National Institute of Child Health and Human Development--Diabetes in Early Pregnancy Study. Am J Obstet Gynecol 1991;164:103–11.

5. Langer O, Conway DL, Berkus MD, Xenakis EM, Gonzales O. A comparison of glyburide and insulin in women with gestational diabetes mellitus. N Engl J Med 2000;343:1134–8.

6. Elliott BD, Langer O, Schenker S, Johnson RF. Insignificant transfer of glyburide occurs across the human placenta. Am J Obstet Gynecol 1991;165:807–12.

7. Hebert MF, Ma X, Naraharisetti SB, Krudys KM, Umans JG, Hankins GD, et al. Are we optimizing gestational diabetes treatment with glyburide? The pharmacologic basis for better clinical practice. Obstetric-Fetal Pharmacology Research Unit Network. Clin Pharmacol Ther 2009;85:607–14.

8. Vanky E, Zahlsen K, Spigset O, Carlsen SM. Placental passage of metformin in women with polycystic ovary syndrome. Fertil Steril 2005;83:1575–8.

9. American College of Obstetricians and Gynecologists. Fetal macrosomia. Practice Bulletin 22. Washington, DC: American College of Obstetricians and Gynecologists; 2000.

10. Rouse DJ, Owen J, Goldenberg RL, Cliver SP. The effectiveness and costs of elective cesarean delivery for fetal macrosomia diagnosed by ultrasound. JAMA 1996; 276:1480–6.

11. Ferrara A, Peng T, Kim C. Trends in postpartum diabetes screening and subsequent diabetes and impaired fasting glucose among women with histories of gestational diabetes mellitus: a report from the Translating Research Into Action for Diabetes (TRIAD) Study. Diabetes Care 2009;32:269–74.

12. Gestational diabetes mellitus. American Diabetes Association. Diabetes Care 2004;27(suppl 1):S88–90.

13. Crowther CA, Hiller JE, Moss JR, McPhee AJ, Jeffries WS, Robinson JS. Effect of treatment of gestational diabetes mellitus on pregnancy outcomes. Australian Carbohydrate Intolerance Study in Pregnant Women (ACHOIS) Trial Group. N Engl J Med 2005;352:2477–86.

14. Gestational diabetes. ACOG Practice Bulletin No. 30. American College of Obstetricians and Gynecologists. Obstet Gynecol 2001;98:525–38.

15. Metzger BE, Lowe LP, Dyer AR, Trimble ER, Chaovarindr U, Coustan DR, et al. Hyperglycemia and adverse pregnancy outcomes. HAPO Study Cooperative Research Group. N Engl J Med 2008;358:1991–2002.

16. Coustan DR. Pharmacological management of gestational diabetes: an overview [published erratum appears in Diabetes Care 2007;30:3154]. Diabetes Care 2007;30(suppl 2): S206–8.

17. Rowan JA, Hague WM, Gao W, Battin MR, Moore MP. MiG Trial Investigators. Metformin versus insulin for the treatment of gestational diabetes. N Engl J Med 2008; 358:2003–15.

18. Brown FM, Jovanovic LB. Insulin therapy. In: Kitzmiller JL, Jovanovic L, Brown F, Coustan DR, Reader DM, editors. Managing preexisting diabetes and pregnancy: technical reviews and consensus recommendations for care. Alexandria (VA): American Diabetes Association; 2008. p. 89–96.

19. Kjos SL, Henry OA, Montoro M, Buchanan TA, Mestman JH. Insulin-requiring diabetes in pregnancy: a randomized trial of active induction of labor and expectant management. Am J Obstet Gynecol 1993;169:611–5.

20. Reinblatt SL, Morin L, Meltzer SJ. The importance of a postpartum 75 g oral glucose tolerance test in women with gestational diabetes. J Obstet Gynaecol Can 2006;28:690–4.

21. Knowler WC, Barrett-Connor E, Fowler SE, Hamman RF, Lachin JM, Walker EA, et al. Reduction in the incidence of type 2 diabetes with lifestyle intervention or metformin. Diabetes Prevention Program Research Group. N Engl J Med 2002;346:393–403.

Thyroid Diseases

Brian M. Casey

The impact of pregnancy on maternal thyroid physiology is substantial. Especially relevant is the intimate relationship between maternal and fetal thyroid function, particularly during the first half of pregnancy. The fetal thyroid gland begins concentrating iodine and synthesizing thyroid hormone after 12 weeks of gestation. Any need for thyroid hormones before this time is accommodated by the mother, and it is during this time that thyroid hormones are most important to fetal brain development. However, significant fetal brain development continues beyond the first trimester, making thyroid hormone important later in gestation. Although overt maternal thyroid failure during the first half of pregnancy has been associated with several pregnancy complications and intellectual impairment in offspring, it is currently less clear whether milder forms of thyroid dysfunction have similar effects on pregnancy and infant outcomes (1).

Hypothyroidism

Overt hypothyroidism complicates between 1 in 1,000 and 3 in 1,000 pregnancies and is characterized by vague, nonspecific signs or symptoms that often are insidious in onset and easily confused with symptoms attributable to pregnancy itself. Initial symptoms include fatigue, constipation, cold intolerance, and muscle cramps. These may progress to insomnia, weight gain, hair loss, voice changes, and intellectual slowness. Women in areas of endemic iodine deficiency or those with chronic autoimmune (Hashimoto) thyroiditis are much more likely to have a goiter. Other signs of hypothyroidism include periorbital edema, dry skin, and prolonged relaxation phase of deep tendon reflexes.

The most common cause of primary hypothyroidism in pregnancy is Hashimoto thyroiditis, painless inflammation with progressive enlargement of the thyroid gland that is characterized by diffuse lymphocytic infiltration, fibrosis, parenchymal atrophy, and eosinophilic change. Other important causes of primary hypothyroidism include endemic iodine deficiency, a history of ablative radioiodine therapy, or thyroidectomy. Secondary hypothyroidism is pituitary in origin. For example, Sheehan syndrome from a history of obstetric hemorrhage is characterized by pituitary ischemia and necrosis with subsequent deficiencies in some or all pituitary hormones. Lymphocytic hypophysitis and hypophysectomy also cause secondary hypothyroidism. Tertiary or hypothalamic hypothyroidism is very rare. Central hypothyroidism refers to inadequate stimulation of the thyroid gland because of a defect at the level of the pituitary or hypothalamus and is characterized by a normal or slightly low thyrotropin level with a low thyroxine (T_4) level.

Women with overt hypothyroidism are at an increased risk of pregnancy complications, such as early pregnancy failure, preeclampsia, placental abruption, infants with low birth weight, and stillbirth. Treatment of women with overt hypothyroidism has been associated with improved pregnancy outcomes.

Diagnosis

Clinical hypothyroidism during pregnancy is particularly difficult to diagnose because many of the signs or symptoms are common to pregnancy. Thyroid testing should be performed on symptomatic women or those with a personal or close family history of thyroid disease, type 1 diabetes mellitus, or other autoimmune conditions.

The mainstay for diagnosis of thyroid disease is the measurement of serum thyrotropin. If the thyrotropin level is abnormal, then evaluation of free T_4 is recommended. Serum thyrotropin is more sensitive than free T_4 for detecting hypothyroidism and hyperthyroidism. Disadvantages of this thyrotropin-first strategy include the potential impact of interfering substances on the thyrotropin assay itself, and unusual thyroid conditions, such as central hypothyroidism, characterized by discordant thyrotropin and free T_4 level measurements, may go undetected. The diagnosis of overt hypothyroidism generally is established by an elevated serum thyrotropin level and a low serum free T_4 level. The reference range for serum thyrotropin concentrations in nonpregnant individuals is 0.45–4.5 mIU/L, but pregnancy-specific nomograms are available.

The impact of changes in free T_4 levels during normal pregnancy has been the subject of much controversy, particularly with the advent of more sensitive and automated immunoassays. The diagnostic accuracy of these free T_4 tests are dependent on protein binding, especially given the physiologic changes in thyroid-binding globulin and other proteins during pregnancy (2). Though there is a significant decrease in free T_4 levels in late gestation when compared with nonpregnant women or those in the first trimester, overall, free T_4 concentrations remain within the reference range (0.7–1.8 ng/dL) throughout pregnancy. Therefore, using nonpregnant free T_4 level thresholds for diagnosis of hypothyroidism is recommended until pregnancy specific free T_4 level thresholds are available (3).

Finally, it may be helpful to confirm the presence of antimicrosomal antibodies in pregnant women with hypothyroidism. The presence of antithyroid antibodies may identify a population of women at particular risk of pregnancy complications, postpartum thyroid dysfunction, or progression to symptomatic disease. Results of one study revealed that 50% of women identified with thyroid peroxidase antibodies at 16 weeks of gestation developed postpartum thyroid dysfunction and one in four of these patients progress to permanent overt hypothyroidism within a year (4).

Treatment

Women with a history of hypothyroidism before conception should have a serum thyrotropin level evaluation at their first prenatal visit. Approximately one half of these women will require an increase in thyroid replacement during pregnancy. This has led some authors to recommend that levothyroxine be routinely increased by 30% at the time that pregnancy is confirmed (5). However, this practice has not been shown to be beneficial and, because there is potential for overtreatment in approximately 25% of such women, thyroid treatment should be guided by results of thyroid function studies performed at initiation of prenatal care. The goal of treatment in pregnant women with overt hypothyroidism is clinical and biochemical euthyroidism. Levothyroxine is the treatment of choice for routine management of hypothyroidism. The starting dose usually ranges from 1–2 micrograms/kg/day to approximately 100 micrograms/kg/day. Thyrotropin level is then measured at 6–8 week intervals and levothyroxine dose adjusted in 25–50 microgram increments. The therapeutic goal is a thyrotropin level between 0.5 and 2.5 microinternational units/L (6). In women with well-controlled thyroid disease, it is recommended that thyroid function studies be repeated during each trimester. Notably, several drugs can interfere with levothyroxine absorption (eg, cholestyramine, ferrous sulfate, and aluminum hydroxide antacids) or its metabolism (eg, phenytoin, carbamazepine, and rifampin). Breastfeeding is not contraindicated in women treated for hypothyroidism. Levothyroxine is excreted into breast milk but at levels too low to alter thyroid function in infants.

Subclinical Hypothyroidism

Reports suggesting increased fetal wastage or subsequent neurodevelopmental complications in offspring of women with mild hypothyroidism have prompted recommendations that levothyroxine be prescribed to restore the thyrotropin level to the reference range (7). However, there are no published intervention trials specifically assessing the efficacy of such treatment to improve neuropsychological performance in off-

spring of women with subclinical hypothyroidism (ie, elevated thyrotropin levels and normal free T_4 levels). As a result, routine screening and treatment of subclinical hypothyroidism during pregnancy currently is not recommended by the American College of Obstetricians and Gynecologists (8).

Isolated Hypothyroxinemia

Maternal isolated hypothyroxinemia, defined as a normal range thyrotropin level with a low free T_4 level, also has been implicated in impaired fetal neurodevelopment. Isolated hypothyroxinemia has been associated with iodine insufficiency and also may be indicative of central hypothyroidism. However, laboratory error from technical interference should be contemplated when discordant thyroid test results are encountered. There are no reports suggesting that treatment of such isolated hypothyroxinemia is beneficial for either the mother or her offspring. Therefore, treatment of such women, in the absence of central hypothyroidism, is unwarranted and should be considered experimental.

Hyperthyroidism

Overt hyperthyroidism complicates approximately 2 in 1,000 pregnancies. As with hypothyroidism, clinical features of hyperthyroidism can be easily confused with those typical of pregnancy. Suggestive symptoms include nervousness, heat intolerance, palpitations, thyromegaly, failure to gain weight or weight loss, and exophthalmos. The most common cause of overt hyperthyroidism is Graves disease, an organ-specific autoimmune process whereby thyroid-stimulating autoantibodies attach to and activate thyrotropin receptors. Other causes of overt hyperthyroidism include functioning adenoma or toxic nodular goiter, thyroiditis, and excessive thyroid hormone intake.

There is a unique form of hyperthyroidism associated with pregnancy called *gestational transient thyrotoxicosis*. It typically is associated with hyperemesis gravidarum, and can be caused by high levels of human chorionic gonadotropin (hCG) resulting from molar pregnancy. These high hCG levels lead to thyrotropin receptor stimulation and temporary hyperthyroidism. Serum free T_4 levels usually normalize in parallel with the decline in hCG concentrations as pregnancy progresses beyond the first trimester. Women with gestational transient thyrotoxicosis rarely are symptomatic, and treatment with antithyroxine drugs has not been shown to be beneficial.

Pregnant women with hyperthyroidism are at increased risk for spontaneous pregnancy loss, congestive heart failure, thyroid storm, preterm birth, preeclampsia, fetal growth restriction, and associated increased perinatal morbidity and mortality. Treatment of hyperthyroid women to achieve adequate metabolic control has been associated with improved pregnancy outcome. Gestational transient thyrotoxicosis has not been associated with poor pregnancy outcomes.

Diagnosis

The diagnosis of overt hyperthyroidism can be reliably confirmed by evaluating serum thyrotropin levels and free T_4 levels. In women with depressed serum thyrotropin levels (less than 0.45 mIU/L), clinical hyperthyroidism is confirmed by an elevation of free T_4 levels (greater than 1.8 ng/dL). However, as is true when diagnosing hypothyroidism during pregnancy, the impact of gestational age on the measurement of thyrotropin levels must be considered. For example, the 2.5th percentile for thyrotropin level during the first half of pregnancy in results of one study fell below 0.1 mIU/L (9). Rarely, symptomatic hyperthyroidism is caused by an abnormally high serum triiodothyronine (T_3) level in women with a normal free T_4 level (T_3 thyrotoxicosis).

Treatment

Thyrotoxicosis during pregnancy can nearly always be controlled by the use of thioamide drugs. Some clinician's prefer propylthiouracil because it partially inhibits the conversion of T_4 and T_3 and crosses the placenta less readily than methimazole. Although not proved, methimazole used in early pregnancy has been associated with esophageal and choanal atresia as well as aplasia cutis in the fetus (10). The dose of thioamide is empirical. In nonpregnant women, the American Thyroid Association recommends an initial daily dose of 100–600 mg for propylthiouracil or 10–40 mg for methimazole (11). Many women with overt hypothyroidism diagnosed during pregnancy though, require a higher average daily propylthiouracil dose, prompting a starting dose of at least 300 mg each day (12). Transient leukopenia occurs in approximately 10% of pregnant women treated with thioamides but usually does not require cessation of therapy. However, in approximately 0.2% of these women, agranulocytosis develops suddenly and mandates discontinuation of the drug. Therefore, women taking thioamide drugs should discontinue the use of this medication immediately if they develop a fever or sore throat until complete evaluation for agranulocytosis can be performed.

The goal of treatment during pregnancy is to maintain free T_4 levels in the upper normal range, using the lowest possible dose of thioamide. Improvement in free T_4 levels generally is seen in 2–4 weeks and the median time to normalization of the thyrotropin concentration is 6–8 weeks. Caution against overtreatment is recommended because it may result in maternal or fetal hypothyroidism.

Alternatives for treatment of overt hyperthyroidism are rarely undertaken during pregnancy. For example, thyroidectomy typically is reserved for treatment outside of pregnancy. Occasionally however, women who cannot adhere to medical therapy or in whom therapy is toxic may benefit from surgical management. Ablative radioactive iodine is contraindicated in pregnancy because it can destroy the fetal thyroid. It has been recommended that women avoid pregnancy for a period of 6 months after radioablative therapy (13).

Thioamides are excreted in breast milk but propylthiouracil is largely protein bound and does not seem to pose a significant risk to the breastfed infant. Methimazole has been found in breastfed infants of treated women in amounts sufficient to cause thyroid dysfunction, but at low doses (10–20 mg/d) it does not appear to pose a major risk to the nursing infant. The American Academy of Pediatricians considers both compatible with breastfeeding.

Thyroid Storm and Heart Failure

Thyroid storm is an acute, life-threatening exacerbation of thyrotoxicosis. The classic findings are fever, tachycardia, tremor, nausea, vomiting, diarrhea, dehydration, and delirium or coma. Thyroid storm is rare in pregnancy and is a clinical diagnosis in women with laboratory test results consistent with overt hyperthyroidism. Heart failure caused by cardiomyopathy from excessive T_4 levels in women with controlled hyperthyroidism is more common to pregnant women (14). Treatment of thyroid storm or thyrotoxic heart failure is similar. Such cases should be treated as medical emergencies in an intensive care setting (15). Specific treatment consists of 1g of propylthiouracil, given orally or crushed and placed through a nasogastric tube. Propylthiouracil treatment should be continued every 6 hours. One hour after initial propylthiouracil dosing, iodide should be given intravenously as sodium iodide, orally as supersaturated solution of potassium iodide, or as Lugol solution every 8 hours. In women with histories of iodine-induced anaphylaxis, lithium carbonate is given instead. Most authorities also recommend dexamethasone be given intravenously every 6 hours for four doses to block peripheral conversion of T_4 to T_3. Treatment with a β-blocker usually is reserved for heart rates of 120 beats per minute or higher. Propranolol, labetalol, and esmolol have all been used successfully in pregnancy.

Subclinical Hyperthyroidism

Subclinical hyperthyroidism is defined as a serum thyrotropin concentration below the statistically defined lower limit of the reference range when serum free T_4 and free T_3 concentrations are within their reference range (1). Subclinical hyperthyroidism affects 1.7% of pregnant women and has been reported to have long-term adverse sequelae that include osteoporosis, cardiovascular morbidity, and progression to overt thyrotoxicosis or thyroid failure (16). During pregnancy, however, the diagnosis of subclinical hyperthyroidism has not been found to be associated with adverse outcomes (16). At present, there is no convincing evidence that treatment is beneficial, and it seems especially unwarranted during pregnancy because antithyroid drugs cross the placenta.

Postpartum Thyroiditis

Transient autoimmune thyroiditis has been identified in up to 10% of women during the first year after childbirth. In clinical practice, postpartum thyroiditis infrequently is diagnosed because it typically develops months after delivery and has vague and nonspecific symptoms. The likelihood of developing postpartum thyroiditis is related to increasing serum levels of thyroid autoantibodies. Women with high antibody titers in early pregnancy are most commonly affected (17).

There are two recognized clinical phases of postpartum thyroiditis. Up to 4 months after delivery, approximately 4% of these women develop transient thyrotoxicosis. Fatigue and palpitations are the most common symptoms. Use of antithyroid medications, such as thioamides, typically is ineffective, and approximately two thirds of patients return to a euthyroid state. A β-blocker may be used temporarily for severe symptoms. Between 4 months and 8 months postpartum, 2–5% of women develop hypothyroidism. Thyromegaly and other symptoms are common and more prominent than during the thyrotoxic phase. Thyroxine replacement frequently is recommended for at least 6–12 months. Most women identified with postpartum thyroiditis will return to the euthyroid state within 12 months of delivery but ultimately have about a 30% risk of developing permanent hypothyroidism.

Nodular Thyroid Disease

Small thyroid nodules detected by sensitive ultrasound methods are common during pregnancy in some populations. Management of palpable thyroid nodules during pregnancy depends on gestational age. Ultrasound examination reliably detects nodules greater than 0.5 cm, and their solid or cystic nature also can be determined. Fine-needle aspiration is an excellent method for assessment and tumor markers and immunostaining are reliable to evaluate for malignancy (18).

Evaluation of thyroid cancer involves a multidisciplinary approach (19). Most thyroid carcinomas are well differentiated and pursue an indolent course. Thus, surgery can be postponed until after delivery. However, several reviews report minimal fetal loss attributed to thyroid cancer surgery performed before 24–26 weeks of gestation.

References

1. Surks MI, Ortiz E, Daniels GH, Sawin CT, Col NF, Cobin RH, et al. Subclinical thyroid disease: scientific review and guidelines for diagnosis and management. JAMA 2004; 291:228–38.

2. Mandel SJ, Spencer CA, Hollowell JG. Are detection and treatment of thyroid insufficiency in pregnancy feasible? Thyroid 2005;15:44–53.

3. Casey BM, Leveno KJ. Thyroid disease in pregnancy. Obstet Gynecol 2006;108:1283–92.

4. Premawardhana LD, Parkes AB, Ammari F, John R, Darke C, Adams H, et al. Postpartum thyroiditis and long-term thyroid status: prognostic influence of thyroid peroxidase antibodies and ultrasound echogenicity. J Clin Endocrinol Metab 2000;85:71–5.

5. Alexander EK, Marqusee E, Lawrence J, Jarolim P, Fischer GA, Larsen PR. Timing and magnitude of increases in levothyroxine requirements during pregnancy in women with hypothyroidism. N Engl J Med 2004;351:241–9.

6. Dickey RA, Wartofsky L, Feld S. Optimal thyrotropin level: normal ranges and reference intervals are not equivalent. Thyroid 2005;15:1035–9.

7. Gharib H, Tuttle RM, Baskin HJ, Fish LH, Singer PA, McDermott MT. Consensus Statement #1: Subclinical thyroid dysfunction: a joint statement on management from the American Association of Clinical Endocrinologists, the American Thyroid Association, and the Endocrine Society. American Association of Clinical Endocrinologists; American Thyroid Association; Endocrine Society. Thyroid 2005;15:24–8; response 32–3.

8. Subclinical hypothyroidism in pregnancy. ACOG Committee Opinion No. 381. American College of Obstetricians and Gynecologists. Obstet Gynecol 2007;110:959–60.

9. Casey BM, Dashe JS, Spong CY, McIntire DD, Leveno KJ, Cunningham GF. Perinatal significance of isolated maternal hypothyroxinemia identified in the first half of pregnancy. Obstet Gynecol 2007;109:1129–35.

10. Barbero P, Valdez R, Rodriguez H, Tiscornia C, Mansilla E, Allons A, et al. Choanal atresia associated with maternal hyperthyroidism treated with methimazole: a case-control study. Am J Med Genet A 2008;146A:2390–5.

11. Singer PA, Cooper DS, Levy EG, Ladenson PW, Braverman LE, Daniels G, et al. Treatment guidelines for patients with hyperthyroidism and hypothyroidism. Standards of Care Committee, American Thyroid Association. JAMA 1995; 273:808–12.

12. Karlsson FA, Axelsson O, Melhus H. Severe embryopathy and exposure to methimazole in early pregnancy. J Clin Endocrinol Metab 2002;87:947–9.

13. Brent GA. Clinical practice. Graves' disease. N Engl J Med 2008;358:2594–605.

14. Sheffield JS, Cunningham FG. Thyrotoxicosis and heart failure that complicate pregnancy. Am J Obstet Gynecol 2004;190:211–7.

15. Zeeman GG, Wendel GD Jr, Cunningham FG. A blueprint for obstetric critical care. Am J Obstet Gynecol 2003;188: 532–6.

16. Casey BM, Dashe JS, Wells CE, McIntire DD, Leveno KJ, Cunningham FG. Subclinical hyperthyroidism and pregnancy outcomes. Obstet Gynecol 2006;107:337–41.

17. Pearce EN, Farwell AP, Braverman LE. Thyroiditis [published erratum appears in N Engl J Med 2003;349:620]. N Engl J Med 2003;348:2646–55.

18. Hegedus L. Clinical practice. The thyroid nodule. N Engl J Med 2004;351:1764–71.

19. Thyroid disease in pregnancy. ACOG Practice Bulletin No. 37. American College of Obstetricians and Gynecologists. Obstet Gynecol 2002;100:387–96.

Hematologic Disorders

Manju Monga

Anemia in pregnant women has been defined as hemoglobin levels of less than 11 g/dL in the first and third trimesters and less than 10.5 g/dL in the second trimester. Anemia during pregnancy may be categorized based on underlying causative mechanism or whether the condition is inherited or acquired. The initial evaluation of women with moderate anemia based on classification by cell size is of practical use in the workup of anemia and is outlined in Figure 18. In individuals of African descent, regardless of the presence or absence of anemia, hemoglobin electrophoresis testing is recommended along with a complete blood count (1).

Iron Deficiency Anemia

The most common causes of anemia during pregnancy and the puerperium are iron deficiency and acute hemorrhage. The iron requirement in a typical pregnancy is approximately 1,000 mg; approximately 300 mg for the fetus and placenta and approximately 500 mg for the expansion of maternal hemoglobin mass. Another 200 mg is shed through the gut, urine, and skin. This considerably exceeds the iron stores of most women. Severe anemia (hemoglobin [Hb] levels of less than 6 g/dL) has been associated with increased low birth weight of

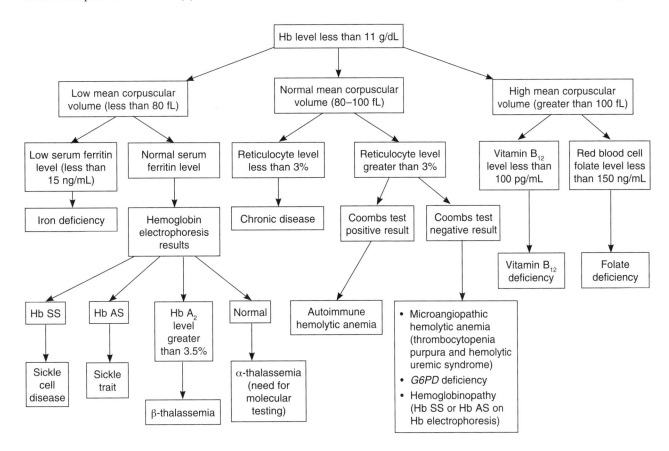

Figure 18. Diagnostic assessment of anemia in pregnancy. Abbreviation: Hb indicates hemoglobin.

infants, induction rates, operative vaginal and cesarean deliveries, and prolonged labor (2) and abnormal fetal oxygenation, nonreassuring fetal heart rate, reduced amniotic fluid volume and fetal cerebral vasodilatation (3), although iron supplementation has not consistently been shown to improve maternal or perinatal outcome (4–6).

To replenish iron stores, oral therapy should be continued for approximately 3 months after the anemia has been corrected (Table 24). After 7–10 days of therapy with an iron compound, reticulocytosis can be seen and hemoglobin concentrations will increase in the following weeks.

In select cases (eg, patients with malabsorption syndromes or those with severe anemia [hemoglobin levels less than 8.5 g/dL] who will not take iron therapy), there is a role for parenteral iron therapy (7, 8). Anaphylaxis is a rare complication (occurring in less than 0.6% of patients) of intravenous iron dextran administration; therefore, a test dose should be administered first. The maximum rate of the full dose is 1 mL/min. In a report of total dose infusion of low molecular dextran in 100 pregnant women with severe anemia, no cases of anaphylaxis were noted (9); however, most case series reporting parenteral iron use during pregnancy are small, and accurate determination of serious adverse event rate is limited (10). Iron sucrose may have a lower rate of anaphylactic reactions and a lower case fatality ratio (11).

Subcutaneous erythropoietin has been administered successfully to correct iron deficiency anemia in pregnancy. In patients with substantial anemia whose treatment with oral iron therapy alone failed to correct anemia, the addition of erythropoietin to oral iron therapy resulted in correction of anemia within 2 weeks in 73% of patients (12–14).

Table 24. Iron Supplements

Preparation	Content
Ferrous fumarate	106 mg of elemental iron per 325-mg tablet
Ferrous sulfate	65 mg of elemental iron per 325-mg tablet
Ferrous gluconate	34 mg of elemental iron per 300-mg tablet
Ferric gluconate	12.5 mg of iron per mL, intravenously only
Iron sucrose	20 mg of iron per mL, intravenously only

From Anemia in Pregnancy. ACOG Practice Bulletin No. 95. American College of Obstetricians and Gynecologists. Obstet Gynecol 2008;112:201–7.

Anemia Associated With Chronic Diseases

Anemia may be associated with chronic diseases, such as inflammatory bowel disease, chronic renal failure, and systemic lupus erythematosus. The etiology of such anemia may result from both decreased production and increased destruction of erythrocytes. The treatment of chronic anemia in pregnancy may be difficult, and treatment response may vary. Besides iron and folic acid supplementation, human recombinant erythropoietin has been used for the treatment of these anemias in pregnant women, especially those associated with chronic renal failure.

Sickle Cell Hemoglobinopathies

The most common maternal morbidity in sickle cell disease is a vasoocclusive episode with severe pain (sickle cell crises) that may be precipitated by dehydration, infection, stress, hypoxemia, or cold. During pregnancy, sickle cell crises may become more frequent. As arterial oxygenation decreases, red blood cells become stiff and less pliable. They become deformed (sickled) and undergo membrane changes that allow an influx of calcium, leakage of potassium, and dehydration. The survival time of these sickled cells is shortened, and they clump together, causing capillary venous occlusion throughout the body. These vasoocclusive episodes frequently are associated with intense pain. Prophylactic red cell transfusion clearly decreases the frequency of pain crises, but it has not been shown to improve the outcome of the pregnancy. Because there are inherent risks of transfusion reactions, alloimmunization, and acquisition of infections, currently it is not routinely recommended to prophylactically treat patients with transfusion during pregnancy.

Most therapeutic regimens include increased fluid intake, the use of potent analgesics, and the use of antibiotics (when necessary for infection). When a pregnant patient with sickle cell disease comes to the emergency room or labor and delivery unit with severe pain, it is important not to overlook the possibility of other causes, such as ectopic pregnancy, spontaneous abortion, placental abruption, appendicitis, and cholecystitis. While these conditions are being evaluated, intravenous hydration should be administered. If the patient has a viable fetus, continuous electronic monitoring should be undertaken. Once other causes are ruled out, aggressive pain management should be instituted using intravenous morphine and preferably patient-controlled analgesia.

Oxygen therapy has not been shown to be effective in decreasing the duration or intensity of the pain crisis, but should be used when there is hypoxemia or fetal distress. Some patients with sickle cell disease develop chronic pain. These patients benefit from seeing a pain specialist and using combination medication for chronic pain.

Acute chest syndrome is characterized by pain, fever, cough, and new pulmonary infiltrates on chest X-ray (15, 16). The exact etiology of this syndrome is unclear, but it has been reported to be associated with infection, microvascular occlusion from sickle hemoglobin, and fat embolism. This is a life threatening condition and requires respiratory support and emergency transfusion (17). Management includes assessment of arterial blood gas and A-a gradient and administration of oxygen in patients who are hypoxemic. Transfusion (simple or exchange) is recommended in patients who are hypoxemic and should not be delayed in patients who are deteriorating. Infection has been associated in up to one third of patients with acute chest syndrome and, therefore, broad-spectrum antibiotics also are recommended.

Special circumstances during pregnancy appreciably increase morbidity among these women. Bacteriuria is common and urinary tract infections, including acute pyelonephritis, are increased substantially. Eradication of asymptomatic bacteriuria is important to prevent most symptomatic infections, and urine culture should be performed monthly. Pneumonia, especially caused by *Streptococcus pneumoniae,* is common, and polyvalent pneumococcal vaccine is recommended for these women. Because of the risk of perinatal mortality and intrauterine growth restriction, fetal surveillance, including ultrasonography for estimated fetal growth and antepartum testing, is recommended, although limited data on their efficacy are reported.

Macrocytic Anemia

Macrocytic anemia may be categorized as megaloblastic or nonmegaloblastic. Macrocytic anemia in pregnancy in the United States most commonly is caused by folic acid deficiency, especially among women with diets lacking in leafy green vegetables, legumes, or animal proteins (3). Folic acid deficiency anemia is characterized by low plasma concentrations of folic acid, low red blood cell folate levels and hypersegmented neutrophils. Severe maternal folate deficiency also may be associated with thrombocytopenia and leukopenia.

Folate requirements increase from 50 micrograms per day in the nonpregnant state to 400 micrograms per day during pregnancy. Supplementation with 1 mg of folic acid daily produces a striking hematologic response with an increase in reticulocyte count within 4–7 days. Multiple gestation is associated with increased folic acid requirement. The use of several drugs, including phenytoin, primidone, paraaminosalicylic acid, and sulfasalazine may decrease serum folate concentrations and cause deficiency.

Vitamin B_{12} deficiency is less commonly seen during pregnancy but may be observed in patients with gastric bypass or Crohn disease. Monthly intramuscular injections of 1,000 micrograms of vitamin B_{12} may be used to treat this deficiency. Neonatal vitamin B_{12} deficiency may result from untreated maternal deficiency and the neonate may manifest with irritability, failure to thrive, anorexia, and developmental regression (18).

Thrombocytopenia

Thrombocytopenia, defined as platelet count of less than 150,000 platelets per microliter, may complicate 7–8% pregnancies. Gestational thrombocytopenia is the most common cause, accounting for up to two thirds of cases.

Gestational Thrombocytopenia

Gestational thrombocytopenia occurs in 5–7% of pregnancies and typically is not associated with maternal, fetal, or neonatal sequelae (19). Platelet count remains greater than 70,000/microliter, and patients remain asymptomatic. Gestational thrombocytopenia may recur during subsequent pregnancies, but there typically is no other history of bleeding or thrombocytopenia. Platelet count usually returns to normal within 2–12 weeks after delivery and, because maternal and fetal hemorrhage rates are not increased, routine obstetric management is recommended.

Idiopathic Thrombocytopenic Purpura

Idiopathic thrombocytopenic purpura (ITP) is an autoimmune disorder characterized by immunoglobulin G (IgG)-mediated destruction of platelets by the reticuloendothelial system (20–22). Platelet destruction leads to maternal thrombocytopenia and, because antiplatelet IgG antibodies cross the placenta, fetal thrombocytopenia may occur. Idiopathic thrombocytopenic purpura is a diagnosis of exclusion. Criteria for ITP include thrombocytopenia, blood smear showing an increased percentage of large platelets, normal coagulation study results, bone marrow with increased size and number of megalokaryocytes, and no other identifiable cause of thrombocytopenia.

Maternal thrombocytopenia may be associated with history of easy bruising, petechiae, epistaxis, or gingival bleeding. Serious hemorrhage usually does not occur unless platelet count is lower than 20,000 per microliter. Pregnancy does not usually exacerbate thrombocytopenia. The management of ITP depends on the severity of maternal thrombocytopenia and gestational age. In the first and second trimester, treatment of thrombocytopenia should be initiated if the maternal platelet count is 30,000–50,000 per microliter or if the patient is symptomatic. Initial treatment consists of steroid administration (1 mg/kg of prednisone per day). Other options for severe thrombocytopenia include the administration of intravenous immunoglobulin (IVIG), with regimens ranging from 400 mg/kg/day for 3 days to higher dose IVIG (for example, 1 g/kg/day). Intravenous immunoglobulin is recommended as first-line therapy for severe thrombocytopenia or bleeding in the third trimester because the use of steroids takes 3–7 days for onset of action, with maximum effect in 2–3 weeks (22). Splenectomy is reserved for the most refractory cases and usually will dramatically improve the thrombocytopenia, although thrombocytopenia can still occur in patients with chronic ITP. Platelet transfusion usually is not indicated unless there is profound thrombocytopenia immediately before surgery. Limited data exist regarding the use of regional analgesia with maternal thrombocytopenia; however, it generally is advised that regional analgesia not be given if the platelet count is less than 50,000/microliter, and consultation with an anesthesiologist is recommended if the platelet count is between 50,000/microliter and 100,000/microliter. Nonsteroidal antiinflammatory drugs should be avoided in the postpartum period.

Thrombocytopenia can occur in neonates born to mothers with ITP. Serial platelet counts in the newborn are required because nadir in platelet count may not occur for several days. The risk of severe neonatal thrombocytopenia (platelet count less than 50×10^9 per liter) occurs in approximately 10% of patients, but the risk of serious morbidity, namely intracranial hemorrhage, occurs in less than 1% of patients. There is no maternal test or characteristic that reliably predicts neonatal thrombocytopenia, and cesarean delivery has not been shown to prevent intracranial hemorrhage; therefore, routine obstetric management is appropriate (23). This is in contradistinction to neonatal alloimmune thrombocytopenia in which the maternal platelet count is normal but maternal alloimmunization to fetal platelets results in profound neonatal thrombocytopenia and 10–20% risk of neonatal intracranial hemorrhage (24).

Microangiopathic Hemolytic Anemias

Thrombotic thrombocytopenic purpura (TTP) and hemolytic uremic syndrome are thrombotic microangiopathic diseases in which intravascular platelet aggregation causes transient ischemia (25). They are characterized by fever, hemolytic anemia, thrombocytopenia, neurologic symptoms, and renal dysfunction. They often are associated with hypertension and frequently can cause multisystem organ failure. The conditions occur in 1 in 25,000 pregnancies. Typically, TTP occurs in women in their 20s and 30s, whereas hemolytic uremic syndrome is primarily a disease of children. Hemolytic uremic syndrome often is preceded by a gastrointestinal illness and is more commonly associated with renal failure than TTP. Thrombocytopenia, bleeding, and neurologic manifestations are more severe in TTP.

The treatment for TTP and hemolytic uremic syndrome is plasmapheresis. Patients with TTP have a progressive deteriorating course, and the disease is fatal (almost 90% of cases) unless treated. Both conditions can occur during and after a normal pregnancy or in association with preeclampsia. In contrast with preeclampsia, there usually is marked thrombocytopenia and elevation of the levels of l-lactate dehydrogenase with TTP. Unlike preeclampsia, TTP and hemolytic uremic syndrome do not typically resolve with delivery, and prompt recognition, diagnosis, and treatment with plasmapheresis are required to limit maternal and perinatal mortality (26). Long-term renal and neurologic sequelae are common and recurrence in subsequent pregnancy may occur in up to 50% of patients (27). Successful management of subsequent pregnancies has been reported in case series in which low dose aspirin, low molecular weight heparin and regular plasma exchange were used (28).

Von Willebrand Disease

Von Willebrand disease is the most common inherited bleeding disorder, affecting up to 1% of the population. Circulating as a series of multimers, von Willebrand factor (vWF) plays an important role in primary hemostasis by binding to both platelets and the endothelium, forming an adhesive bridge (29). Also it acts as a carrier protein for factor VIII. Von Willebrand disease is classified into three major categories:

1. Type I (partial quantitative deficiency)
2. Type II (qualitative deficiency)
3. Type III (total deficiency).

Inheritance and clinical severity vary by type of disease. Von Willebrand disease may be inherited as autosomal dominant or autosomal recessive disease. Management of von Willebrand disease during pregnancy should include assessment of bleeding history, complete blood count, platelet count, measurement of prothrombin time and partial thromboplastin time, and measurement of von Willebrand Factor protein in plasma (vWF:Ag), vWF protein function (ability to interact with normal platelets) that is measured as ristocetin cofactor (vWF:RCo) and vWF's ability to bind and maintain normal factor VIII in plasma (factor VIII coagulant assay). Pregnant women with von Willebrand disease with a history of severe bleeding, or factor VIII levels or VWF:RCo levels less than 50 international units/dL should be managed at a tertiary level center in conjunction with a hematologist and should have the opportunity to discuss the risk of inheritance with a genetic counselor. Prenatal consultation with an anesthesiologist to discuss alternatives to regional anesthesia also is recommended.

Consistent with the increase of most circulating clotting factors, levels of vWF increase during the second and third trimesters of pregnancy to two to three times the baseline. Treatment is not needed during pregnancy in most women with von Willebrand disease. A review of bleeding events and other complications in pregnant women with von Willebrand disease in the United States between 2000 and 2003 indicated that among 4,067 deliveries complicated by von Willebrand disease, there was an increased rate of antepartum bleeding, postpartum hemorrhage, and transfusion (30).

In an effort to decrease the risk of postpartum hemorrhage, it is recommended that factor VIII levels and vWF:RCo levels be checked in the third trimester of pregnancy and that levels greater than 50 international units/dL be achieved before delivery and maintained for at least 3–5 days after delivery (30). Factor VIII levels and vWF:RCo levels may be normalized with the use of desmopressin acetate, which is a synthetic analog of the antidiuretic hormone, vasopressin. Desmopressin acetate can be administered intravenously, by subcutaneous injection, or by intranasal spray, and has been shown to be effective in patients with type I, type IIA, and type IIN von Willebrand disease, but not type IIB or type III. When given intravenously for prophylaxis before invasive procedures or for acute bleeding episodes, a dose of 0.3 microgram/kg (maximum 20 micrograms) is diluted in 50 mL of normal saline solution and infused over 20–30 minutes; the same dose is given with subcutaneous therapy. An increase in vWF levels and factor VIII levels is expected at approximately 30–60 minutes after the infusion, and the response persists for 6–12 hours. A repeat dose may be given at 8–12 hours; subsequent doses often are switched to once daily doses.

Intranasal administration is an excellent choice for patients with mild bleeding. The usual dose is 300 micrograms for adults. The vWF levels achieved with 300 micrograms of intranasal spray (desmopressin) are approximately equivalent to those seen with an intravenous dose of 0.2 microgram/kg. Side effects include facial flushing, headache, and tingling. Hypertension, hypotension, and thrombosis are rare. Tachyphylaxis will occur after repeated administration. Fluid retention and consequent hyponatremia can occur. Concomitant use of nonsteroidal antiinflammatory drugs should be avoided. Other treatment options, especially in women with type IIB or type III von Willebrand disease or in women with acute hemorrhage include factor VIII concentrate and cryoprecipitate.

References

1. Hemoglobinopathies in pregnancy. ACOG Practice Bulletin No. 78. American College of Obstetricians and Gynecologists. Obstet Gynecol 2007;109:229–37.

2. Malhotra M, Sharma JB, Batra S, Sharma S, Murthy NS, Arora R. Maternal and perinatal outcome in varying degrees of anemia. Int J Gynaecol Obstet 2002;79:93–100.

3. Anemia in pregnancy. ACOG Practice Bulletin No. 95. American College of Obstetricians and Gynecologists. Obstet Gynecol 2008;112:201–7.

4. Pena-Rosas JP, Viteri FE. Effects of routine oral iron supplementation with or without folic acid for women during pregnancy. Cochrane Database of Systematic Reviews 2006, Issue 3. Art. No.:CD004736.DOI:10.1002/14651858.CD004736.pub2; 10.1002/14651858.CD004736.pub2.

5. Mungen E. Iron supplementation in pregnancy. J Perinat Med 2003;31:420–6.

6. Scholl TO. Iron status during pregnancy: setting the stage for mother and infant. Am J Clin Nutr 2005;81:1218S–22S.

7. Bashiri A, Burstein E, Sheiner E, Mazor M. Anemia during pregnancy and treatment with intravenous iron: review of the literature. Eur J Obstet Gynecol Reprod Biol 2003;110:2–7.

8. Komolafe JO, Kuti O, Ijadunola KT, Ogunniyi SO. A comparative study between intramuscular iron dextran and oral ferrous sulphate in the treatment of iron deficiency anaemia in pregnancy. J Obstet Gynaecol 2003;23:628–31.

9. Ayub R, Tariq N, Adil MM, Iqbal M, Junaid A, Jaferry T. Efficacy and safety of total dose infusion of low molecular weight iron dextran in the treatment of iron deficiency anemia during pregnancy. J Coll Physicians Surg Pak 2008;18:424–7.

10. Reveiz L, Gyte Gillian ML, Cuervo Luis G. Treatments for iron-deficiency anaemia in pregnancy. Cochrane Database of Systematic Reviews 2007, Issue 2. Art. No.: CD003094. DOI: 10.1002/14651858.CD003094.pub2; 10.1002/14651858.CD003094.pub2.

11. Faich G, Strobos J. Sodium ferric gluconate complex in sucrose: safer intravenous iron therapy than iron dextrans. Am J Kidney Dis 1999;33:464–70.

12. Scott LL, Ramin SM, Richey M, Hanson J, Gilstrap LC 3rd. Erythropoietin use in pregnancy: two cases and a review of the literature. Am J Perinatol 1995;12:22–4.

13. Sifakis S, Angelakis E, Vardaki E, Koumantaki Y, Matalliotakis I, Koumantakis E. Erythropoietin in the treatment of iron deficiency anemia during pregnancy. Gynecol Obstet Invest 2001;51:150–6.

14. Thorp M, Pulliam J. Use of recombinant erythropoietin in a pregnant renal transplant recipient. Am J Nephrol 1998;18:448–51.

15. Stuart MJ, Setty BN. Sickle cell acute chest syndrome: pathogenesis and rationale for treatment. Blood 1999;94:1555–60.

16. Kress JP, Pohlman AS, Hall JB. Determination of hemoglobin saturation in patients with acute sickle chest syndrome: a comparison of arterial blood gases and pulse oximetry. Chest 1999;115:1316–20.

17. Acute chest syndrome and other pulmonary complications. The management of sickle cell disease. National Institutes of Health, National Heart, Lung, and Blood Institute. 4th ed. Bethesda (MD): NHLBI; 2002. p. 103–10.

18. Dror DK, Allen LH. Effect of vitamin B12 deficiency on neurodevelopment in infants: current knowledge and possible mechanisms. Nutr Rev 2008;66:250–5.

19. Rouse DJ, Owen J, Goldenberg RL. Routine maternal platelet count: an assessment of a technologically driven screening practice. Am J Obstet Gynecol 1998;179:573–6.

20. Webert KE, Mittal R, Sigouin C, Heddle NM, Kelton JG. A retrospective 11-year analysis of obstetric patients with idiopathic thrombocytopenic purpura. Blood 2003;102:4306–11.

21. Sukenik-Halevy R, Ellis MH, Fejgin MD. Management of immune thrombocytopenic purpura in pregnancy. Obstet Gynecol Surv 2008;63:182–8.

22. Gernsheimer T, McCrae KR. Immune thrombocytopenic purpura in pregnancy. Curr Opin Hematol 2007;14:574–80.

23. Gill KK, Kelton JG. Management of idiopathic thrombocytopenic purpura in pregnancy. Semin Hematol 2000;37:275–89.

24. Arnold DM, Smith JW, Kelton JG. Diagnosis and management of neonatal alloimmune thrombocytopenia. Transfus Med Rev 2008;22:255–67.

25. Esplin MS, Branch DW. Diagnosis and management of thrombotic microangiopathies during pregnancy. Clin Obstet Gynecol 1999;42:360–7.

26. Martin JN Jr, Bailey AP, Rehberg JF, Owens MT, Keiser SD, May WL. Thrombotic thrombocytopenic purpura in 166 pregnancies: 1955-2006. Am J Obstet Gynecol 2008;199:98–104.

27. Dashe JS, Ramin SM, Cunningham FG. The long-term consequences of thrombotic microangiopathy (thrombotic thrombocytopenic purpura and hemolytic uremic syndrome) in pregnancy. Obstet Gynecol 1998;91:662–8.

28. Scully M, Starke R, Lee R, Mackie I, Machin S, Cohen H. Successful management of pregnancy in women with a history of thrombotic thrombocytopaenic purpura. Blood Coagul Fibrinolysis 2006;17:459–63.

29. Rodeghiero F. von Willebrand disease: still an intriguing disorder in the era of molecular medicine. Haemophilia 2002;8:292–300.

30. The diagnosis, evaluation, and management of von Willebrand Disease. National Institutes of Health, National Heart, Lung, and Blood Institute. Bethesda (MD): National Heart, Lung, and Blood Institute; 2007. Available at: http://www.nhlbi.nih.gov/guidelines/vwd/vwd.pdf. Retrieved September 15, 2009.

Renal Disease

David C. Jones

With careful management of related conditions, such as hypertension, most women with chronic renal disease have a good chance of a successful pregnancy outcome. The primary predictor of the interplay between renal disease and pregnancy is the degree of renal insufficiency, although the etiology of the renal insufficiency is related as well. It is important to consider renal disease as a primary condition and secondary to systemic diseases. In general, the impact of renal insufficiency on pregnancy is related to the serum creatinine level (1). In women with minimal renal insufficiency (serum creatinine levels of less than 1.4 mg/dL), fetal mortality only is mildly increased, and the underlying disease is not irreversibly worsened. However, as the serum creatinine level increases, so does the risk to the mother and fetus (2). When the preconception serum creatinine level is 2 mg/dL or higher, the risk of a rapid decline to end-stage renal disease is 33%. The risks of prematurity and growth restriction also increase as creatinine levels increase.

The next important factor to influence pregnancy outcome in women with renal disease is the presence of preconceptional hypertension. Although even controlled hypertension is associated with a higher incidence of preeclampsia and preterm delivery, it is uncontrolled hypertension that is predictive of poor maternal and fetal outcomes. For this reason, control of hypertension is one of the most important aspects of care. Use of angiotensin-converting enzyme inhibitors, among the most widely prescribed antihypertensive medications in this population, is contraindicated in pregnancy because these drugs are associated with oligohydramnios leading to pulmonary hypoplasia.

During pregnancy, the drugs most commonly used for hypertension in patients with renal disease include α-methyldopa, labetalol, and calcium channel blockers. Among calcium channel blockers, nifedipine is the most widely studied in pregnancy, although usually in the role of a tocolytic. However, in patients with nephropathy outside of pregnancy, diltiazem is the calcium channel blocker that is most effective in decreasing proteinuria and preserving renal function (3). This led one group to retrospectively compare pregnancies in women with renal disease who were treated with diltiazem to those not requiring therapy (4). Although results showed a lower rate of intrauterine growth restriction, improved blood pressure control, and less proteinuria in the diltiazem-treated group, the small size of the trial (only four treated patients compared with three controls) did not allow for statistically significant conclusions. Nonetheless, by reminding us of the findings outside of pregnancy, it suggests that the use of diltiazem is an appropriate alternative to angiotensin-converting enzyme inhibitors and possibly the optimal choice.

Another aspect of chronic renal disease that may cause difficulty is a nephrotic level of proteinuria. In these cases, massive protein loss may lead to hypoalbuminemia and significant body edema. In extreme cases, this edema may be very uncomfortable, and small doses of diuretics may be administered. Whether the degree of proteinuria is itself a prognostic indicator for pregnancy outcome is still an open question. Several authors have suggested that proteinuria is not an independent marker for outcome (2); others believe that it is (5).

Primary Renal Disease

Primary renal disease is divided into glomerulonephritis (eg, membranoproliferative glomerulonephritis, immunoglobulin A nephropathy, focal glomerulosclerosis, and congenital nephrosis) and chronic tubulointerstitial disease (eg, reflux, adult polycystic kidney disease, and chronic obstruction). The evidence that pregnancy outcomes vary substantially based on individual disease is lacking, and the outcomes between the two large categories, glomerulonephritis and tubulointerstitial diseases, have not been shown to be clearly different. Indeed, a single-center study of women with renal disease included 46 pregnancies in 38 women with a variety of primary renal diseases, and results indicated that 98% of pregnancies were associated with a healthy infant without severe handicap 2 years after delivery (6).

Diabetic Nephropathy

The pregnancy outcomes for women with diabetic nephropathy have improved dramatically over the past two decades, although their outcomes are not as favorable as those of diabetic women without nephropathy. Despite an increased risk for preterm birth (greater than 50%), intrauterine growth restriction (15%), preeclampsia (50%), and cesarean delivery (70%), perinatal survival exceeds 95% (7).

Prepregnancy renal function is predictive of obstetric outcome. In a series of 72 pregnancies in 58 women, results demonstrated that a high-serum creatinine level was associated with preterm delivery before 32 weeks of gestation, infants with very low birth weight, and neonatal hypoglycemia (8). These findings were independent of total urinary protein excretion or glycemic control. In a study that evaluated the influence of proteinuria, results indicated that it was of some prognostic value, with patients with less than 1 g proteinuria before 20 weeks

of gestation having a substantially lower risk of pregnancy complications and long-term deterioration in renal function (9). The investigators suggested this was most likely because this group represented a cohort of women with microalbuminuria in whom pregnancy exacerbated protein excretion, resulting in the diagnosis of nephropathy. Thus, until there is a measurable increase in serum creatinine levels, proteinuria is the best predictor of renal function. Once renal function deterioration is indicated by an increased serum creatinine level, then the serum creatinine level becomes most predictive of outcome. It appears that, in general, fetal outcomes are not specifically influenced by the particular etiology of the maternal renal disease (10).

Lupus Nephritis

Although many women with lupus do not have renal involvement, those who do may become exceptionally ill during pregnancy and have perinatal morbidity and mortality exceeding those of other nephropathies. Results from a review of the risks of pregnancy in women with lupus nephritis pointed out the most critical determinants of outcome were quiescence of disease for at least 6 months before conception and the presence of antiphospholipid antibodies (8). For instance, in results from a representative study, fetal loss was noted in 83% of patients with antiphospholipid antibodies compared with 13% in whom no antibodies were detected (11). Investigators noted that proteinuria and hypertension also were independent predictors of adverse fetal outcome. One of the difficulties in these patients is distinguishing pregnancy-induced hypertension from a lupus nephritis flare, and women with lupus nephritis have an increased risk of developing pregnancy-induced hypertension (12). Although being sure of the correct diagnosis may be difficult, an increasing serum uric acid level is suggestive of preeclampsia, whereas hematuria, or cellular casts, or both are more suggestive of lupus nephritis. Increasing anti-DNA antibody levels and decreasing complement levels (note that these may be in the normal range for nonpregnant women, because C3 and C4 increase during pregnancy) also point towards lupus nephritis. It is reassuring that a pregnancy does not appear to increase the frequency of exacerbations of lupus nephropathy or a deterioration of renal function (13).

Renal Dialysis

Although most women undergoing dialysis treatment have irregular or absent menses, pregnancy can occur and be maintained while undergoing dialysis treatment. The lack of regular menstruation is problematic because gestation is frequently quite advanced by the time pregnancy is recognized. Results from early studies were somewhat pessimistic, but recent literature has increasingly shown that successful pregnancy is more likely than not. One review looked at a single center experience pooled with published data (14). The authors found that prematurity was common with the mean gestational age at delivery of 31 weeks of gestation. In the study, women undergoing hemodialysis had a higher success rate (70.9%) than those undergoing peritoneal dialysis (64.2%); however, the mean birth weight was similar in both groups (1529 g plus or minus 132 g with hemodialysis and 1567 g plus or minus 617 g with peritoneal dialysis). However, the consensus has been that there is largely no difference in outcomes between the two modes of dialysis. A very encouraging early report has shown that dramatically increasing the time of dialysis may both increase fertility and decrease pregnancy complications (15). A group of 45 women undergoing nocturnal hemodialysis was studied. They had a 15.6% fertility rate, much higher than that of patients in older reports (only 2.2%). The authors reported that in those seven pregnancies in five women treated with nocturnal hemodialysis, six infants survived (the seventh was terminated because of the suspicion of a molar pregnancy, although pathology ultimately established it had been a normal pregnancy). The average dialysis time was 36 h/wk before conception and 48 h/wk during pregnancy. The mean gestational age at delivery was 36.2 weeks plus or minus 3 weeks with mean birth weight of 2417.5 g plus or minus 657 g. Although the women in this study represented a somewhat selected group (eg, none had diabetes mellitus), if these results are reproduced, women undergoing dialysis may be more optimistic about their ability to conceive and much more optimistic about their ability to successfully carry a child if they do.

The obstetric management of these patients is not substantially altered with the exception of taking great care to avoid magnesium toxicity if magnesium sulfate is chosen as a tocolytic or used for seizure prophylaxis because of preeclampsia. Also, indomethacin should be used cautiously because it may have an effect on any residual renal function a patient may have, increasing their need for dialysis. As with any chronic medical conditions that pose a high risk of stillbirth and intrauterine growth restriction, patients should be monitored with early fetal surveillance. With regard to the route of delivery, cesarean deliveries are reserved for routine obstetric indications (16). For patients undergoing peritoneal dialysis who must undergo cesarean delivery, the abdomen should be drained preoperatively and the surgery performed extraperitoneally, if possible. Peritoneal dialysis may be resumed 24 hours postoperatively, but if transperitoneal cesarean delivery is required and leakage occurs, hemodialysis should be substituted for 2 weeks.

The goals of dialysis during pregnancy do not differ substantially from goals in the nonpregnant state; however, certain modifications are necessary. The minimum goal for dialysis is to maintain the blood urea nitrogen level below 80 mg/dL, and a blood urea nitrogen level below 50–60 mg/dL is much preferred. To limit hypotension and decreased uterine perfusion, the volume of exchanges must be limited. In most pregnant women undergoing hemodialysis, exchanges occur daily or on 6 of 7 days per week by the start of the third trimester. Increasing the number of hours of hemodialysis to 20 or more results in a decreased rate of prematurity and improved infant survival. Women undergoing dialysis often are anemic and may require transfusions. In order to maintain the hematocrit and reduce the need for transfusion, erythropoietin has been used in pregnancy for a number of conditions, including renal anemia, and appears to be well tolerated. It may increase the hematocrit to more than 30% in most patients. It is important to note that because dialysis increases the removal of water-soluble vitamins, pregnant women should take supplements. In particular, it is recommended that folic acid intake be increased fourfold.

Renal Transplantation

The first baby born to a renal transplant patient was delivered in 1958. In the 50 years since then, over 14,000 pregnancies have been reported among women with transplanted organs, of which renal transplants are by far the most common. Pregnancies conceived after renal transplantation that proceed beyond the first trimester are successful more than 90% of the time. It has been shown that the graft undergoes the same functional and anatomic changes seen in the normal kidney in relation to its preconceptional function. Results from numerous case series have shown that renal function is not affected by pregnancy when the graft has been previously stable, but there is an increased risk of deterioration in cases in which there is preexisting chronic rejection, proteinuria, or decreased renal function (serum creatinine level of 2.5 mg/dL or greater).

Biopsy-proven acute rejection complicates 2–4% of pregnancies, depending on calcineurin inhibitor exposure, but it appears that long-term graft survival is unaffected by pregnancy, regardless of the number of pregnancies a woman carries (17). Serial assessment of renal function is appropriate to monitor for graft rejection, and the onset of fever, oliguria, renal enlargement, or tenderness should prompt an evaluation for rejection. The onset or exacerbation of hypertension should be treated aggressively and the diagnosis of preeclampsia must be considered because these pregnancies are complicated by hypertension, preeclampsia, or both, in 30% of cases. Another common maternal complication is urinary tract infection, which is seen in 40% of cases. For this reason, monthly urine cultures are appropriate to screen for asymptomatic bacteriuria.

Also, anemia may occur more often and with greater severity in these women. Erythropoietin therapy is helpful in increasing the hematocrit. As might be expected, fetal survival and maternal course were better for women whose serum creatinine level was less than or equal to 1.4 mg/dL. Nonetheless, even though fetal survival was 96% with serum creatinine levels less than or equal to 1.4 mg/dL, it was still 75% in the group with moderate renal insufficiency.

The chief perinatal risk is prematurity, which is seen in approximately 40% of infants of women with renal transplants. Preterm births are the primary cause of low birth weight infants, with a birth weight of less than 2,500 g seen in almost 50% of patients and a birth weight of less than 1,500 g in approximately 15% of patients. Although many series report high cesarean delivery rates, women with transplants are candidates for vaginal delivery because the graft does not obstruct labor, and renal function is not affected by the mode of delivery (Box 26).

The mainstay of immunosuppression during pregnancy for renal transplants has been the calcineurin inhibitors cyclosporine and tacrolimus. Cyclosporine is not an animal teratogen and does not appear to be harmful to the fetus, but it has been associated with an increased risk of infants born with low birth weight (49.5%) and very low birth weight (17.8%) compared with infants born to women taking only azathioprine and prednisone (39.1% and 7.7%, respectively). However, those observations may be explained by a higher incidence of pregestational hypertension, a higher mean creatinine level, and shorter mean interval from transplant to pregnancy in the cyclosporine group. Cyclosporine levels have been reported both to increase and to decrease in pregnancy. Given the difficulty in predicting how levels will be affected in any given patient, levels should be checked frequently. Tacrolimus is a stronger calcineurin inhibitor than cyclosporine. It is an abortifacient in rats, rabbits, and mice, but this has not been seen in human exposures. There also is a dose-related teratogenicity noted in rabbits, but so far, human data has not suggested teratogenicity in humans.

Azathioprine is another commonly used immunosuppressant. Although it readily crosses the placenta, the fetal liver lacks the enzyme required for conversion to the active form. Consequently, the fetus is relatively protected from the drug. Most authors have reported no evidence of teratogenicity, although there may be an increased risk of intrauterine growth restriction.

Prednisone also is a mainstay of therapy, particularly when an acute rejection occurs. It does not cross the placenta efficiently, with the fetal concentration approximately one tenth of the maternal concentration. Although there have been reports of adrenal insufficiency and thymic hypoplasia in infants of women taking high doses of prednisone during pregnancy, the risk is quite small when the dose is less than or equal to 15 mg/d. Most reports have not suggested prednisone is a teratogen; however, results from one meta-analysis of epidemiologic studies associated the use of corticosteroids in the first trimester with a small increase in major malformations, and results from case–control studies showed a significant association with oral clefts (18). Although this risk should be discussed with a patient, this association should not lead one to withhold the use of prednisone when it is the appropriate therapy.

There are other, newer immunosuppressants for which only limited data on use during pregnancy are available. The use of mycophenolate mofetil outside of pregnancy has increased dramatically over the past decade. Studies identified a characteristic mycophenolate mofetil phenotype in humans, mirroring abnormalities noted in animal models, in multiple reports (19). Consequently, the use of mycophenolate mofetil should be discontinued before conception, and other immunosuppressants should be used. Other immunosuppressants, such as muromonab and sirolimus, have been studied less widely.

Urolithiasis

Urolithiasis, although not common, is one of the most common painful and nonobstetric causes for hospitalization of pregnant women. Its importance is not only the pain that it causes the pregnant women; it has been associated with an 80% increase in the risk of preterm delivery (20).

Urinalysis is helpful when it reveals microscopic hematuria, but definitive diagnosis requires imaging studies. The main modality used in pregnancy is ultrasonography. Standard abdominal ultrasonography has been quoted to have a sensitivity of 34–60%. However, several techniques may enhance sensitivity. Although intravenous urography is superior to ultrasonography, the exposure of the fetus to radiation has moved this

---

Box 26

Characteristics of Patients Who May Best Qualify for Pregnancy After Kidney Transplantation

- Good health and at least 2 years since transplantation
- No (or minimal) proteinuria
- No hypertension
- No evidence of graft rejection
- Stable renal function
- Using maintenance immunosuppression

study to a secondary modality during pregnancy. A limited, three-film study including a scout, a 30-second film, and a 20-minute film has a greater than 90% sensitivity to identify a stone. Radiation exposure to the fetus can be limited by shielding the contralateral, unaffected side and obtaining the films in a prone position helps limit exposure (21). Magnetic resonance imaging has not been shown to add much to our ability to diagnose stones during pregnancy.

Once the diagnosis is made, initial therapy consists of hydration and analgesics. Approximately 80% of stones up to 4 mm will pass spontaneously. Pain should be managed with narcotics. A urine culture also should be obtained with appropriate antibiotic administration if a urinary tract infection is diagnosed. For patients who do not have spontaneous stone passage, the most common intervention is placement of internal stents, usually under ultrasound guidance. Stents will provide symptomatic relief, but they can cause complications themselves. Stent encrustation may occur on long-indwelling stents, and stent migration has been reported (more common with a double-J stent than a pigtail stent). It is recommended that stents be changed every 4–8 weeks to manage encrusting. In cases of a stone in the distal ureter, ureteroscopy with stone extraction by mini-basket or disintegration by ultrasonography has been used successfully. More recently, the use of uteroscopy with holmium laser lithotripsy during pregnancy has been reported with encouraging results. It does not carry the same risks as traditional lithotripsy because the penetration is only 0.5–1 mm from the probe tip, and the sound intensity is decreased, lowering concerns regarding fetal hearing. A theoretical concern that persists is the production of cyanide from the destruction of uric acid stones, but systemic absorption is thought to be minimal. Finally, placement of a percutaneous nephrostomy has been shown to be safe during pregnancy; however, it carries ongoing risks of dislodgement, discomfort, and increased risk of infection.

References

1. Ramin SM, Vidaeff AC, Yeomans ER, Gilstrap LC 3rd. Chronic renal disease in pregnancy. Obstet Gynecol 2006;108:1531–9.

2. Jones DC, Hayslett JP. Outcome of pregnancy in women with moderate or severe renal insufficiency. N Engl J Med 1996;335:226–32.

3. Griffin KA, Picken MM, Bakris GL, Bidani AK. Class differences in the effects of calcium channel blockers in the rat remnant kidney model. Kidney Int 1999;55:1849–60.

4. Khandelwal M, Kumanova M, Gaughan JP, Reece EA. Role of diltiazem in pregnant women with chronic renal disease. J Matern Fetal Neonatal Med 2002;12:408–12.

5. Hemmelder MH, de Zeeuw D, Fidler V, de Jong PE. Proteinuria: a risk factor for pregnancy-related renal function decline in primary glomerular disease? Am J Kidney Dis 1995;26:187–92.

6. Bar J, Ben-Rafael Z, Padoa A, Orvieto R, Boner G, Hod M. Prediction of pregnancy outcome in subgroups of women with renal disease. Clin Nephrol 2000;53:437–44.

7. Landon MB. Diabetic nephropathy and pregnancy. Clin Obstet Gynecol 2007;50:998–1006.

8. Khoury JC, Miodovnik M, LeMasters G, Sibai B. Pregnancy outcome and progression of diabetic nephropathy. What's next? J Matern Fetal Neonatal Med 2002;11:238–44.

9. Gordon M, Landon MB, Samuels P, Hissrich S, Gabbe SG. Perinatal outcome and long-term follow-up associated with modern management of diabetic nephropathy. Obstet Gynecol 1996;87:401–9.

10. Fischer MJ. Chronic kidney disease and pregnancy: maternal and fetal outcomes. Adv Chronic Kidney Dis 2007;14:132–45.

11. Moroni G, Quaglini S, Banfi G, Caloni M, Finazzi S, Ambroso G, et al. Pregnancy in lupus nephritis. Am J Kidney Dis 2002;40:713–20.

12. Ruiz-Irastorza G, Khamashta MA. Lupus and pregnancy: ten questions and some answers. Lupus 2008;17:416–20.

13. Tandon A, Ibanez D, Gladman DD, Urowitz MB. The effect of pregnancy on lupus nephritis. Arthritis Rheum 2004;50:3941–6.

14. Chou CY, Ting IW, Lin TH, Lee CN. Pregnancy in patients on chronic dialysis: a single center experience and combined analysis of reported results. Eur J Obstet Gynecol Reprod Biol 2008;136:165–70.

15. Barua M, Hladunewich M, Keunen J, Pierratos A, McFarlane P, Sood M, et al. Successful pregnancies on nocturnal home hemodialysis. Clin J Am Soc Nephrol 2008;3:392–6.

16. Hou S. Conception and pregnancy in peritoneal dialysis patients. Perit Dial Int 2001;21 (suppl 3):S290–4.

17. Mastrobattista JM, Gomez-Lobo V. Pregnancy after solid organ transplantation. Society for Maternal-Fetal Medicine. Obstet Gynecol 2008;112:919–32.

18. Park–Wyllie L, Mazzotta P, Pastuszak A, Moretti ME, Beique L, Hunnisett L, et al. Birth defects after maternal exposure to corticosteroids: prospective cohort study and meta-analysis of epidemiological studies. Teratology 2000;62:385–92.

19. Perez-Aytes A, Ledo A, Boso V, Saenz P, Roma E, Poveda JL, et al. In utero exposure to mycophenolate mofetil: a characteristic phenotype? Am J Med Genet A 2008;146A: 1–7.

20. Swartz MA, Lydon-Rochelle MT, Simon D, Wright JL, Porter MP. Admission for nephrolithiasis in pregnancy and risk of adverse birth outcomes. Obstet Gynecol 2007;109:1099–104.

21. Biyani CS, Joyce AD. Urolithiasis in pregnancy. I: pathophysiology, fetal considerations and diagnosis. BJU Int 2002;89:811–8; quiz i–ii.

Immunologic Disorders

Donna S. Dizon-Townson and Cara C. Heuser

The immunologic disorders affecting pregnancy may be classified as either autoimmune or alloimmune. Auto-immune diseases likely to be encountered by the obstetrician include rheumatoid arthritis, systemic lupus erythematosus, antiphospholipid antibody syndrome, systemic sclerosis, and myasthenia gravis. Other rare autoimmune diseases less likely to be encountered include Sjögren syndrome, ankylosing spondylitis, and mixed connective tissue disease. Alloimmune disorders are the result of an immune response to antigens of different individuals of the same species. Alloimmune diseases of significant obstetric consequence include hematologic alloimmunization and alloimmune thrombocytopenia. Because these important alloimmune conditions are reviewed in other sections, the current sections focuses on autoimmune disorders.

Rheumatoid Arthritis

Rheumatoid arthritis is a chronic debilitating disease characterized by symmetrical polyarthritis of the small joints of the hands and feet. Most individuals affected by rheumatoid arthritis are women, and its onset is frequently during childbearing years. Overall, rheumatoid arthritis complicates pregnancy in approximately 1 in 1,000–2,000 cases. Although the etiology of rheumatoid arthritis is unknown, it probably is secondary to environmental exposure on an underlying genetic predisposition. Rheumatoid arthritis does not appear to have adverse effects on pregnancy. In fact, secondary to the hormonal and immunologic changes of pregnancy, approximately 75% of women with rheumatoid arthritis improve during pregnancy. However, 10% of pregnant women may experience worsening of their symptoms. A relapse of rheumatoid arthritis is observed within 3–6 months after delivery in approximately 90% of women (1). Disease characteristics, including duration and functional class, do not appear to be predictive of a patient's remission status during pregnancy (2). There are conflicting data on the remission-enhancing effects of greater maternal–fetal human leukocyte antigen mismatches.

Goals of therapy should include reduction of inflammation and pain and preservation of joint function. Analgesics and antiinflammatory agents are the first-line therapy. The primary therapeutic agents during pregnancy are acetaminophen for simple analgesia and aspirin and other nonsteroidal antiinflammatory drugs (NSAIDs) for antiinflammatory action. Contraindications for chronic use of NSAIDs include late pregnancy (greater than 28 weeks of gestation), aspirin-induced asthma, congestive heart failure, and renal dysfunction. Corticosteroids may be used in the short term during acute exacerbations, or chronically in low doses. The risk of neonatal adrenal suppression after maternal treatment with hydrocortisone or prednisolone is very low, probably secondary to the placental metabolism of these corticosteroids. If possible, corticosteroids should be avoided during the first trimester of pregnancy while the hard palate is forming, secondary to a possible association with cleft palate (3). Intraarticular steroids also may be used during pregnancy.

Other medications that can be used with caution by pregnant women with rheumatoid arthritis include hydroxychloroquine, sulfasalazine, gold salts, cyclosporine, and d-penicillamine. Methotrexate and cyclophosphamide use should be avoided in pregnancy and breastfeeding because of the potential mutagenic and teratogenic effects. There is minimal data regarding use of tumor necrosis factor α therapy (ie, infliximab, rituximab, and etanercept) in pregnancy, although there are results from case reports linking these agents with VACTERL association in exposed fetuses. The most experience in pregnancy has been found with the use of infliximab, which is associated with live-born rates consistent with the general population (4). Nonpharmacologic therapy, including rest, appropriate use of heat and cold, assistive devices, and physical therapy, also are important components of caring for pregnant women with rheumatoid arthritis.

Systemic Lupus Erythematosus

Systemic lupus erythematosus (SLE) is an idiopathic chronic inflammatory disease that affects multiple organ systems. It occurs predominantly in women, and for pregnant women, its prevalence is 1 in 2,000–3,000 (5). The prevalence of SLE is greater among minority women, including African-American, Hispanic, and Native-American women. Patients may present with vague constitutional symptoms, with fatigue being the most common. Weight loss, fever, arthralgia, myalgias, and a malar (butterfly) rash or other cutaneous symptoms occur in 80% or more of patients. Fertility does not appear to be affected by SLE.

The diagnosis of SLE is suspected by the clinical presentation and confirmed by the presence of circulation autoantibodies (Box 27). The American College of Rheumatology criteria for the diagnosis of SLE published in 1997 are still valid today (Box 28).

Systemic Lupus Erythematosus Antibodies

- Antinuclear antibody: initial screening test
- Anti-double-stranded DNA: most specific for systemic lupus erythematosus, found in 80–90% of untreated patients, may be related to disease activity
- Anti-single-stranded DNA: less specific
- Anti-Sm antigen
- Antinuclear ribonucleoprotein: mixed connective tissue disease
- Anti-SS-A: specific for Sjögren syndrome and systemic lupus erythematosus, associated with nephritis, congenital heart block, and neonatal lupus
- Anti-SS-B: associated with neonatal lupus
- Anticardiolipin: vascular thromboses and recurrent pregnancy loss

Box 28

Revised Criteria for Classification of Systemic Lupus Erythematosus

To be classified as having systemic lupus erythematosus, an individual must have at least 4 of 11 items of the following criteria simultaneously or serially:

- Malar rash
- Discoid rash
- Photosensitivity
- Oral ulcers
- Arthritis (nonerosive arthritis involving two or more peripheral joints)
- Serositis (pleuritis or pericarditis)
- Renal disorders (proteinuria greater than 0.5 g/d or 3+ if quantitation not performed or cellular casts)
- Neurologic disorders (seizures or psychosis or other central or peripheral neuropsychiatric syndrome)
- Hematologic disorders (hemolytic anemia, leukopenia, lymphopenia, or thrombocytopenia)
- Immunologic disorders (Anti-DNA or Anti-Sm antibodies or positive findings of antiphospholipid antibodies: an abnormal serum level of immunoglobulin G or immunoglobulin M anticardiolipin antibodies; lupus anticoagulant; or false-positive serologic test result for syphilis)
- Antinuclear antibody

Data from Hochberg MC. Updating the American College of Rheumatology revised criteria for the classification of systemic lupus erythematosus [letter]. Arthritis Rheum 1997;40:1725 and Tan EM, Cohen AS, Fries JF, Masi AT, McShane DJ, Rothfield NF, et al. The 1982 revised criteria for the classification of systemic lupus erythematosus. Arthritis Rheum 1982;25:1271–7.

Clinically obvious renal disease occurs in 50% of patients with SLE and is directly related to pregnancy outcome. Proteinuria is the most common presentation and usually worsens in pregnancy. Four basic histologic and clinical categories of lupus nephropathy exist. Diffuse proliferative glomerulonephritis is the most common and most severe lesion. Hypertension, moderate to heavy proteinuria, nephrotic syndrome, hematuria, pyuria, casts, hypocomplementemia, and circulation immune complexes often are seen at the same time. Focal proliferative glomerulonephritis, membranous glomerulonephritis, and mesangial nephritis are progressively less severe.

The effects of SLE on pregnancy outcome are related to the presence of hypertension, renal impairment, active disease, and the presence of antiphospholipid antibody syndrome. If none of these disorders are present, the probability of a normal pregnancy outcome is enhanced. The presence and degree of renal impairment and hypertension antedating pregnancy is related to the frequency of superimposed preeclampsia. Overall, 20–30% of pregnant women with SLE have complications of pregnancy-induced hypertension.

Women with SLE are more likely to have other complications during pregnancy as well. Results from one study found that the risk of maternal mortality was increased 20-fold in patients with SLE (6). Risks of thrombosis, infection, thrombocytopenia, and transfusion were threefold to sevenfold higher than those for the general population. These patients also are at increased risk for cesarean delivery, intrauterine growth restriction, and preterm labor. The increased incidence of preeclampsia and eclampsia in these patients is well established. Furthermore, up to one third of lupus patients will have some degree of pulmonary hypertension, and even mild pulmonary hypertension can be very dangerous during pregnancy. These complications underscore the need for close monitoring of these patients by maternal–fetal medicine and rheumatology specialists during pregnancy.

Whether pregnancy predisposes women to increased SLE disease flares remains controversial. Flares may be related to disease activity at the outset of pregnancy. The rate of disease flare is lower if the disease is under good control for at least 6 months before conception. Approximately 15–60% of women with SLE have an exacerbation during pregnancy or the postpartum period. Most SLE exacerbations during pregnancy are treated with low to moderate doses of corticosteroids, which may be given for 4–6 weeks. There is no evidence that prophylactic corticosteroids will prevent SLE disease flares. Distinguishing an exacerbation of SLE involving active nephritis from preeclampsia may be difficult because each may present with proteinuria, hypertension, and evidence of multiorgan dysfunction. Elevated levels of anti–double-stranded DNA, low levels of classical pathway complement components, and active urinary sediment with cellular casts and hematuria suggest a lupus flare. This is a critical distinction because the management of preeclampsia may involve immediate delivery regardless of gestational age, whereas the management of a lupus flare does not. In addition to hypertensive flare, other manifestations of worsening SLE include cerebritis, carditis, nephritis, and pneumonitis.

Neonatal lupus erythematosus occurs in less than 5% of pregnant patients with SLE. It is characterized by dermatologic, cardiac, or hematologic abnormalities. It results from transplacental passage of maternal anti-SS-A immunoglobulin (Ig)G, anti-SS-B IgG, or both that cause fetal tissue damage. The lesions appear within the first several weeks after delivery and may last up to 6 months. The cardiac lesion associated with neonatal lupus erythematosus is congenital complete heart block from fibrosis and disruption of the conduction system, which occurs in 2% of affected pregnancies. The usual clinical presentation is fixed fetal bradycardia in the range of 60–80 beats per minute detected between 16 weeks of gestation and 25 weeks of gestation in a structurally normal heart. Ultrasound evaluation shows atrioventricular dissociation. Hydrops fetalis and even fetal death may occur. New onset congenital heart block rarely develops after the 30th week of pregnancy. In pregnancies where heart block is detected, steroid treatment with either dexamethasone (4 mg daily) or betamethasone (2–3 mg daily) has shown some promise in improving outcomes, especially if only incomplete heart block exists (7). Most experts recommend a trial of steroid administration when incomplete heart block is newly diagnosed. However, if heart block does not improve after several weeks, continued therapy is unlikely to be beneficial. The role of more frequent ultrasound examinations in patients who test positive for anti-SS-A IgG and anti-SS-B IgG to evaluate the P–R interval or other early markers preceding congenital heart block is still being elucidated (8). Among mothers with SLE and anti-SS-A IgG, the risk of dermatologic manifestations of neonatal lupus erythematosus is approximately 15%. Recurrence risk is 25% for dermatologic manifestations and 10% for congenital heart block. Optimally, women should receive preconception counseling and a thorough discussion of potential maternal and fetal risks during pregnancy (Box 29). Pregnant patients should be seen at least every 2 weeks and instructed to be alert to the signs and symptoms of preeclampsia. After 18–20 weeks of gestation, ultrasonography should be performed every 4–6 weeks to assess fetal growth.

Therapy for SLE should include reduction of inflammation and pain and preservation of joint and organ function. Therefore, drugs most frequently used are analgesics, such as acetaminophen and NSAIDs. More

---

Box 29
Preconception Counseling of Women With Systemic Lupus Erythematosus

Discussion About Potential Risks
- Pregnancy loss, including spontaneous miscarriage and later fetal death
- Preterm delivery
- Pregnancy-induced hypertension
- Intrauterine growth restriction

Physical and Laboratory Evaluation
- General physical examination, including blood pressure measurement
- Complete blood count
- Urinalysis
- Serum creatinine level assessment
- 24-hour urine collection for creatinine clearance and total protein
- Antiphospholipid antibodies (LA and aCL)
- Anti-SS-A, anti-SS-B

---

severe cases require the use of antimalarials, corticosteroids, and cytotoxic agents. Use of antimalarials, specifically hydroxychloroquine, appear to be safe for the fetus. Results from several studies have demonstrated the safety of hydroxychloroquine use in pregnancy and have shown an increase in disease activity and adverse outcome when hydroxychloroquine use was stopped during pregnancy (9, 10). However, antimalarial use has not been shown to be effective in the treatment of fever, SLE nephritis, or neurologic or hematologic disease manifestations. Corticosteroid use is another acceptable alternative therapy for treatment for SLE during pregnancy. The use of systemic corticosteroids are indicated for life-threatening symptoms of SLE, such as nephritis or neurologic or hematologic manifestations. Most experts recommend that stress-dose steroids (hydrocortisone, 100 mg every 6–8 hours) be given during labor or at the time of cesarean delivery to all patients who have been treated with steroids within 1 year. Other medications used to treat SLE, such as azathioprine, methotrexate, and cyclophosphamide, are best avoided during pregnancy. Women with SLE who test positive for antiphospholipid antibodies should be treated as detailed in the section "Antiphospholipid Antibody Syndrome."

Antiphospholipid Antibody Syndrome

Antiphospholipid antibody syndrome is an autoimmune condition characterized by the production of moderate to high levels of antiphospholipid antibodies and specific clinical features. Approximately 70% of patients with antiphospholipid antibody syndrome are female. Clinical manifestations of the syndrome include pregnancy loss (fetal death or recurrent pregnancy loss) and arterial or venous thrombosis (see the section "Deep Vein Thrombosis and Pulmonary Embolism"). Autoimmune thrombocytopenia, a false-positive test result for syphilis, livedo reticularis, and other features also may be seen. Antiphospholipid antibodies are found in as many as 50% of patients with SLE but also may occur in patients without overt lupus. Furthermore, antiphospholipid antibodies of the IgG and IgM classes have been reported to be present in 1.8% and 4%, respectively, of otherwise healthy pregnant women. A diagnosis of antiphospholipid antibody syndrome is based on very specific criteria and requires that the patient have at least one clinical feature of the syndrome along with confirmatory laboratory testing (Box 30). It should be noted that there are a number of clinical and laboratory entities mentioned in this section, including livedo reticularis, thrombocytopenia, neurologic manifestations, IgA antiphospholipid antibodies, and others, that have been associated with antiphospholipid antibody syndrome but that are not included in the revised diagnostic criteria. These clinical manifestations should not be used to diagnose antiphospholipid antibody syndrome but should not be disregarded as irrelevant (11).

Testing

Testing for lupus anticoagulant, anticardiolipin antibodies, and antibodies to β_2-glycoprotein should be done when the diagnosis of antiphospholipid antibody syndrome is considered. Routine screening of healthy pregnant women is not recommended. Possible indications for testing are shown in Box 31. The following tests are used for initial screening, verification of results, and confirmation of specific phospholipid specificity:

- Combination of two phospholipid-dependent clotting assays (ie, activated partial thromboplastin time, dilute Russell viper venom time, or kaolin clotting time)

- Mixing of the patient's plasma with an equal volume of normal plasma to differentiate between the presence of a circulating inhibitor, such as lupus anticoagulant, and the presence of a clotting factor deficiency

- Enzyme-linked immunosorbent assay using purified cardiolipin as the antigen

- Enzyme-linked immunosorbent assay to detect antibodies to β_2-glycoprotein I

The lupus anticoagulant assays will have a result of either present or absent. A present result, along with one of the clinical features of the syndrome is sufficient for diagnosis. In contrast, the diagnosis based on anticardiolipin antibodies or anti-β_2-glycoprotein is more complex.

Low positive anticardiolipin antibodies levels (less than 40 GPL/MPL) should not be used to establish the diagnosis and are of questionable significance. Immunoglobulin A anticardiolipin antibodies also are of questionable significance and should not be used to establish the diagnosis. Only moderate to high levels of anticardiolipin antibodies IgG or IgM (greater than 40 MPL/GPL) should be used to establish the diagnosis, always in conjunction with clinical criteria. Antibodies to β_2-glycoprotein should be at a titer of greater than 99th percentile for either IgG

Box 30

Diagnostic Criteria for Antiphospholipid Antibody Syndrome Based on International Society for Thrombosis and Haemostasis Guidelines

At least one item of the following clinical criteria and one item of the laboratory criteria must be met for the diagnosis of antiphospholipid antibody syndrome:

Clinical Criteria

1. Vascular thrombosis, including one or more clinical episodes of arterial, venous, or small vessel thrombosis in any tissue or organ; must be confirmed by objective validated criteria (ie, unequivocal findings of appropriate imaging studies or histopathology)

2. Pregnancy Morbidity

   A. One or more unexplained death of a morphologically normal fetus at or beyond 10 weeks of gestation

   B. One or more premature births of a morphologically normal fetus at less than 34 weeks of gestation because of eclampsia, severe preeclampsia, or placental insufficiency

   C. Three or more unexplained consecutive spontaneous abortions before the 10th week of gestation after exclusion of other causes

Laboratory Criteria (Must be Present on Two or More Occasions at Least 12 Weeks Apart)

1. Presence of lupus anticoagulant

2. Anticardiolipin antibodies (immunoglobulin G or immunoglobulin M) in medium or high titer (greater than 40 GPL/MPL or greater than 99th percentile) by enzyme-linked immunosorbent assay test

3. Anti-β_2-glycoprotein-I antibody (immunoglobulin G or immunoglobulin M) in titer greater than 99th percentile

Miyakis S, Lockshin M, Atsumi T, Branch DW, Brey RL, Cervera R, et al. International consensus statement on an update of the classification criteria for definite antiphospholipid antibody syndrome (APS). J Thromb Haemostas 2006;4:295–306. Copyright Wiley-Blackwell.

or IgM to suffice as laboratory criteria for diagnosis. Furthermore, positive laboratory test results should be confirmed on two occasions at least 12 weeks apart.

Maternal Risks

Maternal risks include thrombosis, stroke, preeclampsia, postpartum syndrome, and catastrophic antiphospholipid antibody syndrome. More than one half of thrombotic episodes occur in relation to pregnancy or during the use of combination oral contraceptives. Two prospective studies in pregnant women with the syndrome showed a rate of thrombosis and stroke of 5% and 12%, respectively (12, 13).

The high incidence (20–50%) of preeclampsia in patients with antiphospholipid antibody syndrome contributes to a high rate of preterm birth. The rate of preeclampsia does not appear to be markedly reduced by treatment with either low-dose aspirin or heparin. Patients with severe, early-onset preeclampsia at less than 34 weeks of gestation have an increased rate of antiphospholipid antibodies (11–17%).

During the immediate postpartum period, complications that may represent an autoimmune exacerbation may occur. These may include fever, pulmonary infiltrates, pleural effusions, thrombosis, and cardiomyopathy. Renal insufficiency and pulmonary hypertension also may accompany this syndrome.

Box 31

Possible Indications for Testing for Antiphospholipid Antibodies

- Recurrent spontaneous abortion (three or more spontaneous abortions with no more than one live birth)
- Unexplained second-trimester or third-trimester fetal death
- Severe early-onset preeclampsia (less than 34 weeks of gestation)
- Unexplained venous or arterial thrombosis
- Unexplained stroke
- Unexplained transient ischemic attack or amaurosis fugax
- Systemic lupus erythematosus or other connective tissue disease
- Autoimmune thrombocytopenia
- Autoimmune hemolytic anemia
- Livedo reticularis
- Chorea gravidarum
- False-positive serologic test result for syphilis
- Unexplained prolongation in clotting assay
- Unexplained severe intrauterine growth restriction

Catastrophic antiphospholipid antibody syndrome, an accelerated form of antiphospholipid antibody syndrome resulting in multiorgan failure, occurs rarely. Patients have high titers of antiphospholipid antibodies and a rapid, deteriorating course of malignant hypertension, pulmonary hypertension, renal insufficiency, widespread thrombosis, and disseminated intravascular coagulopathy. The associated mortality is high; thus, the condition should be considered an emergency.

Fetal Risks

The fetal risks of antiphospholipid antibody syndrome include death and intrauterine growth restriction. Fetal death appears to be more specific to antiphospholipid antibody syndrome than does early embryonic loss. Recurrent first-trimester pregnancy loss is fairly common, affecting approximately 1% of the general population. Its link to antiphospholipid antibody syndrome, however, must be carefully assessed. Only patients who also meet the laboratory criteria should be considered to have the syndrome.

Antiphospholipid antibodies may be associated with fetal growth impairment. Even with treatment, the rate of fetal growth impairment among liveborn infants approaches 30%. Nonreassuring fetal heart tracings also appear to be more common in pregnancies complicated by antiphospholipid antibody syndrome. Treatment has not been shown to decrease the rate of these complications.

Management

The treatment of antiphospholipid antibody syndrome during pregnancy should focus on improving maternal and fetal outcomes by reducing known complications of this disorder. Preconception counseling in women with antiphospholipid antibody syndrome should cover the potential maternal and fetal risks. Patients should undergo baseline studies assessing the presence of anemia, thrombocytopenia, and underlying renal disease (complete blood count, urinalysis, serum creatinine, and 24-hour urine for creatinine clearance and total protein).

During pregnancy, women with antiphospholipid antibody syndrome may be seen by a physician at least every 2 weeks in the first and second trimesters and weekly thereafter. These patients should be educated about the signs and symptoms of thrombosis, thromboembolism, transient ischemic attacks, amaurosis fugax, and preeclampsia. Serial antiphospholipid antibody determinations are not useful in terms of establishing prognosis or managing therapy. Maternal surveillance for the development of hypertension and proteinuria is crucial. The fetus can be assessed for intrauterine growth restriction with ultrasonography starting at 18–20 weeks of gestation. Antenatal surveillance should be considered after 32 weeks of gestation, or earlier if growth restriction is present.

Heparin, including unfractionated heparin and low molecular weight heparin, and low-dose aspirin, have become the most widely accepted methods of treatment during pregnancy. Heparin therapy is recommended because it may reduce the incidence of pregnancy loss in patients with antiphospholipid antibody syndrome. Furthermore, heparin also is used for prevention of pregnancy-related thrombotic events. Treatment has not been shown to prevent other adverse outcomes during pregnancy, such as preeclampsia, utero–placental insufficiency, preterm birth, and abnormal heart rate tracings.

The dosing of either low molecular weight heparin or unfractionated heparin depends on the patient's clinical history. Furthermore, use of both low molecular weight heparin and unfractionated heparin may have less predictable pharmakinetics during pregnancy secondary to physiologic changes, such as increased weight gain, increased renal clearance, and increased volume of distribution. Therefore, most experts recommend monitoring the partial thromboplastin time when unfractionated heparin is used and anti-Xa levels when low molecular weight heparin is used. Both of these measurements should be taken 4 hours after the administration of the medication. Most laboratories will have a nomogram or protocol for dose adjustments.

For women who have not had a thrombotic event, most experts recommend prophylactic treatment. Usually, this consists of the use of low molecular weight heparin (enoxaparin, 40–80 mg daily, or dalteparin, 5,000 international units daily) or the use of unfractionated heparin (twice daily dosing of 15,000–20,000 units daily) with or without low-dose aspirin during pregnancy and the postpartum period.

Treatment should be started as soon as the diagnosis of pregnancy is made. Delivery often is scheduled to allow for discontinuation of anticoagulation at an appropriate time interval. During the postpartum period, patients may be transitioned to warfarin. Patients should be monitored by an internist or a hematologist to assess the need for anticoagulation therapy outside of pregnancy and the postpartum period. Furthermore, the use of estrogen containing contraceptives should be avoided.

Prompt recognition of the signs and symptoms is essential in cases of postpartum syndrome or catastrophic antiphospholipid antibody syndrome. Medical therapies must be individualized, and the optimal treatment is not known; however, certain guidelines are useful. First, precipitating factors, such as infection, should be identified and treated. Other goals include control of blood pressure, prevention and treatment thrombotic events, and suppression of the excessive cytokine activity. The most commonly described treatments include the use of intravenous heparin followed by the use of oral anticoagulation, corticosteroids, plasma exchange, intravenous gamma globulins and, if associated with SLE, cyclophosphamide.

Systemic Sclerosis

Systemic sclerosis, also known as scleroderma, is characterized by localized or diffuse fibrosis of connective tissue and a progressive obliterative vasculopathy. It is a rare disease, with an annual incidence of only approximately 1–2 per 100,000 individuals, and its effects on fertility remain unknown. In the localized form, the disease usually is limited to the skin in the hands and is associated with Raynaud phenomenon. Raynaud phenomenon is intermittent bilateral ischemia of the fingers, toes, and sometimes ears and nose. It presents as decreased or absent skin color with numbness or pain, and is triggered by cold temperatures or emotional stress. Systemic sclerosis can be either limited (80%) or diffuse (20%). Women with systemic sclerosis are thought to be at an increased risk for spontaneous abortion, and perhaps for intrauterine growth restriction as well. Other effects of this disease on pregnancy are not well described secondary to its uncommon occurrence. Neonatal involvement with skin sclerosis has been reported.

Pregnancy probably is safest among patients with scleroderma without obvious renal, cardiac, or pulmonary disease. Patients with early diffuse scleroderma (duration less than 5 years) are at particularly high risk of developing renal crisis, a condition that may be lethal. Patients in scleroderma renal crisis usually present with thrombocytopenia and daily increases in serum creatinine levels. Whether pregnancy increases the risk for renal crisis is controversial; however, renal crisis can be especially severe and carries a high mortality rate in pregnancy. These patients should be treated with intensive medical support, including dialysis and fetal monitoring, usually in an intensive care unit setting. Women with moderate to severe renal disease and hypertension also have a substantial risk for developing preeclampsia, which can be difficult to distinguish from renal crisis.

Patients with diffuse scleroderma should take a cautious and considered approach to pregnancy. Special attention should be directed to the assessment of renal, cardiac, and pulmonary involvement. In addition, coexisting antiphospholipid antibody syndrome should be ruled out. Unfortunately, there is no satisfactory treatment for scleroderma. Oral vasodilators for the prevention and treatment of Raynaud phenomenon may be used. Systemic corticosteroid use may be continued. Pregnant women with scleroderma should be seen frequently by their obstetricians, with close observation for preeclampsia and growth restriction.

Sjögren Syndrome

Sjögren syndrome is a rare autoimmune disorder characterized by the sicca syndrome, including dryness of the eyes (keratoconjunctivitis sicca), mouth (xerostomia), and other mucosal surfaces. There is a female predominance, with 90% of cases occurring in women aged between 40 years and 60 years. Several autoantibodies are associated with Sjögren syndrome, including anti-SS-A, anti-SS-B, and antinuclear antibodies. Treatment is based on symptoms and includes the use of oral and ocular topicals. The use of low-dose corticosteroids may decrease inflammation of the conjunctival surface. An increase in fetal loss and congenital heart block has been reported in pregnant women with Sjögren syndrome (14).

Ankylosing Spondylitis

Ankylosing spondylitis is a chronic inflammatory condition predominantly involving the spine. It is characterized by progressive, ascending stiffening and limitation of back motion and chest expansion. Often, spinal involvement begins at the level of the sacroiliac joints. Peripheral arthritis and uveitis are additional clinical manifestations. This is a rare autoimmune condition characterized by a male predominance.

During pregnancy, ankylosing spondylitis has been reported to worsen in one third of patients, improve in another one third of patients, and remain stable in the remaining one third of patients (15). Sixty percent of women experienced postpartum flares within 6 months following delivery. The use of general anesthesia is potentially difficult in these individuals because of ankylosis of the cervical spine and temporomandibular joints. Moreover, the use of regional anesthesia also may prove difficult because of calcification and ankylosis of the vertebral column. Consultation with an anesthesiologist early in pregnancy is recommended. Treatment for ankylosing spondylitis is similar to that for rheumatoid arthritis.

Mixed Connective Tissue Disease

Mixed connective tissue disease should be considered in an patient who has a heterogeneous clinical presentation and does not fit into definite criteria for another connective tissue disease. The disease is characterized by overlapping features of different rheumatologic diseases. It has a 16:1 female predominance. Antibodies to ribonucleoprotein often are present. Antiphospholipid antibody syndrome also should be ruled out in affected patients. Pregnancy outcome and management in women with mixed connective tissue disease is similar to that in patients with SLE.

References

1. Ostensen M. Sex hormones and pregnancy in rheumatoid arthritis and systemic lupus erythematosus. Ann N Y Acad Sci 1999;876:131–43; discussion 144.

2. Nelson JL, Ostensen M. Pregnancy and rheumatoid arthritis. Rheum Dis Clin North Am 1997;23:195–212.

3. Park-Wyllie L, Mazzotta P, Pastuszak A, Moretti ME, Beique L, Hunnisett L, et al. Birth defects after maternal exposure to corticosteroids: prospective cohort study and meta-analysis of epidemiological studies. Teratology 2000; 62:385–92.

4. Katz JA, Antoni C, Keenan GF, Smith DE, Jacobs SJ, Lichtenstein GR. Outcome of pregnancy in women receiving infliximab for the treatment of Crohn's disease and rheumatoid arthritis. Am J Gastroenterol 2004;99:2385–92.

5. Yasmeen S, Wilkins EE, Field NT, Sheikh RA, Gilbert WM. Pregnancy outcomes in women with systemic lupus erythematosus. J Matern Fetal Med 2001;10:91–6.

6. Clowse ME, Jamison M, Myers E, James AH. A national study of the complications of lupus in pregnancy. Am J Obstet Gynecol 2008;199:127.e1–127.e6.

7. Saleeb S, Copel J, Friedman D, Buyon JP. Comparison of treatment with fluorinated glucocorticoids to the natural history of autoantibody-associated congenital heart block: retrospective review of the research registry for neonatal lupus. Arthritis Rheum 1999;42:2335–45.

8. Friedman DM, Kim MY, Copel JA, Davis C, Phoon CK, Glickstein JS, et al. Utility of cardiac monitoring in fetuses at risk for congenital heart block: the PR Interval and Dexamethasone Evaluation (PRIDE) prospective study. Circulation 2008;117:485–93.

9. Levy RA, Vilela VS, Cataldo MJ, Ramos RC, Duarte JL, Tura BR, et al. Hydroxychloroquine (HCQ) in lupus pregnancy: double-blind and placebo-controlled study. Lupus 2001;10:401–4.

10. Clowse ME, Magder L, Witter F, Petri M. Hydroxychloroquine in lupus pregnancy. Arthritis Rheum 2006;54:3640–7.

11. Miyakis S, Lockshin MD, Atsumi T, Branch DW, Brey RL, Cervera R, et al. International consensus statement on an update of the classification criteria for definite antiphospholipid syndrome (APS). J Thromb Haemost 2006;4:295–306.

12. Branch DW, Silver RM, Blackwell JL, Reading JC, Scott JR. Outcome of treated pregnancies in women with antiphospholipid syndrome: an update of the Utah experience. Obstet Gynecol 1992;80:614–20.

13. Lima F, Khamashta MA, Buchanan NM, Kerslake S, Hunt BJ, Hughes GR. A study of sixty pregnancies in patients with the antiphospholipid syndrome. Clin Exp Rheumatol 1996; 14:131–6.

14. Julkunen H, Kaaja R, Kurki P, Palosuo T, Friman C. Fetal outcome in women with primary Sjogren's syndrome. A retrospective case-control study. Clin Exp Rheumatol 1995;13:65–71.

15. Ostensen M, Ostensen H. Ankylosing spondylitis--the female aspect. J Rheumatol 1998;25:120–4.

Infection

David E. Soper

Hepatitis

Viral hepatitis is one of the most common and potentially serious infections that can occur in pregnant women. Six forms of viral hepatitis have now been identified, two of which, hepatitis A and hepatitis B, can be prevented effectively through vaccination (1). Detailed discussion of hepatitis and its ramifications in pregnancy can be found in the section "Liver and Alimentary Tract Diseases."

Cytomegalovirus

Cytomegalovirus infection is caused by a double-stranded DNA herpes virus. The incidence of primary cytomegalovirus (CMV) infection in pregnant women in the United States varies from 1% to 3%. Approximately 50–85% of adults have serologic evidence of previous CMV infection by age 40 years. The virus has been shown to spread in households and among young children in day care centers through infected bodily fluids; simple hand washing with soap and water is effective in removing the virus from the hands. Infection also may be transmitted by sexual contact and blood transfusion. Most CMV infections in adults are subclinical. Symptomatic patients typically present with a mononucleosislike illness.

Cytomegalovirus remains an important cause of congenital viral infection in the United States. The morbidity of CMV congenital infection appears to be almost exclusively associated with primary CMV infection during pregnancy. Even in this case, two thirds of the infants will not become infected, and only 10–15% of the remaining third will have symptoms at the time of birth. Neonatal symptoms suggesting generalized infection range from moderate enlargement of the liver and spleen (with jaundice) to fatal illness. Of those neonates, 80–90% will have complications within the first few years of life that may include hearing loss, vision impairment, and varying degrees of mental retardation. After recurrent maternal CMV infection, only 10% of infants become infected, usually without symptoms at birth, but subsequently may have varying degrees of hearing and mental or coordination problems.

There appears to be little risk of CMV-related complications for women who have been infected at least 6 months before conception. For this group, which makes up 50–80% of the women of childbearing age, the rate of newborn CMV infection is 1%, and these infants appear to have no significant illness or abnormalities. The virus also can be transmitted to the infant at delivery from contact with genital secretions or later in infancy through breast milk. However, these infections usually result in little or no clinical illness in the infant.

The most significant risk factor for the development of a primary CMV infection during pregnancy is frequent and prolonged exposure to young children. Susceptible women may be exposed at home or in day care, and 50% of them will acquire CMV within a year. Although routine screening for CMV infection is still not recommended, this group of women may be considered for serologic screening with anti-CMV immunoglobulin (Ig)G and IgM antibody test. A gravid woman with test results that are positive for anti-CMV IgM antibodies should have subsequent IgG avidity testing. Avidity is an indirect measure of the tightness of antibody binding to its target antigen and increases the first weeks and months after primary infection. Currently, apart from IgG seroconversion, the combination of anti-CMV IgM and low-avidity anti-CMV IgG is the best way to diagnose a primary maternal infection (2).

Fetal CMV infection should be suspected when ultrasound examination results demonstrate fetal anomalies, such as abdominal and liver calcifications, echogenic bowel, hepatosplenomegaly, periventricular calcifications, ventriculomegaly, hydrops, and ascites (3). Confirmation of fetal infection is best determined by detection of CMV in amniotic fluid by polymerase chain reaction or culture.

Susceptible pregnant women can decrease their risk of infection by engaging in protective behaviors, such as frequent hand washing and reducing contact with the saliva and nasal secretions from young children. A preliminary report shows that fetuses of those gravidas diagnosed with a primary CMV infection appear to benefit from monthly CMV hyperimmune globulin administration until their IgG avidity increases (4). Because fetal CMV infections also are associated with a diffuse placental infection, follow-up ultrasound evaluations for placental thickness are appropriate. Work is in progress to develop vaccines against CMV.

Toxoplasmosis

Toxoplasmosis is caused by infection with the protozoan parasite *Toxoplasma gondii*. In the United States, an estimated 23% of adolescents and adults have laboratory evidence of infection with *T gondii*. Although these infections usually are either asymptomatic or associated with self-limited symptoms (eg, fever, malaise, and lymphadenopathy), infection in immunosuppressed persons can be severe. In addition, infections in pregnant women can cause serious health problems in the fetus if the parasites are transmitted and cause severe sequelae in the infant (eg, mental retardation, blindness, and epilepsy). Although congenital toxoplasmosis is not a nationally reportable disease and no national data are available regarding its occurrence, extrapolation from regional studies indicates that an estimated 400–4,000 cases occur in the United States each year (5).

Congenital toxoplasmosis can occur if the mother develops a primary infection during pregnancy (Box 32 and Box 33). Approximately one third of infants born to mothers with primary infection will be affected. The frequency of fetal infection is higher when maternal infection occurs in the third trimester (60–65%) than when it occurs in the first trimester (15–20%). However, the severity of infection is greater when the mother is infected during the first trimester.

Approximately one third of infected neonates have evidence of clinical disease at birth. The characteristic triad of congenital toxoplasmosis is intracerebral calcification, chorioretinitis, and hydrocephalus. Other findings may include anemia, jaundice, splenomegaly, generalized lymphadenopathy, seizures, microcephaly, mental retardation, and hearing impairment.

Box 32

Routes of Transmission of *Toxoplasma gondii* to Humans

- Ingestion of raw or inadequately cooked infected meat (primarily pork and lamb)
- Ingestion of oocysts, an environmentally resistant form of the organism that cats pass in their feces, with exposure of humans occurring through exposure to cat litter or soil (eg, from gardening or from unwashed fruits or vegetables)
- A newly infected pregnant woman passing the infection to her fetus

---

Box 33

Prevention of Toxoplasma Infection

- Cook meat to a safe temperature
- Peel or thoroughly wash fruits and vegetables before eating
- Clean cooking surfaces and utensils after they have contacted raw meat, poultry, seafood, or unwashed fruits or vegetables
- Pregnant women should avoid changing cat litter or, if no one else is available to change the cat litter, they should use gloves and then wash their hands thoroughly
- Do not feed raw or undercooked meat to cats and keep cats inside to prevent acquisition of toxoplasma by eating infected prey

---

The mainstay of diagnosis is serologic testing. Antibodies may be detected by indirect immunofluorescence or enzyme-linked immunosorbent assays. Patients with acute infection typically have positive assay results for IgM antibody, and their IgG antibody test results show seroconversion. Titers for IgM may remain positive for several months after acute infection.

Clinicians should be aware that serologic testing for toxoplasmosis is not well standardized, and only a few reference laboratories consistently provide reliable test results. When primary toxoplasmosis during pregnancy is suspected, serum specimens should be forwarded to one of these recognized referral centers for confirmation. State health departments and the Centers for Disease Control and Prevention can provide the names of qualified reference laboratories and should be contacted to obtain medications for treatment.

Several methods have been used to diagnose fetal infection with *T gondii*. A competitive polymerase chain reaction test for *T gondii* can be performed on amniotic fluid obtained by amniocentesis at 18 weeks of gestation (optimal time) or later. Fetal blood can be aspirated by cordocentesis and cultured. Fetal blood also can be assayed for total IgM concentration and IgM-specific antibodies after 21–23 weeks of gestation. However, although these measures may indicate that *T gondii* is present in the fetal and placental circulation, they do not precisely define the severity of fetal infection. Ultrasound findings that are consistent with severe fetal infection include microcephaly, ventriculomegaly, growth restriction, visceromegaly, and hydrops.

If acute fetal infection is documented, patients may be offered pregnancy termination or antibiotic treatment. A multidrug regimen, including the use of spiramycin, pyrimethamine, and sulfadiazine, can eradicate microorganisms in the placenta and fetus (6).

Herpes Simplex Virus

The clinical diagnosis of genital herpes is both insensitive and nonspecific. The typical painful multiple vesicular or ulcerative lesions are absent in many infected women. Both herpes simplex virus (HSV)-1 and HSV-2 can result in vertical transmission to the neonate (7).

Because false-negative HSV culture results are common, especially in patients with recurrent infection or with healing lesions, type-specific serologic tests are useful in confirming a clinical diagnosis of genital herpes. Additionally, such tests can be used to diagnose persons with unrecognized infection and to treat sex partners of persons with genital herpes. Although serologic assays for HSV-2 should be available for persons who request them, screening for HSV-1 or HSV-2 infection in the general population is not indicated.

Most mothers of infants who acquire HSV neonatally lack histories of clinically evident genital HSV. The risk for transmission to the neonate from an infected mother is high (30–50%) among women who acquire genital HSV near the time of delivery and is low (less than 1%) among women with histories of recurrent genital herpetic lesions at term or who acquire genital HSV during the first half of pregnancy. Prevention of neonatal HSV infection depends both on preventing acquisition of genital HSV infection during late pregnancy and avoiding exposure of the infant to herpetic lesions during delivery.

Pregnant women without known orolabial HSV should be advised to avoid cunnilingus with partners known or suspected to have orolabial HSV. Type-specific serologic tests may be used to clarify the gravida's risk for HSV infection and to guide counseling with regard to the risk of acquiring genital HSV during pregnancy. Such testing and counseling may be especially important when a woman's sex partner has HSV infection.

At the onset of labor, all women should be questioned carefully about symptoms of genital HSV, including prodrome, and all women should be examined carefully for herpetic lesions. Women without symptoms or signs of genital HSV or its prodrome can deliver vaginally, but use of invasive monitors should be limited. Women with recurrent genital herpetic lesions or prodromal symptoms at the onset of labor should have cesarean delivery to prevent neonatal HSV infection (8).

Oral antiviral therapy (acyclovir, valacyclovir, or famciclovir) should be considered for women at or beyond 36 weeks of gestation whose first episode of HSV occurred during the current pregnancy as well as for women at risk for recurrent HSV to decrease the likelihood of HSV shedding and need for cesarean delivery. Investigators have monitored more than 1,100 pregnancies in which women were exposed to acyclovir or valacyclovir and have found no evidence of adverse effects on the fetus (9).

Varicella

Varicella zoster virus (VZV), like other herpes viruses, has the capacity to exist in the body after primary infection in a latent state. Primary infection results in chickenpox, whereas reactivation can lead to herpes zoster (shingles). It is highly contagious, with up to 90% of susceptible household contacts becoming infected (10). Pregnant women should not be vaccinated, and vaccinated women should be advised to avoid pregnancy for 1 month after each dose because of concern about possible fetal effects. Women who do not have varicella immunity should receive the first dose of VZV vaccine in the postpartum period before hospital or birth center discharge. Surveillance data to date on fetal outcomes after inadvertent vaccine exposures, however, have not found any cases of fetal varicella syndrome. A pregnant household member is not a contraindication to vaccination of a child (11).

The onset of maternal varicella from 5 days before to 2 days after delivery may result in an overwhelming infection in the neonate, with fatality rates as high as 30% (10). This severe infection is believed to result from fetal exposure to the virus without benefit of passively acquired maternal antibody. For this reason, varicella-zoster immune globulin (VZIG) should be administered to these infants following delivery. Primary varicella infection during the first 20 weeks of pregnancy is associated with a variety of abnormalities in the newborn, including low birth weight, hypoplasia of an extremity, skin scarring, localized muscular atrophy, encephalitis, cortical atrophy, chorioretinitis, and microcephaly. The risk of congenital varicella zoster syndrome is low (approximately 1%).

Varicella zoster virus infection usually is diagnosed clinically, but confirmation by culture of the vesicular fluid and enzyme-linked immunosorbent assay testing for antibodies is available in most institutions. Primary VZV infection during pregnancy is associated with an increased risk for pneumonitis. For this reason, susceptible pregnant women with substantial exposure (live in the same house or have had more than 5 minutes face-to-face contact or have had indoor contact longer than 1 hour with infected individuals) should receive VZIG. If given within 96 hours of exposure, 80% of clinical chickenpox can be prevented, compared with a 90% rate of clinical chickenpox if no VZIG is provided. Administration of VZIG will not necessarily prevent maternal viremia and fetal infection. Pregnant women with clinical chickenpox need to be evaluated and should be monitored for symptoms and signs of varicella pneumonia. Risk factors for this serious complication include smoking, steroid use, and chronic obstructive pulmonary disease. Patients, especially in the third trimester, with an extensive rash, particularly if it is hemorrhagic in nature and involving the mucous membranes, also are at risk, and hospitalization should be considered. If symptoms suggest pneumonia, a chest X-ray and arterial blood gas measurement should be obtained. If the chest X-ray result is abnormal or the pO_2 is less than 80 mm Hg, admission and parenteral therapy with acyclovir is in order. If the patient has been determined to have uncomplicated chickenpox and has presented within 24 hours of rash onset, the use of oral acyclovir is appropriate, and she can be treated as an outpatient, reassessing her status every 24–48 hours.

On October 27, 2004, the Advisory Committee on Immunization Practices was informed that the only company making VZIG had discontinued production. The supply of the licensed VZIG product is now nearly depleted. In February 2006, an investigational (not licensed) VZIG product became available under an investigational new drug application submitted to the U. S. Food and Drug Administration. This product can be requested from the sole authorized U.S. distributor for the indications noted earlier. There have been periodic shortages of VZV vaccine. Current information regarding vaccine availability may be found at the Centers for Disease Control and Prevention web site (see "Resources").

Human Parvovirus B19

Human parvovirus B19 is the causative agent of erythema infectiosum (fifth disease). The clinical manifestations of this virus include a macular rash with a "slapped-cheek" appearance that spreads to the trunk and proximal extremities and symmetrical arthralgias. The viral syndrome, which also is associated with a low-grade fever, malaise, and upper respiratory symptoms, lasts less than 3 weeks. Risk factors for infection include exposure to children and working in an elementary school; however, up to 60% of adults are seropositive, suggesting childhood disease (3). Only 3% of susceptible school employees seroconvert each year. The highest risk for infection occurs in women whose children develop the disease; nursery school teachers have the highest occupational risk.

The rate of intrauterine infection ranges from 25% to 51%, but the risk of an adverse fetal outcome is less than 5%, with the greatest risk occurring before 20 weeks of gestation (8). Exposed women should have serology for IgM and IgG antibodies drawn. A positive result for IgG antibodies and a negative result for IgM antibodies confirms a state of immunity. Approximately 50–65% of individuals exhibit immunity as evidenced by the presence of an IgG antibody. If the period since exposure is unknown, a baseline IgG titer should be obtained and repeated in 4 weeks. A fourfold increase in IgG antibody titer indicates maternal infection; an assay result that is positive for IgM antibodies after this interval also is indicative of maternal infection, although the rate of false-positive results is high at many commercial laboratories.

The theoretic risk for the development of hydrops fetalis ranges from 0% to 8% of cases. Hydrops fetalis is believed to result from transient suppression of the erythroid cell lines of the fetal bone marrow, as well as from myocarditis. If maternal parvovirus infection is suspected, the patient should be followed by weekly ultrasound assessments for hydrops fetalis, which typically presents as fetal ascites with or without scalp edema or pleural effusion. Doppler assessment of the peak middle cerebral artery systolic velocity will detect fetal anemia before the onset of frank hydrops. Hydrops fetalis has been reported to occur as late as 10 weeks after maternal disease; therefore, assessments should be continued during this period after maternal infection. Significant hydrops can be treated with cordocentesis and intrauterine transfusion after 18 weeks of gestation. Detection of human parvovirus B19 DNA in fetal blood confirms the diagnosis. Follow-up with these infants has not revealed any long-term sequelae of infection.

Influenza

During influenza season (defined as when influenza viruses are circulating within the community) the diagnosis of influenza should be considered in women with the acute onset of fever and upper respiratory symptoms. Nasopharyngeal aspirates and swabs are the preferred specimens to be sent for influenza testing. Rapid influenza tests include reverse transcription-polymerase chain reaction (results available in 4–6 hours), immunofluorescence, and antigen detection (results available in 10–30 minutes, but these tests are less sensitive) tests. Viral culture also can be performed. Treatment is recommended for pregnant women with a positive influenza test result, regardless of vaccination status and severity of illness, and is best initiated within 48 hours of symptom onset. Oseltamivir (preferred because of its systemic absorption) or zanamivir are recommended for the treatment of influenza in pregnancy, including the novel influenza A (H1N1), which may be more severe in pregnant women than in the general population (12). Concomitant antipyretic therapy is important. Because of the increased risk of severe complications, pregnant women in close contact with a person who has a confirmed case of influenza should receive a 10-day course of oseltamivir or zanamivir as chemoprophylaxis. Breastfeeding is not contraindicated in women infected with influenza but infection control measures, such as handwashing and covering the mouth and nose with a tissue when sneezing, should be emphasized (13). For more details on influenza during pregnancy see the section "Pulmonary Disorders."

Acute Pyelonephritis

Approximately 70–75% of cases of pyelonephritis are right-sided, approximately 10–15% are left-sided, and 10–15% are bilateral. Bacteremia may be present in as many as 10% of infected patients, and 1–2% of patients actually develop septic shock. A similar percentage also may manifest signs of adult respiratory distress syndrome. In patients with pyelonephritis, microscopic examination of urine typically shows leukocyte casts and bacteria. The urine culture result will be positive unless the patient previously has received antibiotic treatment.

Infected patients should be hospitalized and treated with parenteral antibiotics. In some cases, outpatient management may be considered (14). Patients should be carefully selected for this approach. A third-generation cephalosporin, such as ceftriaxone, is an excellent empirical choice because of its uniform activity against the major uropathogens and its minimal toxicity. Patients who appear to be critically ill or who are particularly likely to have a resistant organism should be treated initially with both ampicillin and gentamicin, or with aztreonam, until sensitivity tests are completed.

The use of parenteral antibiotics should be continued until the patient has been afebrile and asymptomatic for 24–48 hours. Once this criterion is met, the patient may be discharged from the hospital and treated with an appropriate oral antibiotic for 7–10 days. The patient's condition subsequently needs to be assessed with periodic urine cultures.

Approximately 75% of obstetric patients with pyelonephritis become afebrile within 48 hours. Almost 95% are afebrile within 72 hours. Patients who have a poor response to therapy are likely to have either a resistant organism or a urinary tract obstruction. If the latter condition is suspected, the patient should be evaluated with renal ultrasonography or intravenous pyelography. If obstruction is demonstrated, urologic consultation is indicated.

Group B Streptococci

Early-onset neonatal sepsis caused by group B streptococci (GBS) remains a leading cause of morbidity and mortality despite the widespread acceptance of intrapartum antibiotic prophylaxis. Current recommendations are that all women with GBS bacteriuria during their current pregnancy or who previously had an infant with early-onset GBS disease are candidates for intrapartum antibiotic prophylaxis. Screening for vaginal and rectal GBS colonization should be done by culture at 35–37 weeks of gestation, and the laboratory should use selective enrichment broth to maximize the isolation of GBS and avoid overgrowth of other organisms (15). The culture should be obtained by swabbing both the lower vagina and rectum (ie, through the anal sphincter). Cultures of samples obtained from the cervix are not considered adequate.

Women with GBS colonization should be offered intrapartum antibiotics at the time of labor. Women with asymptomatic rectal–vaginal GBS colonization should not be treated before the intrapartum period. However, women with GBS bacteriuria should receive appropriate treatment at the time of diagnosis and then should also receive intrapartum prophylaxis. Women with negative vaginal and rectal GBS screening results within 5 weeks of delivery do not require intrapartum antimicrobial prophylaxis for GBS even if obstetric risk factors develop. However, if intrauterine infection is suspected in labor, broad-spectrum antibiotics should be given. Intrapartum antibiotic prophylaxis is not recommended for women undergoing planned cesarean delivery in the absence of labor or amniotic membrane rupture. However, culture results should still be obtained at 35–37 weeks of gestation because some of these women will enter labor or present with membrane rupture before the time of scheduled surgery.

Women without available culture results at the time of delivery should be treated according to the risk-based approach. Risk factors that should lead to intrapartum antibiotic prophylaxis include preterm delivery before 37 weeks of gestation, membrane rupture for 18 hours or longer, and maternal temperature of 38°C (100.4°F) or greater.

A complete copy of the 2002 Revised Guidelines for the Prevention of Perinatal GBS Disease is available on the CDC's web site (see Appendix A). The guidelines also provide an algorithm for the management of patients with threatened preterm delivery (Figure 19).

Ampicillin and penicillin are the agents of choice for intrapartum prophylaxis and treatment of GBS bacteriuria. It is important that health care providers pay special attention to women with a history of penicillin allergy. For penicillin-allergic women who are not at high risk for anaphylaxis, cefazolin is the agent of choice for treatment. For penicillin-allergic women who are at high risk for anaphylaxis, a sensitivity-based approach should be used. At the time of rectal and vaginal culture, the laboratory should be informed of the patient's allergy, and those with positive GBS results should have the isolates evaluated for susceptibility to clindamycin and erythromycin if feasible (16, 17). Clindamycin or erythromycin can be given for intrapartum GBS prophylaxis if the GBS isolate is susceptible to both. If the patient is at high risk for anaphylaxis and susceptibility studies reveal resistance to clindamycin or erythromycin, or if susceptibility results are unavailable, treatment with vancomycin is recommended.

Human Immunodeficiency Virus Infection

The management of human immunodeficiency virus (HIV) infection continues to evolve at a rapid pace. In recognition of this fact, a web site has been created by the U.S. Department of Health and Human Services (see Appendix A).

Up to 20% of women infected with HIV, however, do not initiate prenatal care. Given that data confirm the efficacy of intrapartum and early neonatal prophylaxis in reducing the risk of vertical transmission, efforts should be made during labor for rapidly determining the serostatus of those women using a commercially available rapid test, usually an enzyme-linked immunosorbent assay, so that these preventive measures can be undertaken (18).

Use of highly active antiretroviral therapy during pregnancy should be discussed with and provided to all women infected with HIV, regardless of their HIV RNA level. The cornerstones of monitoring remain viral loads and CD4 cell counts. Determinations of CD4 cells should be performed at baseline and every 3 months or after changes in therapy (11). Plasma HIV RNA levels should be monitored monthly until undetectable and then at least every 2 months. Particularly important is a level drawn between 34 weeks of gestation to 36 weeks

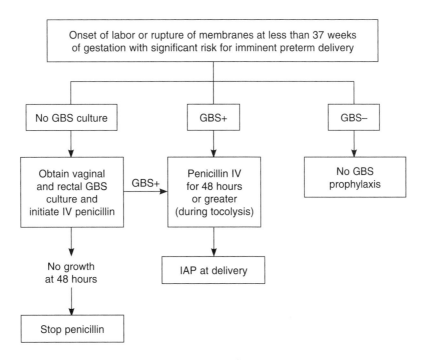

Figure 19. Sample algorithm for group B streptococci prophylaxis for women with threatened preterm delivery. Abbreviations: GBS indicates group B streptococci; IAP, intrapartum antibiotic prophylaxis; IV, intravenous. This algorithm is not an exclusive course of management. Variations that incorporate individual circumstances or institutional preferences may be appropriate. (Schrag S, Gorwitz R, Fultz-Butts K, Schuchat A. Prevention of perinatal group B streptococcal disease. Revised guidelines from CDC. MMWR Recomm Rep 2002;51(RR-11):1–22.)

of gestation on which the decision for mode of delivery is based. Vertical transmission is linked to viral loads, and cesarean deliveries scheduled at 38 weeks gestation are recommended for women whose viral loads exceed 1,000 copies/mL. With appropriate therapy, viral loads should decrease by more than one log within the first month of therapy and should eventually become undetectable. Failure to meet this goal suggests treatment failure and probable emerging resistance. For this reason, resistance testing (phenotypic and genotypic) has become a standard component of HIV care.

The combination of antepartum, intrapartum, and early neonatal therapy is optimal in preventing the vertical transmission of HIV. Initiation of therapy should occur in consultation with an expert. Adherence to therapy is crucial. The antiretroviral regimen recommended depends on the treatment status of the patient when she presents for care and whether there are indications for therapy of her HIV infection. The use of zidovudine, which crosses the placental wall, should be used whenever possible as a component of highly active antiretroviral therapy regimens. Monitoring for complications of antiretroviral drugs during pregnancy should be based on what is known about the side effects of the drugs that the patient is receiving.

It is estimated that 70% of mother-to-child transmissions occur at delivery and about 30% in utero. Approximately two of three in utero transmissions occur in the last 14 days before delivery. Factors other than

viral load that have been linked to vertical transmission include prolonged rupture of membranes, vaginal delivery, prematurity, drug use, and breastfeeding.

Breastfeeding is not recommended for women infected with HIV (including those receiving highly active antiretroviral therapy) in the United States where safe, affordable, and feasible alternatives are available and culturally acceptable.

Syphilis

Syphilis is a systemic disease caused by the spirochete *Treponema pallidum*. Patients with syphilis may seek treatment for signs or symptoms of primary infection (ulcer or chancre at site of infection), secondary infection (manifestations that include rash, mucocutaneous lesions, and adenopathy), or tertiary infection (cardiac, neurologic, ophthalmic, auditory, or gummatous lesions). However, most infections are detected during the latent stage by serologic testing. All women should be screened serologically for syphilis as early as possible in pregnancy (19). In populations with high syphilis prevalence and in patients at high risk, serologic testing should be repeated at the beginning of the third trimester and again at delivery. Any woman who delivers a stillborn infant after 20 weeks of gestation should be tested for syphilis. The serologic status of an infant's mother should be determined during pregnancy before the infant is discharged from the hospital.

All women with syphilis should be offered testing for HIV infection.

The specificity of serologic testing is high if both a nontreponemal screening test (Venereal Disease Research Laboratory test or rapid plasma reagent test) and a subsequent treponemal serologic test (fluorescent treponemal antibody absorption test or microhemagglutination–*T pallidum* test) produce reactive results. Nontreponemal test antibody titers usually correlate with disease activity, and results should be reported quantitatively. Microscopic dark-field and histologic examinations for spirochetes are most reliable when lesions are present. Seropositive pregnant women should be considered infected unless treatment history is clearly documented in a medical or health department record and sequential serologic antibody titers have declined appropriately.

The use of penicillin is effective for preventing transmission to the fetus and for treating established infection in the fetus. Treatment during pregnancy should be the use of the penicillin regimen appropriate for the woman's stage of syphilis. Some experts recommend additional therapy 1 week after the initial dose, particularly for women in the third trimester of pregnancy and for those with secondary syphilis during pregnancy. Nontreponemal test results usually become nonreactive with time after treatment; however, in some women, nontreponemal antibodies can persist at a low titer for a long period of time, sometimes for the life of the patient. This response is referred to as a serofast reaction. Most women with reactive treponemal tests will have reactive tests for the remainder of their lives, regardless of treatment or disease activity.

Women who are treated for syphilis during the second half of pregnancy are at risk for uterine contractions, preterm labor, or nonreassuring fetal heart rate tracings if their treatment precipitates the Jarisch–Herxheimer reaction. These women should be advised to seek medical attention after treatment if they notice any change in fetal movements or if they have contractions (20). Stillbirth is a rare complication of treatment; however, because therapy is necessary to prevent further damage, this concern should not delay treatment.

Serologic titers should be checked monthly until the adequacy of treatment has been ensured. There are no proven alternatives to the use of penicillin. Skin testing is helpful in most patients with a dubious history of penicillin allergy. A pregnant woman with a penicillin allergy should be treated with penicillin after desensitization. The use of tetracycline and doxycycline is contraindicated during pregnancy.

Bacterial Vaginosis

Bacterial vaginosis is a complex alteration of the vaginal flora characterized by a replacement of the normal H_2O_2-producing *Lactobacillus* species with high concentrations of anaerobic bacteria (eg, *Prevotella* species or *Mobiluncus* species), *Gardnerella vaginalis*, and *Mycoplasma hominis*. Women with bacterial vaginosis report an abnormal vaginal discharge associated with a fishy odor, particularly after unprotected sexual intercourse. The diagnosis of bacterial vaginosis is based on the following composite clinical criteria: homogenous white noninflammatory discharge, clue cells, pH of vaginal fluid greater than 4.5, and a fishy odor of vaginal secretions after the addition of 10% potassium hydroxide (whiff test) (19). Additional methods of diagnosis include Gram stain and a test card for the detection of elevated pH and trimethylamine.

All symptomatic pregnant women should be tested and treated. Bacterial vaginosis has been associated with premature rupture of membranes, preterm labor and delivery, intraamniotic fluid infection, chorioamnionitis, and postcesarean endometritis. Screening for bacterial vaginosis is not recommended because evidence is insufficient to assess the balance of benefits and harm of screening in asymptomatic pregnant women at either low or high risk for preterm delivery (21).

Oral metronidazole is the treatment of choice for bacterial vaginosis. Alternative regimens include topical medications, such as metronidazole gel and oral clindamycin.

Immunizations During Pregnancy

Currently, four types of immunobiologic agents are available for immunization: 1) toxoids, 2) inactivated vaccines, 3) live vaccines, and 4) immune globulin preparations. As a general rule, only live viral or live bacterial vaccines are contraindicated during pregnancy (22). The most commonly used live virus vaccines in the United States are those for measles, mumps, and rubella. Varicella vaccine also is a live attenuated virus preparation.

Ideally, all women of childbearing age should be immune to measles, mumps, rubella, tetanus, pertussis, diphtheria, poliomyelitis, and varicella by virtue of either childhood vaccination or natural infection. Women who are susceptible to any of these infections may receive toxoids or inactivated vaccines (tetanus, pertussis, diphtheria, inactivated polio vaccine), during pregnancy. Live virus vaccinations (eg, measles, mumps, rubella, varicella, or live polio vaccine) should be deferred until after delivery.

Since the 1970s, parents, especially mothers, have been identified as the most important source of infant pertussis. For this reason, the Centers for Disease Control and Prevention Advisory Committee on Immunization Practices recommends that pregnant women who were not vaccinated previously with the tetanus–diphtheria–acellular pertussis vaccine receive the vaccine in the immediate postpartum period before discharge from the hospital or the birthing center.

Varicella vaccine has been available since 1995 and is recommended for all susceptible persons older than 12 months. The Advisory Committee on Immunization Practices of the Centers for Disease Control and Prevention has designated adolescents and adults living in households with children a high-risk group. Susceptible nonpregnant women of childbearing age should receive varicella vaccine and should be advised to use contraception for 1 month. In addition, pregnant women with a negative history for chicken pox, no history of varicella vaccination, and a negative varicella serology, are candidates for postpartum varicella vaccination.

Influenza vaccine, acceptably administered in any trimester, is strongly recommended for all women who are or anticipate being in the second or third trimester of pregnancy during the influenza season (October to May). A recent study showed that maternal inactivated influenza vaccination reduced proven influenza illness by 63% in their infants up to 6 months of age and averted approximately one third of all febrile respiratory illnesses in these mothers and young infants.

Certain patients may merit special consideration for vaccination during pregnancy. Patients with risk factors for hepatitis B virus (see the section "Liver and Alimentary Tract Diseases") should receive the recombinant vaccine. Patients with acute exposure to hepatitis B virus also should receive hepatitis B immune globulin. Patients who live in communities where hepatitis A is endemic should receive the inactivated hepatitis A vaccine. Women who have had a splenectomy, who have sickle cell anemia, or who are immunocompromised should be vaccinated against pneumococcal infection. Pregnant patients who anticipate foreign travel may require special immunizations for infections such as cholera, plague, typhoid, and hepatitis A.

References

1. Viral hepatitis in pregnancy. ACOG Practice Bulletin No. 86. American College of Obstetricians and Gynecologists. Obstet Gynecol 2007;110:941–56.

2. Adler SP, Nigro G, Pereira L. Recent advances in the prevention and treatment of congenital cytomegalovirus infections. Semin Perinatol 2007;31:10–8.

3. American College of Obstetricians and Gynecologists. Perinatal viral and parasitic infections. Practice Bulletin 20. Washington, DC: American College of Obstetricians and Gynecologists; 2000.

4. Nigro G, Adler SP, La Torre R, Best AM. Passive immunization during pregnancy for congenital cytomegalovirus infection. Congenital Cytomegalovirus Collaborating Group. N Engl J Med 2005;353:1350–62.

5. Lopez A, Dietz VJ, Wilson M, Navin TR, Jones JL. Preventing congenital toxoplasmosis. MMWR Recomm Rep 2000;49:59–68.

6. Montoya JG, Remington JS. Management of Toxoplasma gondii infection during pregnancy. Clin Infect Dis 2008;47:554–66.

7. Wald A, Zeh J, Selke S, Ashley RL, Corey L. Virologic characteristics of subclinical and symptomatic genital herpes infections. N Engl J Med 1995;333:770–5.

8. Brown ZA, Wald A, Morrow RA, Selke S, Zeh J, Corey L. Effect of serologic status and cesarean delivery on transmission rates of herpes simplex virus from mother to infant. JAMA 2003;289:203–9.

9. Sheffield JS, Hollier LM, Hill JB, Stuart GS, Wendel GD. Acyclovir prophylaxis to prevent herpes simplex virus recurrence at delivery: a systematic review. Obstet Gynecol 2003;102:1396–403.

10. Nathwani D, Maclean A, Conway S, Carrington D. Varicella infections in pregnancy and the newborn. A review prepared for the UK Advisory Group on Chickenpox on behalf of the British Society for the Study of Infection. J Infect 1998;36 Suppl 1:59–71.

11. American Academy of Pediatrics, American College of Obstetricians and Gynecologists. Guidelines for perinatal care. 6th ed. Elk Grove Village (IL): AAP; Washington, DC: American College of Obstetricians and Gynecologists; 2007.

12. Use of Influenza A (H1N1) 2009 monovalent vaccine. Recommendations of the Advisory Committee on Immunization Practices (ACIP), 2009. MMWR Recomm Rep 2009;58(RR-10):1–8.

13. Harper SA, Bradley JS, Englund JA, File TM, Gravenstein S, Hayden FG, et al. Seasonal influenza in adults and children--diagnosis, treatment, chemoprophylaxis, and institutional outbreak management: clinical practice guidelines of the Infectious Diseases Society of America. Expert Panel of the Infectious Diseases Society of America. Clin Infect Dis 2009;48:1003–32.

14. Mittal P, Wing DA. Urinary tract infections in pregnancy. Clin Perinatol 2005;32:749–64.

15. Schrag SJ, Zell ER, Lynfield R, Roome A, Arnold KE, Craig AS, et al. A population-based comparison of strategies to prevent early-onset group B streptococcal disease in neonates. Active Bacterial Core Surveillance Team. N Engl J Med 2002;347:233–9.

16. Prevention of early-onset group B streptococcal disease in newborns. ACOG Committee Opinion No. 279. American College of Obstetricians and Gynecologists. Obstet Gynecol 2002;100:1405–12.

17. Manning SD, Foxman B, Pierson CL, Tallman P, Baker CJ, Pearlman MD. Correlates of antibiotic-resistant group B streptococcus isolated from pregnant women. Obstet Gynecol 2003;101:74–9.

18. Minkoff H. Human immunodeficiency virus infection in pregnancy. Obstet Gynecol 2003;101:797–810.

19. Workowski KA, Berman SM. Sexually transmitted diseases treatment guidelines, 2006. Centers for Disease Control and Prevention [published erratum appears in MMWR Morb Mortal Wkly Rep 2006;55:997]. MMWR Recomm Rep 2006;55:1–94.

20. Myles TD, Elam G, Park-Hwang E, Nguyen T. The Jarisch-Herxheimer reaction and fetal monitoring changes in pregnant women treated for syphilis. Obstet Gynecol 1998;92:859–64.

21. Screening for bacterial vaginosis in pregnancy to prevent preterm delivery: U.S. Preventive Services Task Force recommendation statement. U.S. Preventive Services Task Force. Ann Intern Med 2008;148:214–9.

22. Update on immunization and pregnancy: tetanus, diphtheria, and pertussis vaccination. ACOG Committee Opinion No. 438. American College of Obstetricians and Gynecologists. Obstet Gynecol 2009;114:398–400.

Chronic Pain and Headache

Rakesh B. Vadhera

Chronic Pain

The U.S. National Center for Health Statistics describes a chronic condition as the one lasting 3 months or more. Thus, pain that lasts 3 months or more beyond the usual course of an acute injury or disease is defined as chronic pain, although some define this period to be 1 month. There are two fundamental types of pain: 1) nociceptive pain (ordinary pain), which is felt in response to a noxious stimulus, and 2) neuropathic pain, which occurs when a pain signal originates within abnormally functioning peripheral or central neurons. Chronic pain usually is a combination of both.

Understanding regarding chronic pain syndromes is just evolving. These syndromes encompass multiple mechanisms operating at different sites in the nervous system and with different temporal profiles in different patients. The initial pain is initiated by the primary injury or disease, but the pain mechanism itself, not the disease or injury, leads to chronic pain (1). Chronic pelvic pain, fibromyalgia, chronic daily headaches, chronic low back pain, compressive neuropathy (Bell palsy, carpel tunnel syndrome, and meralgia paresthetica), chronic sickle cell pain, and cancer pain are examples of chronic pain syndromes.

The management of chronic pain is complex and evolving rapidly as new discoveries are made. Pain medicine is a relatively new and rapidly growing specialty. The current emphasis in pain medicine is to approach chronic pain as a disease state, using pain mechanisms themselves to define the pain state and determine the best treatment regimens. Ideally, a pregnant patient with chronic pain would be managed by close cooperation between her pain physician and her obstetrician.

In most patients with chronic pain, the disease or pathology cannot be treated effectively or cured. The current approach by pain medicine specialists is to consider pain to be a disease and to attempt to identify and treat the mechanisms responsible for the chronic pain. This pain mechanism-based approach is very different from management based primarily on the underlying disease. Women with chronic pain tend to have different experiences during pregnancy. Some women experience increases in pain, whereas others actually feel less pain while pregnant. Treating pregnant women who have chronic pain is complicated by the potential risks to the fetus from treatment medications.

Prepregnancy Planning

The patient's medicines should be reviewed with the risks to the developing fetus in mind. Often it takes months to find the right combination of medications to control chronic pain. The decision to change these medications is a difficult one because the benefits to the patient in terms of pain control and psychologic benefits, including treating or preventing depression, may outweigh the small risks (usually uncertain) to the fetus by remaining on the medication (Table 25).

Treatment of Chronic Pain During Pregnancy

Many of the commonly used pain medications are not safe for use during pregnancy. Other treatments may require alterations.

Acetaminophen remains the safest drug to use for mild to moderate pain during pregnancy and often is effective. Codeine can be added to the treatment for more severe pain and is safe during pregnancy. The use of hydrocodone usually is better tolerated and causes less constipation.

The use of normal-dose aspirin, nonsteroidal antiinflammatory drugs, and over-the-counter medications for prolonged periods should be avoided because of associated risks, such as maternal and fetal bleeding; spontaneous abortion, if taken for more than 7 days at time of conception (2); premature closure of fetal ductus arteriosus, if given after 32 weeks of gestation (3); and gastroschisis (4).

The use of tricyclic antidepressants is considered first-line systemic therapy for many neuropathic pain syndromes, including diabetic neuropathic pain, postherpetic neuralgia, and cancer-related neuropathic pain. The use of selective serotonin reuptake inhibitors (SSRIs) probably is safe. In 2005, GlaxoSmithKline sponsored a retrospective, U.S. epidemiologic study of major malformations after maternal exposure to antidepressant use in the first trimester of pregnancy. The results from this

Table 25. Medications Frequently Used in Chronic Pain Management

Medication	Use in Pregnancy
NSAIDs	Recent evidence points to an increased risk of spontaneous miscarriage if used at the time of conception or for more than 7 consecutive days.*
	Should not be used chronically after 28 weeks of gestation except in rare circumstances; close ultrasound surveillance for amniotic fluid changes is mandatory.
Aspirin	Should not be used at all or only in low doses (81 mg); it has the same risks as other NSAIDs and has been associated with gastroschisis.[†]
Opioids	There are no known teratogenic risks. Physical dependence of the fetus requiring withdrawal is expected if opioids are used throughout the pregnancy.
	For long-term, chronic treatment of pain, opioids can be given transdermally or by long-acting oral formulations. Fentanyl administration by patch has gained wide acceptance by pain physicians.
Tricyclic antidepressants	These agents often are used in pain management. Amitriptyline is the most studied and probably the safest to use during pregnancy.
	Nortriptyline, imipramine, desipramine, and doxepin are less well studied and should be avoided if possible.
SSRIs	Role in chronic pain management is evolving; fluoxetine is the most studied and has been used the most in chronic pain; however, concerns have been raised regarding its teratogenicity and higher incidence of fatal neonatal pulmonary hypertension associated with use when given after 20 weeks of gestation.[‡]
	The exposure to SSRIs late in pregnancy is associated with transient neonatal complications.[§]
Anticonvulsants	Phenytoin is associated with major and minor congenital anomalies and should be avoided.
	Carbamazepine and valproic acid are contraindicated because of the risk of neural tube defects.
	Gabapentin is especially helpful in treating chronic neuropathic pain. Results from a recent study indicated no increased risk for congenital anomalies associated with use, but the numbers were small.[||]

Abbreviations: NSAIDs indicates nonsteroidal antiinflammatory drugs; SSRIs, selective serotonin reuptake inhibitors.

*Li DK, Liu L, Odouli R. Exposure to non-steroidal anti-inflammatory drugs during pregnancy and risk of miscarriage: population based cohort study. BMJ 2003;327:368.

[†]Werler MM, Sheehan JE, Mitchell AA. Maternal medication use and risks of gastroschisis and small intestinal atresia. Am J Epidemiol 2002;155:26–31 and Martinez-Frias ML, Rodriguez-Pinilla E, Prieto L. Prenatal exposure to salicylates and gastroschisis: a case-control study. Teratology 1997;56:241–3.

[‡]Chambers CD, Hernandez–Diaz S, Van Marter LJ, Werler MM, Louik C, Jones KL, et al. Selective serotonin–reuptake inhibitors and risk of persistent pulmonary hypertension of the newborn. N Engl J Med 2006;354:579–87.

[§]Use of psychiatric medications during pregnancy and lactation. ACOG Practice Bulletin No. 92. American College of Obstetricians and Gynecologists. Obstet Gynecol 2008;111:1001–20.

[||]Montouris G. Gabapentin exposure in human pregnancy: results from the Gabapentin Pregnancy Registry. Epilepsy Behav 2003;4:310–7.

study showed a statistically significant increased overall risk of major congenital malformations, with a 1.5-fold increased risk for cardiovascular malformations with the use of paroxetine compared with other antidepressants. The exposure to SSRIs late in pregnancy is associated with transient neonatal complications (5, 6). Results from a second, independent retrospective epidemiological analysis using the Swedish national registry database indicated a twofold increased risk of cardiac defects in infants exposed to paroxetine compared with the general population. The U.S. Food and Drug Administration risk category for paroxetine was subsequently changed from C to D. The use of monoamine oxidase inhibitors may

cause sudden severe increase in blood pressure; hence, their use should be avoided.

The use of all of the opioids is relatively safe in pregnancy. None of them is related to congenital abnormalities. Role of opioid treatment in cancer pain is well established, but opioid treatment for chronic noncancer pain remains controversial. Short-term use of lower doses of opiates seems to be safe and is unlikely to be associated with development of tolerance and addiction, although prolonged use and higher doses may be associated with fetal and maternal dependence and neonatal withdrawal after delivery. Opioid withdrawal can be a problem in patients who were already dependent on opioids before pregnancy. Such patients need to be treated with and receive maintenance therapy with methadone regimen. The antiepileptic agent gabapentin is being used increasingly for chronic neuropathic pain and seems to be safe. Benzodiazepines can be used as an adjunct therapy to reduce anxiety, to treat insomnia, and as muscle relaxant in patients with chronic pain; provided its use is avoided just before delivery and also during first trimester of pregnancy because their use is associated with increased risk of congenital malformation.

There are well-defined strategies used in chronic pain management and some of them can be applied to treatment of pregnant patients:

- One provider should be designated to manage the pain medication. All questions and medication needs should be handled by that provider, who alone should prescribe pain medications. At the same time, there should be a plan in place for treatment of acute exacerbations of pain.

- Analgesics should be given on a fixed-dose schedule around the clock (not on an as-needed basis); this provides more consistent pain relief.

- The lowest dose that is effective should be used.

- Often there is synergy between two medications that allows effective treatment at lower doses for both, thereby minimizing side effects and fetal risks.

- Medications, especially opioids, should be administered in the way most comfortable for the patient: orally, transdermally, or by rectal suppositories.

Adjunctive Therapies in the Treatment of Chronic Pain

Psychoeducational interventions (such as detailed patient education, cognitive–behavioral therapy, relaxation techniques, and psychotherapy) and physical interventions (including gentle stretching and aerobic exercise, physical therapy including massage and ice or heat therapy, acupuncture, and therapeutic massage) are safe and often helpful in the treatment of chronic pain in pregnancy, although rigorous studies are lacking. Electrical stimulation (transcutaneous nerve stimulation) or vibratory stimulation may be helpful in treating low back pain. Alternate therapies, such as biofeedback techniques, can be used to lower the stress and help with chronic pain during pregnancy. Involving the patient in the management of her chronic pain has been shown to increase the effectiveness of the treatment program (7, 8).

Headache

Headaches are the most common recurrent pain problem among adults and a reason 8 million Americans visit primary care physicians, neurologists, and emergency departments every year. Not only is it a major cause of personal suffering and disability, also its impact on society from missed days at work and loss of productivity ($13 billion per year from migraine alone) is enormous (9). Headaches are especially common in women: lifetime incidence is 99%, with tension-type headache occurring in 88% of women and migraine headache in at least 18% of women. Most women will have headaches during their pregnancies, even those who do not have an underlying primary headache disorder. Certain women have a greater risk for headache. Some of the known triggers for headache are shown in Box 34. It is of utmost importance to rule in or out preeclampsia in every pregnant woman with headaches whose pregnancy is beyond 20 weeks of gestation.

Classifying headaches is important because the management of headaches during pregnancy is influenced by the underlying headache type. The International Headache Society formalized the classification and specific diagnostic criteria of primary headache in 1988, and this classification was updated in 2004 (10). Primary headache includes migraine headache, with and without aura, and tension-type headache (often called muscle-contraction headache), cluster headache, and other trigeminal autonomic types of cephalgia. The classification distinguishes primary from secondary headaches, in which the headaches are caused by underlying conditions, such as intracranial vascular or nonvascular lesions, head and neck trauma, substance or its withdrawal, infection and psychiatric and homeostasis disorders. Symptoms of secondary headaches may include the first and worst headache of the patient's life. Such

---

Box 34

Headache Triggers

- Diet—Alcoholic beverages, caffeine, and foods that contain certain substances (eg, nitrates and monosodium glutamate)

- Eating and sleeping patterns—Fasting or skipping meals, too much or too little sleep, or dehydration

- Emotions—Stress, anxiety, excitement, or anger

- Medications—Medications, such as those used to treat chest pain (angina) and high blood pressure

- Environment—Things in the workplace and home, including bright lights, noise, and eyestrain, and inhalation of fumes from substances, such as gasoline, insecticides, or cleaning agents

- Changing hormone levels—Many women notice that headaches occur around their menstrual periods or during pregnancy. Oral contraceptives also can trigger headache.

Silberstein SD. Migraine and other headache disorders. Clin Update Womens Health Care 2009;VIII(5):1–56.

headaches should be evaluated in the emergency room with neurologic consultation and computed tomography or magnetic resonance imaging.

Migraine headaches usually are unilateral, have a pulsating or throbbing quality, are moderate-to-severe in intensity (which inhibits or prohibits daily activities), and are aggravated by walking stairs or similar routine physical activity. Migraines often are accompanied by gastrointestinal (nausea or vomiting), neurologic (photophobia and phonophobia), or autonomic changes. Other family members often have similar headaches. Fortunately, many women with migraines will note improvement during pregnancy (11).

Tension-type headaches are the most common and least defined of the headache syndromes affecting 30–78% of general population. The temporal pattern is vague or inconsistent, and most patients are unable to be precise about time of onset or duration. The pain is mild to moderate, band-like, bilateral, dull, nagging, and persistent and often goes into the neck. Pregnancy does not have the same beneficial effect on tension-type headaches as it does on migraines.

Cluster headache, fortunately rare, is one of the most painful types of headaches. The pain is typically described as sharp, penetrating, or burning, and it always occurs on same side of the head. These attacks occur in cyclical pattern or clusters and bouts of frequent attacks occur over cluster periods, lasting weeks to months followed by complete remission. Cluster headaches are more common in males.

Analgesic rebound headache (also called *transformed migraine headache*) is a recently identified phenomenon that explains much about the cause of the recurrent, daily headaches that beset many patients. These patients begin with occasional migraine attacks and end up years later with chronic daily headaches caused by overuse of prescription and over-the-counter medications (12).

Prepregnancy Issues

Many women with migraine headaches are treated with medications that should not be used during pregnancy. These include ergotamine derivatives, 5-hydroxytryptamine serotonin agonists (triptans), chronic use of nonsteroidal antiinflammatory drugs, and certain medications used for preventive treatment—valproate and methysergide. Women planning pregnancy should discontinue use of these medications before conception. Aspirin use should be avoided during pregnancy (with the exception of low-dose aspirin [81 mg/day] prescribed for specific medical or obstetric indications).

If a woman has analgesic-rebound headaches, she should be referred to a headache specialist for detoxification. This entails stopping the daily use of analgesics, sedative or tranquilizer drugs, ergotamine derivatives, and other prescription or over-the-counter medication,

with inpatient support if necessary during the withdrawal process. Successfully treated, the daily headaches will abate, and medications used to treat migraine episodes will be effective once again.

Good evidence supports the use of nonpharmacologic approaches to headache treatment and prevention: relaxation training, cognitive–behavioral therapy, thermal and electromyographic biofeedback, and acupuncture (13). These techniques could be learned before pregnancy (14). In addition, a patient can decrease migraine attacks by avoiding known triggers, adopting regular sleeping and eating patterns, exercising regularly, and avoiding cigarette smoke.

Treating Headaches During Pregnancy

Initial pharmacotherapy for migraine and tension-type headaches overlaps. The goal is to stop individual attacks or to reduce the severity and duration of symptoms. As soon as the patient is aware of the onset of headache, she should rest in a dark, quiet room, avoid sensory over stimulation, and apply an ice pack to the head. The medications recommended for treatment are listed in Table 26. The patient, with input from her physician, should choose her treatment based on the intensity of the pain, selecting the medications most likely to be effective for that episode with minimal detrimental effect on pregnancy and fetal wellbeing.

Prophylactic Treatment for Migraine and Tension-Type Headaches

Prophylactic treatment should be considered under the following conditions:

- The patient has at least two or three episodes per month.
- The episodes are incapacitating, or of prolonged duration or associated with focal neurologic signs.
- The patient is unable to cope with her headache.
- There are contraindications or adverse reactions to medications used for treatment.
- Attempts at nonpharmacologic prevention have failed.

The goals of preventive treatment are to decrease the frequency and intensity of the headache attacks. Table 27 lists medications that can be used for prophylaxis during pregnancy. Each medication should be given an adequate trial, usually several weeks, starting low and increasing gradually until the desired effect is reached. Use of other medications should be avoided except for treatment of acute attacks. For additional information on the diagnosis and management of headache, see the section "Headache" in *Precis: Primary and Preventive Care*, Fourth Edition.

Table 26. Medications for Treatment of Headaches During Pregnancy

Medication	U.S. Food and Drug Administration Pregnancy Risk Category	Dosages
Mild Intensity		
Acetaminophen with or without caffeine	B	Limit dose to 1 g immediately, 4 g/d for 2–3 days
If Nausea Is Present		
Metoclopramide	B	10 mg at onset of nausea; may be repeated every 6 hours for four times
If Unable to Tolerate Oral Administration		
Promethazine	C	12.5–25 mg at onset of nausea; may be repeated in 4–6 hours, if necessary
Mild–Moderate Intensity		
Ibuprofen	B/D*	800 mg immediately and 400 mg every 4 hours, up to 2,400 mg/d, 2–3 days
Naproxen sodium	B/D*	Three 275-mg tablets initially, two tablets twice daily up to 2–3 days
Mild–Moderate Intensity, Not Responsive to Above		
Acetaminophen–with or without caffeine–butalbital	C/D[†]	Limit dose to 1–2 immediately and repeat in 4 hours; 6 per attack, 24 per month
Mild–Moderate Intensity, Not Responsive to Above		
Isometheptene–acetaminophen Dichloralphenazone	B	2 capsules at onset; then 1 capsule every 30–60 min; maximum of 6 capsules per attack, 2 days per week
Moderate–Severe Intensity		
Acetaminophen–codeine	C/D[†]	Limit dose to 1–2 capsules immediately, repeat every 3–4 hours; 6 capsules per attack, 16 capsules per month
Acetaminophen–hydrocodone	C/D[†]	Limit dose to 1–2 capsules immediately, repeat every 3–4 hours; 6 capsules per attack, 16 capsules per month
Rescue Medication—If Condition Is of Severe Intensity and Unresponsive Other Medication		
Acetaminophen–oxycodone	B/D[†]	Limit dose to 1–2 capsules immediately, repeat every 3–4 hours; 6 capsules per attack, 12 capsules per month
Hydromorphone	B/D[†]	Limit dose to 1–2 capsules immediately, repeat every 3–4 hours; 6 capsules per attack, 12 capsules per month

*Pregnancy risk category D, if used more than 2–3 days in the third trimester or at term

[†]Pregnancy risk category D, if used for prolonged periods or in high doses at term

Table 27. Preventive Medications for Migraines and Tension-Type Headaches During Pregnancy

Medication	U.S. Food and Drug Administration Pregnancy Risk Category	Initial Dosage	Dosage
Propranolol*	C	20 mg orally, 4 times daily	If well tolerated, use long-acting formulation: 80 mg daily, increasing by 80 mg every 2 weeks; ceiling is 240 mg/day
Amitriptyline*	B	10 mg orally at bedtime	Drug of choice for tension-type headache; can be used together with β-antagonist; titrate slowly up to 250 mg/d
Fluoxetine[†]	B	20 mg/d	Works especially well if there is a component of depression present[‡]
Verapamil[†]	C	240 mg/d	Decreases the frequency of attacks, not the intensity; may take 4–6 weeks to show efficacy

*Group 1 in The U.S. Headache Consortium Guidelines: medium to high efficacy, good strength of evidence, with acceptable side effect profile

[†]Group 2 in The U.S. Headache Consortium Guidelines: lower efficacy than Group 1, or limited strength of evidence, and mild to moderate side effects. Silberstein SD. Migraine and other headache disorders. Clin Update Womens Health Care 2009;VIII(5):1–56 and Silberstein SD, Freitag FG. Preventive treatment of migraine. Neurology 2003;60(suppl 2):s38–44.

[‡]d'Amato CC, Pizza V, Marmolo T, Giordano E, Alfano V, Nasta A. Fluoxetine for migraine prophylaxis: a double-blind trial. Headache 1999;39:716–9.

References

1. Ballantyne J, Fishman S, Abdi S, editors. The Massachusetts General Hospital Handbook of Pain Management. 2nd ed. Philadelphia (PA): Lippincott Williams & Wilkins; 2002.

2. Li DK, Liu L, Odouli R. Exposure to non-steroidal anti-inflammatory drugs during pregnancy and risk of miscarriage: population based cohort study. BMJ 2003;327:368.

3. Momma K, Hagiwara H, Konishi T. Constriction of fetal ductus arteriosus by non-steroidal anti-inflammatory drugs: study of additional 34 drugs. Prostaglandins 1984;28:527–36.

4. Werler MM, Sheehan JE, Mitchell AA. Maternal medication use and risks of gastroschisis and small intestinal atresia. Am J Epidemiol 2002;155:26–31.

5. Moses-Kolko EL, Bogen D, Perel J, Bregar A, Uhl K, Levin B, et al. Neonatal signs after late in utero exposure to serotonin reuptake inhibitors: literature review and implications for clinical applications. JAMA 2005;293:2372–83.

6. Einarson A. The safety of psychotropic drug use during pregnancy: a review. MedGenMed 2005;7(4):3.

7. Arnstein P, Caudill M, Mandle CL, Norris A, Beasley R. Self efficacy as a mediator of the relationship between pain intensity, disability and depression in chronic pain patients. Pain 1999;80:483–91.

8. Caudill MA. Managing pain before it manages you. 3rd rev. ed. New York (NY): Guilford Press; 2008.

9. Hu XH, Markson LE, Lipton RB, Stewart WF, Berger ML. Burden of migraine in the United States: disability and economic costs. Arch Intern Med 1999;159:813–8.

10. The International Classification of Headache Disorders: 2nd edition. Headache Classification Subcommittee of the International Headache Society. Cephalalgia 2004;24(suppl 1):9–160.

11. Sances G, Granella F, Nappi RE, Fignon A, Ghiotto N, Polatti F, et al. Course of migraine during pregnancy and postpartum: a prospective study. Cephalalgia 2003;23:197–205.

12. Silberstein SD. Migraine and other headache disorders. Clin Update Womens Health Care 2009;VIII(5):1–68.

13. Linde K, Allais G, Brinkhaus B, Manheimer E, Vickers A, White AR. Acupuncture for migraine prophylaxis. Cochrane Database of Systematic Reviews 2009, Issue 1. Art. No.: CD001218. DOI: 10.1002/14651858.CD001218.pub2; 10.1002/14651858.CD001218.pub2.

14. Silberstein SD. Practice parameter: evidence-based guidelines for migraine headache (an evidence-based review): report of the Quality Standards Subcommittee of the American Academy of Neurology [published erratum appears in Neurology 2000;56:142]. Neurology 2000;55:754–62.

Surgical Complications

J. Gerald Quirk

From 0.5% to 2% of women require surgery during pregnancy. If diagnostic and therapeutic procedures are clearly indicated during pregnancy, they should be undertaken. The challenge is to make a prudent decision regarding the need for surgery and the appropriate approach to disease management. Adverse perinatal outcomes do not appear to be increased in the face of uncomplicated surgery or anesthesia; however, when complications arise, perinatal outcome may be affected adversely.

The largest report of anesthetic and surgical risks during pregnancy came from the Swedish Birth Registry for the years 1973–1981 (1). Nonobstetric surgery was performed on 5,405 of 720,000 pregnant women. Procedures were performed in all trimesters: 41% in the first trimester, 35% in the second trimester, and 24% in the third trimester. Abdominal surgery constituted 25% of procedures and gynecologic and urologic procedures made up another 16%. In this series, laparoscopy to rule out ectopic pregnancy was the most frequently performed procedure in the first trimester of pregnancy, and appendectomy was the most frequently performed procedure in the second trimester of pregnancy. When the authors compared the outcomes in these 5,405 pregnancies with the outcomes for the remainder of the 720,000 pregnancies in the registry, the rate of congenital malformations and stillbirths was not increased significantly. This observation is strengthened by the parallel observation that commonly used anesthetic agents are not teratogenic (2). However, the Swedish study did document an increased occurrence of neonatal death within 7 days of surgery, low birth weight, and preterm delivery in the women who underwent surgery. These outcomes were thought to be secondary to the disease process that necessitated the surgical intervention rather than a direct effect of surgery or anesthesia.

Laparoscopy

The most commonly performed laparoscopic procedure in pregnant women is for diagnosis and treatment of ectopic pregnancy. Whereas appendectomy, performed open or with the laparoscope, is the most commonly performed surgical procedure in established pregnancies, cholecystectomy is the most commonly performed laparoscopic procedure.

Initial reassuring experience with laparoscopy in the first half of pregnancy has resulted in its use later in pregnancy for other indications, such as appendectomy, exploratory surgery, and adnexal surgery. An early review of case series that included 518 women with established pregnancies who underwent laparoscopic surgery for such indications report good outcomes with regard to low

birth weight, preterm labor, and low Apgar scores, but information on long-term outcomes is lacking (3). Results from more recent systematic reviews of laparoscopic surgery for the diagnosis of appendicitis in pregnancy support these initial observations but demonstrate that laparoscopy resulting in removal of a normal appendix is associated with an increased risk of fetal loss (4, 5). Potential advantages and disadvantages of laparoscopic approach to surgery in pregnancy are listed in Box 35.

The Society of American Gastrointestinal Endoscopic Surgeons recognizes that limited experience with surgery in pregnancy and laboratory data suggest caution when choosing the laparoscopic approach and urge that certain maneuvers must be routinely adopted in order to enhance operative safety (6). A summary of their recommendations germane to this discussion is depicted in Box 36.

Box 35

Potential Advantages and Disadvantages of the Laparoscopic Approach to Surgery in Pregnancy

Advantages

- Early mobilization, rapid postoperative recovery, and early return to normal activities, which can be very important because of the higher occurrence of deep vein thrombosis in pregnancy
- Decreased postoperative morbidity
- Small scars and few incisional hernias
- Early return of gastrointestinal activity because of less manipulation of the bowel, which may result in fewer adhesions and less bowel obstruction
- Low rate of fetal depression due to decreased pain and narcotic use

Disadvantages

- Technical difficulty because of the gravid uterus
- Possible injury to the gravid uterus
- Potential decrease in uteroplacental blood flow because of increased intraabdominal pressure (hypothetical risk, because maternal Valsalva, coughing, or straining maneuvers generate similar pressure)
- Effects of carbon dioxide or nitrous oxide pneumoperitoneum on the fetus are unknown

Data from Fatum M, Rojansky N. Laparoscopic surgery during pregnancy. Obstet Gynecol Surv 2001;56:50–9 and Bisharah M, Tulandi T. Laparoscopic surgery in pregnancy. Clin Obstet Gynecol 2003;46:92–7.

Box 36

Guidelines for the Use of Laparoscopy for Surgical Problems During Pregnancy

Surgical Technique

- Diagnostic laparoscopy is safe and effective when used selectively in the workup and treatment of acute abdominal processes in pregnancy.

Patient Selection

- Preoperative decision making—Laparoscopic treatment of acute abdominal processes has the same indications in pregnant and nonpregnant patients.
- Laparoscopy and trimester of pregnancy—Laparoscopy can be safely performed during any trimester of pregnancy.

Treatment

- Patient positioning—Pregnant patients should be placed in the left lateral recumbent position to minimize compression of the vena cava and the aorta.
- Initial port placement—Initial access can be safely accomplished with an open Hassan needle, Veress needle, or optical trocar if the location is adjusted according to fundal height, previous incisions, and experience of the surgeon.
- Insufflation pressure—Carbon dioxide (CO_2) insufflation of 10–15 mm Hg can be safely used for laparoscopy in the pregnant patient. Intraabdominal pressure should be sufficient to allow for adequate visualization.
- Intraoperative CO_2 monitoring—Intraoperative CO_2 monitoring by capnography should be used during laparoscopy in the pregnant patient.
- Venous thromboembolic prophylaxis—Intraoperative and postoperative pneumatic compression devices and early postoperative ambulation are recommended types of prophylaxis for deep vein thrombosis in the pregnant patient.
- Gallbladder disease—Laparoscopic cholecystectomy is the treatment of choice in the pregnant patient with gallbladder disease regardless of trimester.
- Choledocholithiasis—Choledocholithiasis during pregnancy may be managed with preoperative endoscopic retrograde cholangiopancreatography with sphincterotomy followed by laparoscopic cholecystectomy, intraoperative laparoscopic transcystic or choledochotomy common bile duct exploration, or postoperative endoscopic retrograde cholangiopancreatography, depending on local resources and clinical scenario.
- Laparoscopic appendectomy—Laparoscopic appendectomy may be performed safely in any patient with suspected appendicitis.
- Solid organ resection—Laparoscopic adrenalectomy, nephrectomy, splenectomy, and mesenteric cyst excision are safe procedures in pregnant patients when indicated and standard precautions are taken.
- Adnexal mass—Laparoscopy is a safe and effective treatment in pregnant patients with symptomatic cystic masses. Observation is acceptable for all other cystic lesions provided ultrasound results are not indicative of malignancy and tumor markers are normal. Initial observation is warranted for most cystic lesions smaller than 6 cm.
- Adnexal torsion—Laparoscopy is recommended for both diagnosis and treatment of adnexal torsion unless clinical severity warrants laparotomy.

Perioperative Care

- Fetal heart monitoring—Fetal heart monitoring should occur preoperatively and postoperatively in the setting of urgent abdominal surgery during pregnancy.
- Obstetric consultation—Obstetric consultation can be obtained preoperatively, postoperatively, or both based on the acuteness of the patient's disease and availability.
- Tocolytics—Tocolytics should not be used prophylactically but should be considered perioperatively when signs of preterm labor are present in coordination with obstetric consultation.

Yumi H. Guidelines for diagnosis, treatment, and use of laparoscopy for surgical problems during pregnancy: this statement was reviewed and approved by the Board of Governors of the Society of American Gastrointestinal and Endoscopic Surgeons (SAGES), September 2007. It was prepared by the SAGES Guidelines Committee. Guidelines Committee of the Society of American Gastrointestinal and Endoscopic Surgeons. Surg Endosc 2008;22:849–61.

The Acute Abdomen

The most frequent cause of an acute surgical abdomen in pregnancy is appendicitis; less frequent causes include bowel obstruction and cholecystitis. The pregnant woman presents substantial diagnostic dilemmas. Nausea, vomiting, and loss of appetite, common symptoms of an acute abdomen, frequently are pregnancy-related conditions. Early diagnosis of the surgical abdomen and aggressive treatment are the keys to optimal maternal and fetal outcomes.

Appendicitis

Nearly 1 in 1,000 pregnant women undergo appendectomy, and appendicitis is confirmed in two thirds of these cases (1 in nearly 1,500) (1). The physician is faced with a concern that unnecessary surgery may affect outcomes adversely and at the same time recalls the admonition that "the mortality of appendicitis in pregnancy is the mortality of delay" (7). Diagnosing appendicitis in pregnancy can be a challenge. Because the uterus enlarges, the appendix frequently rises with the cecum and rotates to a retrocecal position so that pain may occur in the flank, not in the right lower quadrant. Nausea, vomiting, and anorexia are common symptoms of appendicitis that also often occur in normal pregnancies. Leucocytosis regularly is encountered in normal pregnancy. Other diseases encountered in pregnancy may mimic characteristics of appendicitis, including renal colic, pyelonephritis, degeneration of a myoma, and placental abruption (Box 37). Late in pregnancy, with the enlarged uterus shielding the abdominal wall and the appendix elevated and rotated toward the right flank, classic signs of peritonitis, including cervical motion, rectal tenderness, and rebound tenderness of the abdominal wall, may not be present or they may become prominent findings only late in the course of the disease when an abscess leaks or a viscus ruptures. As a result of these changes, one half of pregnant women with appendicitis have perforative appendicitis with generalized peritonitis, and deaths occasionally occur (8).

Persistent lower abdominal pain with tenderness is observed in 80% of pregnant women with appendicitis. Most pregnant women with appendicitis are afebrile. Similar to nonpregnant patients in whom the diagnosis of appendicitis is considered, both graded compression ultrasonography and helical computed tomography (CT) have been used to assist in diagnosis during pregnancy. Transabdominal ultrasonography is readily available; if a graded compression examination of the right lower quadrant reveals a noncompressible blind-ended tubular structure with a diameter no greater than 6 mm, appendicitis is diagnosed (9). This ultrasound technique has the limitation of being operator dependent and unreliable in the third trimester. Computed tomography also is widely available. In many centers, helical CT has become the imaging modality of choice. With existing protocols that minimize exposure to ionizing radiation, the fetus is exposed to less than 0.003 gray (300 millirad) without compromising the quality of the study (10). Images demonstrate findings of right lower quadrant inflammation, an enlarged nonfilling tubular structure and an appendicolith. Although experience with helical CT in pregnancy is limited, its efficacy is likely to mimic its well-documented utility in the nonpregnant patient (11). Helical CT results should be equally accurate in all three trimesters of pregnancy. Magnetic resonance imaging could be used as an alternative modality (12).

Ultimately, in most cases, appendicitis in pregnancy will be diagnosed clinically. If the diagnosis of appendicitis is seriously considered, immediate surgical exploration is warranted because rupture so frequently is encountered, and generalized peritonitis, besides put-

---

Box 37

Differential Diagnoses of Acute Abdomen

Nonobstetric
- Pyelonephritis
- Urinary calculi
- Cholecystitis
- Cholelithiasis
- Bowel obstruction or perforation
- Pancreatitis
- Gastroenteritis
- Rectus hematoma
- External hernia
- Acute intermittent porphyria
- Perforated duodenal ulcer
- Intraperitoneal hemorrhage
- Pneumonia
- Pulmonary embolism
- Meckel diverticulum
- Toxic megacolon
- Sickle cell crisis
- Diabetic ketoacidosis
- Tuberculous peritonitis

Obstetric or Gynecologic
- Preterm labor
- Abruptio placentae
- Chorioamnionitis
- Adnexal or uterine torsion
- Ectopic or heterotopic pregnancy
- Pelvic inflammatory disease
- Myomatous red degeneration
- Uterine rupture

ting the mother's life in danger, places the pregnancy at high risk of preterm labor and delivery, with all of its attendant implications for the newborn. When surgery is undertaken early, a normal appendix may be found, but most experts agree that it is better to operate unnecessarily than to delay intervention until the pregnant woman has developed generalized peritonitis.

A growing body of evidence supports the safety of the laparoscopic approach to appendectomy in the first half of pregnancy (13). However, recent systematic reviews of retrospective studies comparing laparoscopic appendectomy to laparotomy demonstrated increased fetal losses in pregnant women in the laparoscopic appendectomy group (5.6%) compared with the laparotomy group (3.1%). Interestingly, the preterm delivery rate was much lower in the laparoscopic appendectomy group (2.1%) compared with the laparotomy group (8.1%) (5). If laparotomy is to be performed, the incision should be made over the point of maximum tenderness on the patient's abdominal wall. If there is doubt about the diagnosis, the best approach is either through a right paramedian or vertical midline incision. In all cases, the patient should receive broad-spectrum antibiotics preoperatively, preferably a second-generation cephalosporin or semisynthetic penicillin. Antibiotics should be continued postoperatively if the appendix has ruptured or there is a periappendiceal abscess or other evidence of generalized peritonitis. In preparation for the procedure, the patient should be placed in the lateral tilt position; during the procedure, efforts should be made to maintain blood pressure in the normal range. Both of these maneuvers will optimize uterine blood flow. There is no evidence to demonstrate that continuous fetal heart rate monitoring during surgery improves outcomes, but it seems reasonable to consider its use if the patient is septic or in labor or if there is difficulty in maintaining her blood pressure.

Biliary Tract Disease

Biliary tract disease is the second most common surgical condition encountered in pregnancy after appendicitis. Surgery for biliary tract disease complicates from 1 in 2,000 pregnancies to 1 in 4,000 pregnancies.

By age 40 years, nearly 20% of women in the United States will have gallstones. Among these women, 1–2% per year undergo surgery for symptomatic disease. Cholecystectomy should not be performed for asymptomatic gallstones. In asymptomatic pregnant women, as many as 2.5–10% will have ultrasonographically detectable gallstones. Pregnancy is thought to increase the frequency of symptomatic gallstones because of progesterone's effect on biliary tract smooth muscle.

A consensus has developed that pregnant patients should undergo cholecystectomy while still pregnant if conservative management fails during the initial admission, if symptoms recur upon resumption of oral intake, or if symptoms recur in the same trimester (14). Pregnant women treated medically require rehospitalization during pregnancy in more than one half of cases. As many as one out of three patients will ultimately undergo cholecystectomy while still pregnant. Late in pregnancy, preterm labor is a significant complication in these patients, and cholecystectomy is technically more difficult to perform. Results from most recent reports cite better maternal and neonatal outcomes when a primary surgical approach is used (15). For all these reasons, at most major centers, the pregnant woman with biliary disease caused by gallstones is treated surgically. In a review of 111 reported cases of laparoscopic cholecystectomy performed on pregnant women, fewer spontaneous abortions in the first trimester and a lower frequency of preterm labor in the third trimester were found with laparoscopic cholecystectomy than with the open approach. Reviewers concluded that the laparoscopic approach was safe throughout pregnancy (16).

During pregnancy, gallstones are responsible for virtually all cases of acute pancreatitis. Clinically, the presentation of acute pancreatitis is not altered by pregnancy, but when the patient presents in the third trimester, the differential diagnosis can include severe preeclampsia and fatty liver of pregnancy. The finding of elevated serum lipase may contribute to the diagnosis (Table 28). The cornerstones of management include intravenous hydration with careful electrolyte management, correction of any hypocalcemia and hyperglycemia, the use of analgesics, and restriction of oral intake, with nasogastric suction in severe cases. Patients with fever should be treated with broad-spectrum antibiotics (17). Patients with respiratory insufficiency, shock,

Table 28. Selected Laboratory Values in 43 Pregnant Women With Pancreatitis

Value	Pancreatitis		Normal
	Mean	Range	
Amylase (international units/L)	1,392	111–4,560	30–110
Lipase (international units/L)	6,929	36–41,842	23–208
Total bilirubin (mg/dL)	1.7	0.1–4.9	0.2–1.3
Aspartate transferase (units/L)	120	11–498	3–35
Leucocytes (per mL)	12,000	7,000–14,500	4,100–10,900

Reprinted from Am J Obstet Gynecol, Vol. 173. Ramin KD, Ramin SM, Richey SD, Cunningham FG. Acute pancreatitis in pregnancy. p. 187–91. Copyright 1995, with permission from Elsevier.

need for massive colloid replacement, or whose serum calcium level is less than 8 mg/dL are best served by management in an intensive care setting because combinations of these findings are associated with mortality in up to 70% of cases.

Adnexal Masses

There is no consensus as to the threshold size of an adnexal mass that mandates surgery. The traditional teaching in obstetrics is that pregnant women with adnexal masses of 6 cm or greater should undergo surgery. Removal of the mass may be indicated for three reasons: 1) danger of torsion, 2) risk of malignancy, and 3) possible obstruction of labor. The optimal time for surgery was thought to be in the second trimester, when the risk of abortion was very low and the pregnancy did not depend on a functioning corpus luteum.

Before the development of ultrasonography, adnexal masses were diagnosed by clinical examination in approximately 1 in 600 pregnancies; 3–6% of masses were malignant. In results from more recent studies with variable access to ultrasonography and with variation in the size of the mass included in the study, adnexal masses were diagnosed in 1 in 100 to 1 in 600 pregnancies, and from 3% to 13% were malignant or borderline tumors. Despite newer imaging technologies, in 5–10% of cases the adnexal mass was a leiomyoma. In results from a 12-year experience from North Carolina, adnexal masses were found in 1 in 750 pregnancies, were generally diagnosed in the second trimester, and one half of the masses were benign cystic teratomas. Among the 13% of masses that were malignant, two thirds were of low malignant potential (18). Earlier investigators estimated that up to 15% of adnexal masses underwent torsion during that pregnancy (19).

When masses were diagnosed in the first trimester, about 90% of mobile unilateral noncomplex cysts smaller that 5 cm resolved spontaneously as did 36% of similar cysts larger than 5 cm (20). Thus, it is reasonable to observe these nonsuspicious masses until the second trimester and plan surgery electively. Ultrasound techniques have the same ability as CT and magnetic resonance imaging to differentiate malignant disease from benign disease (21) (Box 38).

Simple protocols for the management of adnexal masses in pregnancy generally ignore the nuance of ultrasound findings, the utility of maternal serum markers, and the presence of symptoms (20). The asymptomatic mass found incidentally at the time of routine ultrasound examination should be evaluated as would one for a premenopausal woman (22). The surgical approach (laparoscopy or open laparotomy) to the symptomatic adnexal mass or the mass likely to be malignant will depend on the size of the mass, the level of suspicion for malignancy, the length of gestation, and the skills of the surgeon.

Box 38

Ultrasound Characteristics Supporting the Diagnosis of Benign and Malignant Masses

Benign

- Anechoic fluid filled cysts with thin walls—follicular or corpus luteum cysts
- Homogeneous low to medium echodensity in a cystic mass—endometrioma
- Internal echoes with a reticular pattern—hemorrhagic cyst
- Markedly hyperechoic nodule with shadowing—benign cystic teratoma (dermoid)

Malignant

- Solid component that is not hyperechoic and is often nodular or papillary
- Septations, if present, that are thick (greater than 2–3 mm)
- Color Doppler or power Doppler image of flow in the solid component
- Presence of ascites (virtually any intraperitoneal fluid in postmenopausal women and more than a small amount of intraperitoneal fluid in premenopausal women is usually abnormal)
- Peritoneal masses, enlarged nodes, or matted bowel (may be difficult to detect by ultrasonography)

Trauma

Approximately two thirds of all traumas during pregnancy result from motor vehicle accidents. Other leading causes of trauma in pregnancy include falls, direct assaults to the abdomen, and gunshot wounds. In the United States, domestic violence has emerged as a major cause of trauma in pregnancy, with a prevalence of 1–7% (23). In urban inner-city environments across the United States, that prevalence is reported to range from 7% to 20%, and 60% of these women report two or more episodes of physical assault during their pregnancy (24).

Accidental or intentional trauma is a leading cause of mortality in reproductive-aged women. In many parts of the United States, injury-related deaths are the leading causes of nonobstetric maternal mortality (25). Fetal losses resulting from trauma can only be estimated. Extrapolations from case series suggest that 1,300 to 3,900 pregnancies are lost as a result of trauma. Life-threatening maternal trauma is reported to be associated with a 40–50% fetal loss rate, whereas minor and non-life-threatening trauma may be associated with a 1–5% loss rate (26). Placental abruption is the direct cause of fetal death in 50% of trauma cases.

Pregnancy is associated with different mechanisms of injury than those found in nonpregnant women. Gestational age at the time of injury affects the pattern of maternal injury and affects the need to assess the fetal condition acutely. As pregnancy advances and the uterus rises out of the pelvis and rises in the abdomen, the uterus functions as a shield protecting the large bowel and great vessels from low abdominal trauma. At the same time, as the small bowel is displaced to the upper abdomen, trauma to the upper abdomen or trauma that displaces the gravid uterus cephalad results in a greater risk of hepatic and splenic rupture and retroperitoneal hematomas. The abdominal wall, uterine myometrium, and amniotic sac serve as buffers to afford a considerable degree of protection to the fetus from direct traumatic injury. In less than 1% of cases, blunt abdominal trauma results in fetal injury. However, indirect injury can occur from rapid compression, deceleration shearing force, or contrecoup effect, all having the potential to cause placental abruption. Although up to 40% of cases of severe maternal blunt trauma may be associated with placental abruption, even minor abdominal trauma is associated with abruption in 2–3% of cases. Uterine rupture infrequently is associated with blunt abdominal trauma. When it occurs, it usually is associated with severe and direct trauma to the uterus (26).

Penetrating trauma is most commonly the consequence of gunshot or stab wounds. Depending on uterine size, the rest of the abdominal viscera are relatively protected from penetrating injury. Maternal outcomes generally are better in pregnant women than in nonpregnant individuals with similar injuries. At the same time, the likelihood of uterine injury is increased, resulting in a very high rate of fetal mortality caused by direct injury or by injury of the placenta or umbilical cord.

Management of the injured pregnant woman is directed initially at primary assessment and resuscitation of the mother followed by assessment of the fetus before conducting a secondary survey of the mother. If assessment of the fetus occurs too early in the process and before the mother is stabilized, serious or life-threatening maternal injuries may be overlooked, and clinical circumstances that can result in poor fetal oxygenation (maternal hypoxia, hypovolemia, or supine hypotension) may be ignored. The primary survey and resuscitation of the mother begins with assurance of a functioning airway, adequate ventilation, effective circulation, and an adequate circulatory volume (Figure 20). Guidelines for airway and ventilatory management are the same as for the nonpregnant trauma patient.

A very important aspect of management is deflection of the gravid uterus from the great vessels by placing the woman in the lateral decubitus position. This simple maneuver maximizes cardiac output and ameliorates the shock state. Because maternal intravascular volume can increase by 25% through the early third trimester,

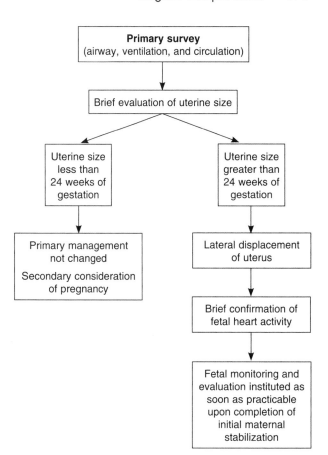

Figure 20. Obstetric aspects of primary trauma management. (Van Hook JW. Trauma in pregnancy. Clin Obstet Gynecol 2002;45:414–24.)

the pregnant woman can lose up to 35% of her blood volume before tachycardia or hypotension occurs. An important mechanism used by the mother to maintain a euvolemic state is to shunt one sixth of her cardiac output that perfuses the uterus into her systemic circulation. Thus, fetal bradycardia and late decelerations of the fetal heart rate can be seen on the fetal monitor. Appropriate initial maneuvers to reverse these processes include rapid infusion of colloid and type-specific blood. Pressors are to be avoided because they further decrease uterine blood flow.

After stabilization, a more detailed secondary assessment of the mother and fetus is undertaken as is done for all trauma patients (27). For the trauma patient who is more than 20 weeks pregnant, the use of electronic fetal heart rate and tocographic monitoring may be predictive in identifying the patient with placental abruption. If the frequency of uterine contractions is less than every 10 minutes during 4 hours of monitoring, placental abruption has not occurred. In contrast, among women contracting more frequently than every 10 minutes, 20% have had an abruption (26). Placental abruption usually occurs during or shortly after the traumatic event. It therefore is recommended that the pregnant trauma victim be placed on electronic fetal monitoring as soon as possible following initial stabilization. No large prospective studies have been published with results that validate any recommendation concerning the length of time a pregnant woman should be observed on electronic fetal monitoring. However, it seems reasonable to recommend that maternal evaluation and fetal monitoring continue so long as uterine contractions continue, a nonreassuring fetal heart pattern persists, any vaginal bleeding continues, rupture of fetal membranes occurs, or the maternal condition remains serious (26).

Ultrasonography has not been demonstrated to be of value in diagnosing or excluding the diagnosis of placental abruption. Fetal to maternal hemorrhage can complicate maternal abdominal trauma and can result in fetal anemia, hydrops, or death. However, there is no evidence that testing for fetal to maternal hemorrhage (as with the Kleihauer–Betke test) can predict adverse immediate sequelae caused by hemorrhage. It is recommended that women who are D-negative receive anti-D immune globulin in quantities sufficient to protect her from D alloimmunization. For more than 90% of women, treatment with 300 micrograms (one vial) will prove sufficient.

References

1. Mazze RI, Kallen B. Appendectomy during pregnancy: a Swedish registry study of 778 cases. Obstet Gynecol 1991;77:835–40.

2. Czeizel AE, Pataki T, Rockenbauer M. Reproductive outcome after exposure to surgery under anesthesia during pregnancy. Arch Gynecol Obstet 1998;261:193–9.

3. Lachman E, Schienfeld A, Voss E, Gino G, Boldes R, Levine S, et al. Pregnancy and laparoscopic surgery. J Am Assoc Gynecol Laparosc 1999;6:347–51.

4. McGory ML, Zingmond DS, Tillou A, Hiatt JR, Ko CY, Cryer HM. Negative appendectomy in pregnant women is associated with a substantial risk of fetal loss. J Am Coll Surg 2007;205:534–40.

5. Walsh CA, Tang T, Walsh SR. Laparoscopic versus open appendicectomy in pregnancy: a systematic review. Int J Surg 2008;6:339–44.

6. Yumi H. Guidelines for diagnosis, treatment, and use of laparoscopy for surgical problems during pregnancy: this statement was reviewed and approved by the Board of Governors of the Society of American Gastrointestinal and Endoscopic Surgeons (SAGES), September 2007. It was prepared by the SAGES Guidelines Committee. Guidelines Committee of the Society of American Gastrointestinal and Endoscopic Surgeons. Surg Endosc 2008;22:849–61.

7. Babler EA. Perforative appendicitis complicating pregnancy: with report of a successful case. J Am Med Assoc 1908;51:1310–4.

8. Tracey M, Fletcher HS. Appendicitis in pregnancy. Am Surg 2000;66:555,9; discussion 559–60.

9. Lim HK, Bae SH, Seo GS. Diagnosis of acute appendicitis in pregnant women: value of sonography. AJR Am J Roentgenol 1992;159:539–42.

10. Wagner LK, Huda W. When a pregnant woman with suspected appendicitis is referred for a CT scan, what should a radiologist do to minimize potential radiation risks? Pediatr Radiol 2004;34:589–90.

11. Terasawa T, Blackmore CC, Bent S, Kohlwes RJ. Systematic review: computed tomography and ultrasonography to detect acute appendicitis in adults and adolescents. Ann Intern Med 2004;141:537–46.

12. Vu L, Ambrose D, Vos P, Tiwari P, Rosengarten M, Wiseman S. Evaluation of MRI for the diagnosis of appendicitis during pregnancy when ultrasound is inconclusive. J Surg Res 2009;156:145–9.

13. Affleck DG, Handrahan DL, Egger MJ, Price RR. The laparoscopic management of appendicitis and cholelithiasis during pregnancy. Am J Surg 1999;178:523–9.

14. Barone JE, Bears S, Chen S, Tsai J, Russell JC. Outcome study of cholecystectomy during pregnancy. Am J Surg 1999;177:232–6.

15. Lee S, Bradley JP, Mele MM, Sehdev HM, Ludmir J. Cholelithiasis in pregnancy: surgical versus medical management [abstract]. Obstet Gynecol 2000;95 (suppl):70s–1s.

16. Graham G, Baxi L, Tharakan T. Laparoscopic cholecystectomy during pregnancy: a case series and review of the literature. Obstet Gynecol Surv 1998;53:566–74.

17. Sainio V, Kemppainen E, Puolakkainen P, Taavitsainen M, Kivisaari L, Valtonen V, et al. Early antibiotic treatment in acute necrotising pancreatitis. Lancet 1995;346:663–7.

18. Sherard GB 3rd, Hodson CA, Williams HJ, Semer DA, Hadi HA, Tait DL. Adnexal masses and pregnancy: a 12-year experience. Am J Obstet Gynecol 2003;189:358–62; discussion 362–3.

19. Hogston P, Lilford RJ. Ultrasound study of ovarian cysts in pregnancy: prevalence and significance. Br J Obstet Gynaecol 1986;93:625–8.

20. Agarwal N, Parul, Kriplani A, Bhatla N, Gupta A. Management and outcome of pregnancies complicated with adnexal masses. Arch Gynecol Obstet 2003;267:148–52.

21. Liu J, Xu Y, Wang J. Ultrasonography, computed tomography and magnetic resonance imaging for diagnosis of ovarian carcinoma. Eur J Radiol 2007;62:328–34.

22. Management of adnexal masses. ACOG Practice Bulletin No. 83. American College of Obstetricians and Gynecologists. Obstet Gynecol 2007;110:201–14.

23. Gazmararian JA, Lazorick S, Spitz AM, Ballard TJ, Saltzman LE, Marks JS. Prevalence of violence against pregnant women. JAMA 1996;275:1915–20.

24. Helton AS, McFarlane J, Anderson ET. Battered and pregnant: a prevalence study. Am J Public Health 1987;77:1337–9.

25. Fildes J, Reed L, Jones N, Martin M, Barrett J. Trauma: the leading cause of maternal death. J Trauma 1992;32:643–5.

26. American College of Obstetricians and Gynecologists. Obstetric aspects of trauma management. Educational Bulletin 251. Washington, DC: American College of Obstetricians and Gynecologists; 1998.

27. American College of Surgeons. ATLS, advanced trauma life support program for doctors. 7th ed. Chicago, IL: ACS; 2004.

Depression*

Katherine M. Sharkey, Teri Pearlstein, and Zachary N. Stowe

Women are at greatest risk of having a first episode of major depression during the childbearing years, and although pregnancy is perceived as a time of emotional well-being, there is little evidence that pregnancy provides protection against psychiatric illness (1). The adverse consequences of depression, including increased maternal morbidity and mortality, poor obstetric outcome, and abnormal child development highlight the need for early identification and intervention.

Unipolar Disorders

The rates of depressive disorders have been examined in pregnant women, with 10–14% of women experiencing a major depressive episode during pregnancy and 25% of pregnant women experiencing an increase in depressive symptoms (2). One study found that more than 25% of pregnant women with psychiatric illness experienced suicidal ideation during pregnancy (3). Nevertheless, despite the prevalence of depressive disorders in obstetric and gynecologic patients and the acknowledgement that recognition and treatment of these disorders is imperative most obstetric and gynecologic patients with depression do not receive a diagnosis (4).

Major Depressive Disorder in Pregnancy

The hallmark symptoms of a major depressive disorder are sustained depressed mood and anhedonia. The diagnostic criteria require that the patient experience at least five of nine symptoms nearly every day for most of the day during the symptomatic period (5). In addition, at least one symptom must be depressed mood or diminished interest and pleasure. Dysthymic disorder, a more chronic unipolar mood disorder, is characterized by fewer symptoms than major depressive disorder, but lasts a minimum of 2 years. Depressive disorders often occur with other psychiatric disorders, resulting in greater morbidity overall. Particularly striking is the comorbidity of depressive disorders with anxiety and substance use disorders. More than 50% of patients with major depressive disorder have a comorbid anxiety disorder, close to 25% have alcohol dependence, and 13% are drug dependent (6).

A number of risk factors are associated with depression during pregnancy (Box 39). Early intervention is critical to minimize the effects of maternal depression. Pregnancy constitutes an ideal time to screen for depression because a woman is likely to have frequent contact with a health care provider. Rating scales, such as the Pregnancy Depression Scale (7), the Edinburgh Postnatal Depression Scale (8), the Postpartum Depression Screening Scale (9), and the Postpartum Depression Checklist (10), can aid in the diagnosis of depression during pregnancy and the postpartum period. These scales minimize the reliance on the presence of symptoms that overlap with pregnancy and the postpartum period, such as sleep changes, appetite changes, and fatigue.

The clinical course of unipolar depression varies in pregnancy, and studies examining prevalence rates during each trimester have yielded inconsistent results regarding which trimester has the highest rates of depression. Depressive symptoms during pregnancy are a strong predictor for postpartum depression. Thus, depression during pregnancy should be treated because of the risk of potential adverse consequences of untreated depression in the mother, including postpartum depression, suicidality, alcohol and substance misuse, miscarriage, and preeclampsia, as well as in the infant (preterm delivery, low birth weight, and abnormal neurobehavioral responses, such as altered heart rate reactivity and sleep disruption).

Postpartum Blues

Postpartum blues affect 50–80% of new mothers and include symptoms of labile mood, anxiety, sleep difficulties, and irritability. The blues occur at such a high

---

Box 39

Risk Factors Associated With Depression During Pregnancy

- History of depressive disorders
- Low social support and high interpersonal conflict
- Financial disadvantage
- Adolescence
- Unmarried status
- Hispanic or African-American race
- Poor social adjustment
- Recent adverse life events
- An unplanned pregnancy or uncertainty about having the child
- A high-risk pregnancy
- Nicotine dependence
- History of intimate partner violence

Data from Pearlstein T. Perinatal depression: treatment options and dilemmas. J Psychiatry Neurosci 2008;33:302–18.

---

*This work reflects a substantial contribution by Megan Smith, MD, in the previous edition.

frequency that it is considered normal sequelae of childbirth. Postpartum blues usually begin within the first days postpartum and start to remit by the second week. Although clinical intervention is not typical, women experiencing the blues appear to be at greater risk of later depression. As many as 20% of women who experience postpartum blues ultimately develop a major depressive episode during the first postnatal year. It is noteworthy that this purportedly normal condition appears to have many of the same risk factors seen for depression (Box 40). The role of the blues as a trigger or representing a brief episode of mood disorder in a vulnerable population warrants further attention.

Postpartum Depression

Postpartum depression is classified as a major depressive disorder with postpartum onset within the first month postpartum, but the depression can occur up to 6 months after birth (11). The rate of major depression in the postpartum period is highly variable with study results citing 8–22% (12, 13). There is evidence that adolescent mothers and mothers living in poverty have higher rates of postpartum depression (Box 41) (14, 15). The symptoms of postpartum depression closely resemble those seen in depression at other times (16), and as with depression during pregnancy, there is considerable overlap between depressive symptoms (alterations in sleep, libido decline, fatigue, and appetite changes) and the normal sequelae of childbirth and the early postpartum period. As discussed earlier, rating scales may be used to help clinicians screen for depression in this population.

The clinical course for women with postpartum major depressive disorder varies. Results from an early study suggested that most women with postpartum depression recover within 6 months (12). In results from another study, it was found that 20% of women experience chronic depression for more than 2 years (17). Long-term follow-up indicates substantial recurrence over the 4 years after delivery, with 50% of women continuing in treatment or again seeking treatment (12).

A particularly dangerous consequence of a mother's postpartum depressive illness is the deleterious effect on her offspring. Postnatal depression has been shown to negatively influence infant behavior (18), cognitive development, and emotional well-being (19).

Postpartum Psychosis

Postpartum psychosis affects 0.2% of postpartum women, with the onset most commonly within the first week after delivery, but by definition within the first 4–6 weeks postpartum (20). Although 80% of women with postpartum psychosis have onset after the birth of their first child (21), it is a highly recurrent illness for women who have another child (22). This disorder is characterized by intense mood lability, obsessive ruminations about the baby, hallucinations, sleep disturbances, and paranoia (20). The strongest risk factors for postpartum psychosis are a history of bipolar disorder or previous episode of postpartum psychosis (21, 23). In the results of one study of 486 women admitted to an inpatient facility with postpartum psychosis, it was found that more than one third had prior diagnoses of bipolar disorder as compared with less than 5% who had a diagnosis of schizophrenia (24).

Treatment consists of the use of antipsychotic and mood stabilizing medications and hospitalization (with the infant, if possible). Patients at high risk should be monitored carefully in the first few weeks, with special attention to obsessive thinking about harming the infant, sleep disorders, and feelings of hopelessness and anhedonia (loss of pleasure in activities previously enjoyed).

Treatment

Depression during the perinatal period should be treated because of the risk of potential adverse consequences

---

Box 40

Possible Characteristics of Women at Risk for Postpartum Blues

- Personal or family history of depression
- Premenstrual dysphoria
- Recent stressful life events or poor social adjustment
- Depression or anxiety during pregnancy
- Excessive fear of labor or view of the pregnancy as emotionally difficult

---

Box 41

Risk Factors for Postpartum Depression

- History of depression
- Family history of depression or anxiety
- Lack of social support
- Negative life events
- Unplanned pregnancy
- Poor marital relations or being unmarried
- Multiple births
- Occupational instability
- Poor outcomes of previous pregnancies (abortion, miscarriage, or sick infant)
- Poor prenatal care
- Malnutrition
- Substance abuse
- Previous suicide attempts
- Pregnancy loss

(25). The type of treatment—psychosocial, psychotherapeutic, or pharmacologic—remains a case-by-case decision. Given that more than 50% of pregnancies are unplanned, most cases of pharmacologic exposure in pregnancy will occur before recognition of the pregnancy. In addition to the patient's psychiatric history, treatment history and fetal exposure to medication should be incorporated in the clinical decision.

PHARMACOTHERAPY

Balancing the risks and benefits of pharmacotherapy during the perinatal period has undergone extensive review (26). There are no risk-free treatment options, and pharmacotherapy decisions should be addressed on an individual basis. The past decade has seen a dramatic increase in the available data on antidepressant medication use during pregnancy. In results from an analysis of eight health care databases, it was found that up to 8% of pregnant women receive a prescription for antidepressants at some point during pregnancy (27). In general, the amount of reproductive safety information available for a particular treatment is proportional to the duration of its use.

The risks of antidepressant use in pregnancy can be broadly categorized as: 1) obstetric complications, 2) birth defects and congenital malformations, 3) neonatal outcomes, and 4) long-term developmental effects. The challenge in using psychotropic medication during pregnancy is to both minimize the risk to the fetus and limit the morbidity of untreated psychiatric illness of the mother. Women with recurrent major depressive disorder taking antidepressants before conception often are advised or choose to discontinue medication before pregnancy or during the first trimester. Although 26% of women who continued to take medications during pregnancy had a relapse of major depression during pregnancy, women who discontinued medication relapsed significantly more in the course of their pregnancy (68–74%) (28, 29). Furthermore, untreated maternal depression has been associated with negative fetal outcomes, such as low birth weight, as well as long-term neurobehavioral consequences (30).

Selective serotonin reuptake inhibitors (SSRIs) and selective serotonin–norepinephrine reuptake inhibitors (SSNRIs) are the first-line treatments for depression. Fetal exposure to antidepressants varies widely among individual medications with the ratio of SSRI concentrations in umbilical cord blood to maternal serum ranging from 0.29 for sertraline to 0.89 for citalopram (31). In results from two recent meta-analyses increased odds ratios of 1.5–1.7 increased relative risk of spontaneous miscarriage with prenatal SSRI exposure were reported (32, 33). Controversy exists surrounding the relationship between the use of SSRIs and preterm delivery and low birth weight. In results from one study, significantly lower gestational age at birth and birth weight among infants exposed to an SSRI in utero compared with those exposed to tricyclic antidepressants (TCAs) or no exposure were found (34). Results from another retrospective chart review revealed that infants of women who received prescriptions for SSRIs during pregnancy had greater risk of low birth weight, preterm birth, fetal death, and seizures compared with infants whose mothers did not receive prescriptions for SSRIs (35). Other studies, however, have not revealed differences in birth weights between infants with exposure to SSRIs versus nonexposed infants (36). The observation that many studies of SSRIs and infant outcomes have not controlled for comorbid illness, untreated depression, and sociodemographic variables known to increase risk of maternal and infant morbidity further complicates the interpretation of these data.

The risk of major congenital malformations in the general population ranges from 1–3%, and SSRI exposure appears to slightly increase this risk, particularly if mothers took SSRIs early in pregnancy. For instance, in results from a study of more than 150,000 births, an increased relative risk of 1.34 for congenital malformations in infants whose mothers took SSRIs during pregnancy was reported (37). The use of paroxetine in particular has been associated with an increased relative risk of 2.2 for congenital malformations (mainly cardiovascular and predominantly ventricular septal defect). As a consequence of these findings, the U.S. Food and Drug Administration (FDA) issued a public health advisory against use of paroxetine in pregnancy and changed its pregnancy category from C to D. Fetal echocardiography may be indicated in pregnancies with early paroxetine exposure.

Selective serotonin reuptake inhibitor use during the third trimester of pregnancy also has been associated with a neonatal behavioral syndrome. This syndrome is alternately felt to represent SSRI withdrawal or toxicity and is estimated to occur in 30% of infants exposed to SSRIs (38). Symptoms include low Apgar scores, respiratory distress, poor muscle tone, jitteriness or irritability, and hypoglycemia. Although the symptoms usually are transient, severity can vary widely. In results of one study, it was demonstrated that more neonates exposed to SSRIs in the third trimester require supportive care in special or intensive care nurseries compared with infants with first trimester SSRI exposure (39). At this time, the neonatal behavioral syndrome has been reported with the use of paroxetine, fluoxetine, venlafaxine, and citalopram (26).

The use of SSRIs after 20 weeks of gestation was demonstrated to increase the risk of persistent pulmonary hypertension of the newborn from 1 per 700 births to 7 per 1000 births (40). Because this syndrome of respiratory distress and hypoxia can be fatal in up to 20% of infants, the FDA has issued a warning regarding this increased risk. Further investigations may elucidate the mechanism of this postnatal complication.

Several prospective controlled studies have been conducted on pregnant women taking TCAs. More than 450 cases of first-trimester exposure to TCAs have been examined through both prospective and retrospective studies. Overall, no significant association between fetal exposure to TCAs and risk of major congenital anomalies was found. Preferred TCAs for use during pregnancy include desipramine and nortriptyline because they are less anticholinergic and least likely to aggravate orthostatic hypotension (41). Behavioral development in children exposed in utero to TCAs or fluoxetine is not adversely affected in terms of global intelligence, language development, or behavioral development, and timing of the antidepressant therapy (first trimester versus the entire pregnancy) does not affect behavioral outcomes (42).

Tricyclic antidepressant dosage requirements increase across gestation, such that during the final trimester the dose required to sustain remission from depression is 1.3–2 times the nonpregnant dose. Therefore, in cases where breakthrough depressive symptoms occur, serum levels should be obtained to ensure appropriate TCA dosage. If depressive symptoms warrant, the dose of TCAs could be tapered during the 2-week period before the estimated delivery date to reduce the fetal drug load at birth. However, taper and discontinuation of any antidepressant before delivery may increase the risk the development of postpartum depression. If a TCA is appropriate for use during pregnancy, nortriptyline is the preferable TCA because of its long use and study. Other benefits of nortriptyline are its low relative anticholinergic activity and the tight relationship between plasma concentration and therapeutic effect (43).

OTHER TREATMENT OPTIONS FOR DEPRESSION

Nonpharmacologic techniques also are available for the treatment of depression among pregnant and postpartum women. They include psychotherapy, such as cognitive-behavior therapy or interpersonal psychotherapy, and electroconvulsive therapy.

Bipolar Disorders

Patients with bipolar disorders may experience mania, hypomania, depression, and mixed states (ie, a combination of manic and depressive symptoms simultaneously). In results of one study of 191 women without previous psychiatric diagnoses, it was found that 11% had significant hypomanic symptoms on postpartum day 5, and 7.6% had significant hypomanic symptoms at 6 weeks, with 21% of the original hypomanic women exhibiting symptoms at both time points (44). A replication and extension in a second group of 258 women demonstrated hypomanic symptoms in 10% on postpartum day 3 and 7% at 6 weeks and also revealed that one half of the new mothers who exhibited hypo-

mania on postpartum day 3 went on to have clinically significant depressive symptoms at 6 weeks postpartum. These data suggest that hypomania during the immediate postpartum period may be related to later development of depressive symptoms. In the general population, women with hypomanic symptoms may not come to the attention of clinicians, but they may be at increased risk of subsequent depression (45).

Treatment

For women with bipolar disorder who elect to take medication during the first trimester, exposure to a single psychotropic agent may be safer than exposure to multiple agents. Furthermore, if a medication proves effective, changing medication to avoid teratogenic risk may jeopardize the woman's psychiatric stability and the pregnancy.

MOOD STABILIZERS

Lithium, antiepileptic medications, and antipsychotic medications can be used during pregnancy to treat bipolar disorder and psychotic symptoms. With lithium treatment, maternal serum levels, which may be affected by vomiting, sodium intake, and fluid shifts, should be closely monitored (46). Risk of cardiac malformations, particularly Ebstein anomaly, increases from 0.05% to 0.1% with first-trimester lithium exposure. A Level II ultrasound examination and fetal echocardiography should be performed. As pregnancy progresses, the dose of lithium may need to be increased because renal lithium excretion increases. The use of lithium during labor requires specific precautions. Some experts advise tapering lithium 1 week before delivery to minimize neonatal toxic effects and to stop the use of lithium on the onset of labor. Treatment with lithium should be resumed immediately after delivery.

Data show that lamotrigine has extensive placental transfer and slow elimination in infants, resulting in neonatal lamotrigine plasma concentrations comparable with those observed during active lamotrigine therapy (47). Pregnancy registry data suggest that infants with in utero exposure to lamotrigine have an increased risk of cleft lip or palate, and in 2006, the FDA issued an alert regarding oral cleft risk with use of lamotrigine in pregnancy. Nevertheless, lamotrigine has a lower reported incidence of major congenital malformations and fetal deaths compared with carbamazepine and phenytoin. Valproate has been associated with fetal anomalies, such as neural tube defects and fetal valproate syndrome, as well as poor neurocognitive outcomes. Adverse fetal and infant effects with valproate appear to be dose related and exposure during the first trimester carries the greatest teratogenic risk. Because of the risk of neural tube defects, women of child-bearing age being treated with carbamazepine or valproate also should take folate.

Antipsychotic medications also are used to control symptoms and maintain mood stability in patients with bipolar disorder. Use of traditional antipsychotics, such as haloperidol and phenothiazines, has been associated with congenital malformations at slightly higher rates than in the general population. In addition, neonatal withdrawal syndromes have been observed. When traditional antipsychotics are used in pregnancy, high-potency antipsychotics (eg, haloperidol and fluphenazine) are preferred to avoid anticholinergic effects (26).

Studies of the use of second-generation atypical antipsychotics (ie, clozapine, olanzapine, risperidone, quetiapine, aripiprazole, and ziprasidone) during pregnancy are limited with respect to teratogenic risk, although congenital malformations and increased and decreased birth weights have been reported. As in men and non-pregnant women, there is a possibility of an increased risk of hyperglycemia in pregnant women who take atypical antipsychotics.

BENZODIAZEPINES

Benzodiazepines, such as lorazepam and clonazepam, are used to treat anxiety and insomnia. Third-trimester exposure to benzodiazepines has resulted in neonatal syndromes such as floppy infant syndrome—characterized by impaired temperature regulation, apnea, and muscle hypotonia—and failure to feed. Infants born to mothers who used benzodiazepines chronically during pregnancy may experience a withdrawal syndrome that includes irritability, hyperreflexia, hypertonia, abnormal sleep, and feeding difficulties.

OTHER TREATMENT OPTIONS FOR BIPOLAR DISORDER

Other options for the treatment of bipolar disorder among pregnant women include the use of electroconvulsive therapy and psychosocial interventions. Electroconvulsive therapy has been shown to have a low rate of complications during pregnancy; however, fetal cardiac monitoring during electroconvulsive therapy allows for detection of arrhythmias and their correction. Agents routinely given in nonpregnant electroconvulsive therapy patients to reduce bradycardia and decrease secretions should not be given during pregnancy because they increase the risk of gastric reflux.

References

1. Bebbington PE, Dunn G, Jenkins R, Lewis G, Brugha T, Farrell M, et al. The influence of age and sex on the prevalence of depressive conditions: report from the National Survey of Psychiatric Morbidity. Psychol Med 1998;28:9–19.

2. Evans J, Heron J, Francomb H, Oke S, Golding J. Cohort study of depressed mood during pregnancy and after childbirth. BMJ 2001;323:257–60.

3. Newport DJ, Levey LC, Pennell PB, Ragan K, Stowe ZN. Suicidal ideation in pregnancy: assessment and clinical implications. Arch Womens Ment Health 2007;10:181–7.

4. Kelly R, Zatzick D, Anders T. The detection and treatment of psychiatric disorders and substance use among pregnant women cared for in obstetrics. Am J Psychiatry 2001;158:213–9.

5. American Psychiatric Association. Diagnostic and statistical manual of mental disorders: DSM-IV-TR. 4th ed., text revision ed. Washington, DC: American Psychiatric Association; 2000.

6. Kessler RC, Nelson CB, McGonagle KA, Liu J, Swartz M, Blazer DG. Comorbidity of DSM-III-R major depressive disorder in the general population: results from the US National Comorbidity Survey. Br J Psychiatry Suppl 1996;(30):17–30.

7. Altshuler LL, Cohen LS, Vitonis AF, Faraone SV, Harlow BL, Suri R, et al. The Pregnancy Depression Scale (PDS): a screening tool for depression in pregnancy. Arch Womens Ment Health 2008;11:277–85.

8. Cox JL, Holden JM, Sagovsky R. Detection of postnatal depression. Development of the 10-item Edinburgh Postnatal Depression Scale. Br J Psychiatry 1987;150:782–6.

9. Beck CT, Gable RK. Comparative analysis of the performance of the Postpartum Depression Screening Scale with two other depression instruments. Nurs Res 2001;50:242–50.

10. Beck CT. Screening methods for postpartum depression. J Obstet Gynecol Neonatal Nurs 1995;24:308–12.

11. Stowe ZN, Hostetter AL, Newport DJ. The onset of postpartum depression: implications for clinical screening in obstetrical and primary care. Am J Obstet Gynecol 2005;192:522–6.

12. Kumar R, Robson KM. A prospective study of emotional disorders in childbearing women. Br J Psychiatry 1984;144:35–47.

13. O'Hara MW, Zekoski EM, Philipps LH, Wright EJ. Controlled prospective study of postpartum mood disorders: comparison of childbearing and nonchildbearing women. J Abnorm Psychol 1990;99:3–15.

14. Hobfoll SE, Ritter C, Lavin J, Hulsizer MR, Cameron RP. Depression prevalence and incidence among inner-city pregnant and postpartum women. J Consult Clin Psychol 1995;63:445–53.

15. Troutman BR, Cutrona CE. Nonpsychotic postpartum depression among adolescent mothers. J Abnorm Psychol 1990;99:69–78.

16. Suri R, Burt VK. The assessment and treatment of postpartum psychiatric disorders. J Pract Psychiatry Behav Health 1997;3:67–77.

17. England SJ, Ballard C, George S. Chronicity in postnatal depression. Eur J Psychiatry 1994;8:93–6.

18. Campbell SB, Cohn JF, Meyers T. Depression in first-time mothers: mother-infant interaction and depression chronicity. Dev Psychol 1995;31:349–57.

19. Murray D, Cox JL, Chapman G, Jones P. Childbirth: life event or start of a long-term difficulty? Further data from

the Stoke-on-Trent controlled study of postnatal depression. Br J Psychiatry 1995;166:595–600.

20. Muller C. On the nosology of post-partum psychoses. Psychopathology 1985;18:181–4.

21. McNeil TF. A prospective study of postpartum psychoses in a high-risk group. 2. Relationships to demographic and psychiatric history characteristics. Acta Psychiatr Scand 1987;75:35–43.

22. Davidson J, Robertson E. A follow-up study of post partum illness, 1946-1978. Acta Psychiatr Scand 1985;71:451–7.

23. Marks MN, Wieck A, Checkley SA, Kumar R. Life stress and post-partum psychosis: a preliminary report. Br J Psychiatry Suppl 1991;(10):45–9.

24. Kendell RE, Chalmers JC, Platz C. Epidemiology of puerperal psychoses [published erratum appears in Br J Psychiatry 1987;151:135]. Br J Psychiatry 1987;150:662–73.

25. Bonari L, Pinto N, Ahn E, Einarson A, Steiner M, Koren G. Perinatal risks of untreated depression during pregnancy. Can J Psychiatry 2004;49:726–35.

26. Pearlstein T. Perinatal depression: treatment options and dilemmas. J Psychiatry Neurosci 2008;33:302–18.

27. Andrade SE, Raebel MA, Brown J, Lane K, Livingston J, Boudreau D, et al. Use of antidepressant medications during pregnancy: a multisite study. Am J Obstet Gynecol 2008;198:194.e1–194.e5.

28. Cohen LS, Altshuler LL, Stowe ZN, Faraone SV. Reintroduction of antidepressant therapy across pregnancy in women who previously discontinued treatment. A preliminary retrospective study. Psychother Psychosom 2004;73:255–8.

29. Cohen LS, Altshuler LL, Harlow BL, Nonacs R, Newport DJ, Viguera AC, et al. Relapse of major depression during pregnancy in women who maintain or discontinue antidepressant treatment. JAMA 2006;295:499–507.

30. Oberlander TF, Warburton W, Misri S, Aghajanian J, Hertzman C. Neonatal outcomes after prenatal exposure to selective serotonin reuptake inhibitor antidepressants and maternal depression using population-based linked health data. Arch Gen Psychiatry 2006;63:898–906.

31. Hendrick V, Stowe ZN, Altshuler LL, Hwang S, Lee E, Haynes D. Placental passage of antidepressant medications. Am J Psychiatry 2003;160:993–6.

32. Rahimi R, Nikfar S, Abdollahi M. Pregnancy outcomes following exposure to serotonin reuptake inhibitors: a meta-analysis of clinical trials. Reprod Toxicol 2006;22:571–5.

33. Hemels ME, Einarson A, Koren G, Lanctot KL, Einarson TR. Antidepressant use during pregnancy and the rates of spontaneous abortions: a meta-analysis. Ann Pharmacother 2005;39:803–9.

34. Simon GE, Cunningham ML, Davis RL. Outcomes of prenatal antidepressant exposure. Am J Psychiatry 2002;159:2055–61.

35. Wen SW, Yang Q, Garner P, Fraser W, Olatunbosun O, Nimrod C, et al. Selective serotonin reuptake inhibitors and adverse pregnancy outcomes. Am J Obstet Gynecol 2006;194:961–6.

36. Suri R, Altshuler L, Hendrick V, Rasgon N, Lee E, Mintz J. The impact of depression and fluoxetine treatment on obstetrical outcome. Arch Womens Ment Health 2004;7: 193–200.

37. Wogelius P, Norgaard M, Gislum M, Pedersen L, Munk E, Mortensen PB, et al. Maternal use of selective serotonin reuptake inhibitors and risk of congenital malformations. Epidemiology 2006;17:701–4.

38. Levinson-Castiel R, Merlob P, Linder N, Sirota L, Klinger G. Neonatal abstinence syndrome after in utero exposure to selective serotonin reuptake inhibitors in term infants. Arch Pediatr Adolesc Med 2006;160:173–6.

39. Malm H, Klaukka T, Neuvonen PJ. Risks associated with selective serotonin reuptake inhibitors in pregnancy. Obstet Gynecol 2005;106:1289–96.

40. Chambers CD, Hernandez-Diaz S, Van Marter LJ, Werler MM, Louik C, Jones KL, et al. Selective serotonin-reuptake inhibitors and risk of persistent pulmonary hypertension of the newborn. N Engl J Med 2006;354:579–87.

41. Nonacs R, Cohen LS. Depression during pregnancy: diagnosis and treatment options. J Clin Psychiatry 2002;63 (suppl 7):24–30.

42. Nulman I, Rovet J, Stewart DE, Wolpin J, Gardner HA, Theis JG, et al. Neurodevelopment of children exposed in utero to antidepressant drugs. N Engl J Med 1997;336:258–62.

43. Szigethy EM, Wisner KL. Psychopharmacological treatment of mood and anxiety disorders during pregnancy. In: Steiner M, Yonkers KA, Eriksson E, editors. Mood disorders in women. London: Martin Dunitz; 2000. p. 295–311.

44. Glover V, Liddle P, Taylor A, Adams D, Sandler M. Mild hypomania (the highs) can be a feature of the first postpartum week. Association with later depression. Br J Psychiatry 1994;164:517–21.

45. Heron J, Craddock N, Jones I. Postnatal euphoria: are 'the highs' an indicator of bipolarity? Bipolar Disord 2005;7:103–10.

46. Newport DJ, Viguera AC, Beach AJ, Ritchie JC, Cohen LS, Stowe ZN. Lithium placental passage and obstetrical outcome: implications for clinical management during late pregnancy. Am J Psychiatry 2005;162:2162–70.

47. Ohman I, Vitols S, Tomson T. Lamotrigine in pregnancy: pharmacokinetics during delivery, in the neonate, and during lactation. Epilepsia 2000;41:709–13.

INTRAPARTUM MANAGEMENT

Labor Stimulation

Andrew J. Satin

The goal of labor stimulation is to effect uterine activity that is sufficient to produce cervical change and fetal descent, while avoiding abnormal fetal heart rate patterns. Labor stimulation includes induction and augmentation. Induction of labor implies stimulation of uterine contractions previously absent, with or without ruptured fetal membranes, and augmentation refers to stimulation of uterine contractions when spontaneous contractions have failed to result in progressive cervical dilation or descent of the fetus or both. The overall rate of induction of labor in the United States has more than doubled since 1990 to 22.5% in 2006 (1). Common indications for labor induction are listed in Box 42. Before initiating labor induction, a diagnosis should be established by performing a pelvic examination documenting whether the cervix is favorable and estimated fetal weight.

Purely elective induction of labor is associated with an increase in rates of abdominal and operative vaginal delivery compared with spontaneous labor and is not recommended. If initiated, elective induction should not be performed before 39 weeks of gestation or before documentation of pulmonary maturity of the fetus.

Box 42

Common Indications for Labor Stimulation

- Abruptio placentae
- Chorioamnionitis
- Fetal demise
- Gestational hypertension
- Premature rupture of membranes
- Postterm pregnancy
- Maternal medical conditions (eg, diabetes mellitus, renal disease, chronic pulmonary disease, and chronic hypertension)
- Fetal compromise (eg, severe intrauterine growth restriction and isoimmunization)
- Preeclampsia and eclampsia
- Logistical reasons (risk of rapid labor, distance from hospital, and psychosocial indications), provided term gestation is confirmed or fetal lung maturity is established

Induction of labor. ACOG Practice Bulletin 107. American College of Obstetricians and Gynecologists.Obstet Gynecol 2009;114:386-97.

Labor Induction and Augmentation

Techniques for induction of labor may be surgical or medical. Medical techniques include the use of oxytocin infusion or prostaglandins. Surgical techniques include amniotomy or stripping of membranes. Labor augmentation typically is performed with oxytocin infusion, although prostaglandin therapy can be used for this purpose if the fetus is not potentially viable.

Oxytocin

Continuous oxytocin infusion remains the mainstay of medical therapy for labor augmentation and for induction of labor when the cervix is favorable. Factors affecting the dose response to oxytocin induction include initial cervical dilation, parity, and gestational age (2). Higher doses of oxytocin generally are required in preterm nulliparous women with an unfavorable cervix. However, the prediction of an individual's oxytocin requirement is not possible. The principles of oxytocin administration for labor augmentation are the same as those for induction. Because oxytocin augmentation typically is prescribed in women with more advanced cervical dilation and effacement, it is not surprising that the maximum required infusion rate typically is lower than that needed for induction (2).

Oxytocin should be administered by means of an infusion pump according to established departmental protocols. The fetal heart rate, resting uterine tone, and frequency and duration of contractions should be monitored appropriately by electronic monitoring or by palpation and auscultation every 15 minutes during the first stage of labor and every 5 minutes during the second stage of labor.

Numerous protocols regarding the initial dose, dose increments, and time intervals between dose increases have been studied. Low-dose regimens (starting dose 0.5–2 mU/min with increments of 1–2 mU/min every 15–40 minutes) were developed based on the knowledge that it takes oxytocin 40–60 minutes to reach a steady-state concentration in maternal serum. Low-dose protocols are associated with a lower incidence of uterine tachysystole. High-dose protocols (starting doses 3–6 mU/min with increments of 3–6 mU/min every 15–40 minutes) have been credited with shortening the duration of labor and reducing the number of cesarean deliveries resulting from labor dystocia (3). The advantages of high-dose protocols appear to be more profound when used for augmentation than for induction of labor. The clinical success of high-dose regimens may be because cervical dilation and uterine contraction pressures do not correlate with serum oxytocin levels (4). To date, no clinical trials have compared dosing protocols with outcome measures focused primarily on patient safety. Most clinical trials investigating the utility of more aggressive oxytocin regimes generally reflect shorter times from admission to delivery, but a higher need for cessation of infusion. Applying safety theory to oxytocin administration, it stands to reason that labor and delivery units should establish protocols that prescribe indications for cessation of the infusion and ongoing monitoring of compliance. The optimal protocol used on a given unit may be influenced by the patient population and hospital environment.

Artificial Rupture of the Membranes

Amniotomy may be used for labor induction, particularly if the condition of the cervix is favorable. However, the interval to the onset of contractions after artificial membrane rupture is unpredictable, and this technique can result in prolonged membrane rupture, which is associated with an increased risk of chorioamnionitis. If the fetal head is not well applied to the cervix, amniotomy can result in prolapse of the umbilical cord or fetal parts. The combination of initial amniotomy and the use of oxytocin has been shown to result in a shorter time to delivery than amniotomy alone (5).

Membrane Stripping

Stripping or sweeping of the fetal membranes involves bluntly separating the chorioamnionic membrane from the lower uterine segment above the internal cervical os. This practice does not induce labor, per se, but likely initiates the process through local release of prostaglandins and phospholipases (6). Stripping of membranes increases the likelihood of spontaneous labor within 48 hours and reduces the need for subsequent labor induction (7, 8). Potential risks of membrane stripping include infection, bleeding from undiagnosed placenta previa or low-lying placenta, and accidental rupture of membranes. There are insufficient data to guide practice regarding membrane stripping for women within a positive group B streptococci culture result.

Prostaglandins

Prostaglandin E_2 (PGE$_2$), Prostaglandin $F_{2\alpha}$ (PGF$_{2\alpha}$) and Prostaglandin E_1 (PGE$_1$) may be used for induction of labor at term and also in early and middle pregnancy when the uterus can be more refractory to oxytocin. Prostaglandins also can be used for preinduction cervical ripening, and this treatment can result in labor; the line between cervical ripening and labor induction

can be somewhat blurred. Although systemic or local administration of prostaglandins have been widely used and is often successful, prostaglandin use may be associated with unwanted side effects, such as tachysystole (greater than five contractions in 10 minutes) with fetal heart rate decelerations (9).

Prostaglandin E_2 can be given orally, or intravaginally as a suppository or gel (Table 29). In results from a comprehensive review of 57 studies involving 10,039 women, it was found that the use of vaginal PGE$_2$ compared with placebo shortened the time to delivery and reduced the likelihood of failure to achieve vaginal delivery within 24 hours (18% versus 99%; relative risk [RR], 0.19; 95% confidence interval [CI], 0.14–0.25). The risk of cesarean delivery was not decreased, but tachysystole with fetal heart rate abnormalities was more common (4.6% versus 0.51%; RR, 4.14; 95% CI, 1.91–8.9) with the use of PGE$_2$ (10). In the results of the same review, the use of vaginal PGF$_{2\alpha}$, was associated with less frequent need for oxytocin augmentation (53.9% versus 89.1%; RR, 0.65; 95% CI, 0.53–0.8) and fewer operative vaginal deliveries, with no differences in cesarean delivery rates (5.8% versus 10.2%; RR, 0.58; 95% CI, 0.29–1.18).

Misoprostol, a synthetic PGE$_1$ analog, has been marketed for the prevention of peptic ulcers in the United States since 1988. The advantages of the use of misoprostol over PGE$_2$ derivatives include lower cost, ease of storage, and stability at room temperature. These have led to its widespread use for induction of labor in women with an unfavorable cervix. In results of a systematic review of vaginal misoprostol for cervical ripening and induction of labor, which included 70 trials, vaginal misoprostol use was found to be more effective than conventional methods (11). Compared with the use of vaginal PGE$_2$, intracervical PGE$_2$ and oxytocin, the use of vaginal misoprostol was associated with less failure to achieve vaginal delivery within 24 hours and less epidural analgesia use, but with more frequent uterine tachysystole. Compared with the use of intracervical or vaginal PGE$_2$, oxytocin augmentation was less common after misoprostol therapy, but meconium-stained amni-

Table 29. Prostaglandin Ripening Agents

Agents	Dose	Route
Dinoprostone (prostaglandin E$_2$)	0.5 mg in 2.5 mL of gel	Intracervically
Dinoprostone (prostaglandin E$_2$)	10 mg (0.3 mg/h)	Intravaginally
Prostaglandin E$_2$	2.5-mg gel	Intravaginally
Misoprostol (PGE$_1$)	25–50 micrograms*	Intravaginally

*Available as 100-microgram and 200-microgram tablets that must be broken to provide a 25-microgram or a 50-microgram dose

otic fluid was more common. Lower doses of misoprostol were associated with less frequent tachysystole than were higher doses but resulted in a greater need for oxytocin augmentation. No studies have produced results that have indicated that intrapartum exposure to misoprostol (or other prostaglandin cervical ripening agents) has any long-term adverse health consequences to the fetus in the absence of fetal heart rate abnormalities. Although the optimal dosing regimen has not been established, general guidelines for misoprostol use exist (Box 43).

Recent studies have assessed alternate routes of misoprostol administration for labor induction. In results from a systematic review, which included 5,096 women assigned to use oral or vaginal misoprostol in 26 trials, the authors concluded that oral misoprostol use is more effective than placebo, is as effective as the use of vaginal misoprostol, and results in fewer cesarean deliveries than vaginal dinoprostone (12). They suggested that 20–25 micrograms of misoprostol in solution administered every 2 hours may be an optimal dose but cautioned that further studies are needed to assess its safety, efficacy, and optimal dose and dosing intervals. In results of another recent review of three studies, the use of sublingual misoprostol was found to be as

effective as the use of oral misoprostol (13). In theory, buccal or sublingual administration may avoid first pass hepatic metabolism associated with oral ingestion and may increase bioavailability. However, the use of sublingual or buccal misoprostol cannot be recommended until optimal dosage and safety have been established by larger trials.

In results of a retrospective cohort study involving 20,095 women with a previous cesarean delivery, the risk of uterine rupture was significantly higher with prostaglandin-induced labor than with spontaneous or non–prostaglandin-induced labor (14). Misoprostol should not be used in term pregnancies in women with previous cesarean deliveries or uterine scars because there is an increased risk of uterine rupture (15).

Preinduction Cervical Ripening

If induction is indicated and the cervix is unfavorable, the use of agents for cervical ripening can reduce the rate of failed induction and the need for and duration of oxytocin administration. Intracervical mechanical devices provide cervical ripening with the advantages of low cost, less tachysystole, lack of systemic side effects, and easy reversibility. Mechanical dilation methods for cervical ripening include synthetic or natural hygroscopic dilators, and the Foley catheter (14–26 French) or double balloon device with or without extra amniotic saline infusion. Disadvantages of mechanical cervical ripening techniques can include an increased risk of infection, disruption of a low-lying placenta, and maternal discomfort with cervical manipulation. Prostaglandin formulations that have been used for cervical ripening include intracervical and intravaginal PGE_2, intravaginal PGE_1, and oral PGE_1. Local administration of prostaglandin to the posterior fornix of the vagina or into the endocervical canal has become the preferred route because the frequency of side effects is reduced while maintaining an acceptable clinical response (7).

Foley Catheter

To insert a Foley catheter, the cervix is examined with the aid of a sterile speculum and cleansed with a povidone–iodine solution. Ring forceps are used to pass a deflated catheter (number 16 French, with a 30–80 mL balloon, and the tip removed) through the internal os. The balloon is distended with sterile water or saline and retracted against the internal os. Although attaching a weight to the end of the catheter to apply traction has been described, it has not been proved to enhance cervical ripening. Results from randomized trials generally, but not consistently, have reported use of a balloon catheter to be as effective as the use of prostaglandins for cervical ripening (7). Results of a systematic review comparing mechanical methods of cervical

---

Box 43

General Principles for Misoprostol Use for Cervical Ripening or Labor Induction

- If misoprostol is to be used for cervical ripening or labor induction in the third trimester, one quarter of a 100-microgram tablet (ie, approximately 25 micrograms) should be considered for the initial dose. The use of higher doses (50 micrograms every 6 hours) may be appropriate in some situations, although increasing the dose appears to be associated with uterine tachysystole, fetal heart rate decelerations, and an increase in meconium-stained amniotic fluid.

- Doses should not be administered more frequently than every 3–6 hours.

- Oxytocin should not be administered less than 4 hours after the last misoprostol dose.

- Patients undergoing cervical ripening or labor induction with the use of misoprostol should undergo fetal heart rate monitoring and uterine activity monitoring in a hospital setting.

- The use of misoprostol in women with prior cesarean delivery or major uterine surgery has been associated with an increase in uterine rupture and, therefore, should be avoided in the third trimester.

Data from Induction of labor. ACOG Practice Bulletin 107. American College of Obstetricians and Gynecologists. Obstet Gynecol 2009;114:386–97.

ripening with the use of vaginal PGE$_2$ indicated more frequent failure to achieve delivery within 24 hours (73% versus 42%; RR, 1.74; 95% CI, 1.21–2.49) but a decrease in tachysystole with fetal heart rate changes with mechanical methods. There appears to be no difference in the risk of cesarean delivery with mechanical methods versus the use of prostaglandins (8).

Extra amniotic saline infusion involves insertion of a 22–25 gauge Foley catheter into the cervical canal, with the balloon passed through the internal os and inflated with 30–40 mL of sterile water or saline. A normal saline solution is infused through the catheter at a constant rate of 30–60 mL/h by infusion pump, resulting in stripping of the fetal membranes from the uterine wall. The catheter is spontaneously expelled with cervical dilation or removed at rupture of membranes or after a predetermined time. The combination of the use of extra amniotic saline infusion plus a balloon catheter does not appear to offer an advantage over the use of a Foley catheter alone. Furthermore, results of a comparison of the use of extra amniotic infusion with any prostaglandins indicated that women undergoing mechanical cervical ripening were more likely not to achieve vaginal delivery within 24 hours (57% versus 42%; RR, 1.33; 95% CI, 1.02–1.75) and had an increased risk of cesarean delivery (31% versus 22%; RR, 1.48; 95% CI, 1.14–1.9) without a reduction in the risk of tachysystole (8).

Prostaglandins

Two PGE$_2$ preparations are commercially available for cervical ripening—a vaginal insert containing 10 mg of dinoprostone and a gel in a 2.5 mL syringe containing 0.5 mg of dinoprostone in 2.5 mL gel. Both are approved by the U.S. Food and Drug Administration for the use of cervical ripening at or near term. Side effects of vaginally administered prostaglandins are uncommon and include vomiting, diarrhea, and fever. The vaginal insert releases prostaglandin at a slower rate (0.3 mg/h) than does the gel and is left in place until labor begins or for up to 12 hours. Oxytocin may be administered 30–60 minutes after its removal. The use of intracervical gel can be repeated in 6–12 hours if there is inadequate cervical change and minimal uterine activity after administration of the first dose. The manufacturer of the intracervical gel recommends a maximum of three doses (1.5 mg of dinoprostone) within a 24-hour period. Most physicians advocate delaying oxytocin administration for 3–12 hours after prostaglandin-induced ripening. Vaginal PGE$_2$ used for cervical ripening or induction of labor compared with placebo or no treatment results in a higher likelihood of vaginal delivery within 24 hours and no difference in cesarean delivery rates, but a higher risk of uterine tachysystole with fetal heart rate changes (11). Similarly, results of a review of the use of intracervical

PGE$_2$ versus placebo showed a reduction in the number of women who did not achieve vaginal delivery within 24 hours (RR, 0.61; 95% CI, 0.47–0.79) (16). Results of an analysis of 29 trials involving 3,881 women, in which the use of intracervical and intravaginal PGE$_2$ were compared, suggested that failure to achieve vaginal delivery within 24 hours was more common with the use of intracervical PGE$_2$ (RR, 1.26; 95% CI, 1.12–1.41) without an increase in the rates of cesarean delivery or tachysystole. The authors concluded that the use of intravaginal PGE$_2$ was superior.

As noted previously, misoprostol has been shown to be an effective agent for use in cervical ripening but does have more potential for uterine tachysystole and also the risk of uterine rupture when there has been prior uterine surgery. Many women treated with misoprostol for cervical ripening will progress into labor without the need for additional oxytocin infusion, and misoprostol is significantly cheaper that the two commercially available agents. In comparison with placebo, the use of vaginal PGF$_{2\alpha}$ also has been associated with improved cervical scores and reduced need for oxytocin augmentation, but similar cesarean delivery rates.

References

1. Martin JA, Hamilton BE, Sutton PD, Ventura SJ, Menacker F, Kimeyer S, et al. Births: final data for 2006. Natl Vital Stat Rep 2009;57(7):1–104.

2. Satin AJ, Leveno KJ, Sherman ML, McIntire DD. Factors affecting the dose response to oxytocin for labor stimulation. Am J Obstet Gynecol 1992;166:1260–1.

3. Dystocia and augmentation of labor. ACOG Practice Bulletin No. 49. American College of Obstetricians and Gynecologists. Obstet Gynecol 2003;102:1445–54.

4. Perry RL, Satin AJ, Barth WH, Valtier S, Cody JT, Hankins GD. The pharmacokinetics of oxytocin as they apply to labor induction. Am J Obstet Gynecol 1996;174:1590–3.

5. Moldin PG, Sundell G. Induction of labour: a randomised clinical trial of amniotomy versus amniotomy with oxytocin infusion. Br J Obstet Gynaecol 1996;103:306–12.

6. McColgin SW, Bennett WA, Roach H, Cowan BD, Martin JN Jr, Morrison JC. Parturitional factors associated with membrane stripping. Am J Obstet Gynecol 1993; 169:71–7.

7. Wing D. Induction of labor. In: Basow DS, editor. UpToDate. Wellesley (MA): UpToDate; 2009.

8. Boulvain M, Kelly AJ, Lohse C, Stan CM, Irion O. Mechanical methods for induction of labour. Cochrane Database of Systematic Reviews 2001, Issue 4. Art. No.: CD001233. DOI: 10.1002/14651858.CD001233; 10.1002/14651858.CD001233.

9. Intrapartum fetal heart rate monitoring: nomenclature, interpretation, and general management principles. ACOG Practice Bulletin No. 106. American College of Obstetricians and Gynecologists. Obstet Gynecol 2009;114:192–202.

10. Kelly AJ, Kavanagh J, Thomas J. Vaginal prostaglandin (PGE2 and PGF2a) for induction of labour at term. Cochrane Database of Systematic Reviews 2003, Issue 4. Art. No.: CD003101. DOI: 10.1002/14651858.CD003101; 10.1002/14651858.CD003101.

11. Hofmeyr GJ, Gulmezoglu AM. Vaginal misoprostol for cervical ripening and induction of labour. Cochrane Database of Systematic Reviews 2003, Issue 1. Art. No.: CD000941. DOI: 10.1002/14651858.CD000941; 10.1002/14651858.CD000941.

12. Alfirevic Z, Weeks A. Oral misoprostol for induction of labour. Cochrane Database of Systematic Reviews 2006, Issue 2. Art. No.: CD001338. DOI: 10.1002/14651858.CD001338.pub2; 10.1002/14651858.CD001338.pub2.

13. Muzonzini G, Hofmeyr GJ. Buccal or sublingual misoprostol for cervical ripening and induction of labour. Cochrane Database of Systematic Reviews 2004, Issue 4. Art. No.: CD004221. DOI: 10.1002/14651858.CD004221. pub2; 10.1002/14651858.CD004221.pub2.

14. Lydon-Rochelle M, Holt VL, Easterling TR, Martin DP. Risk of uterine rupture during labor among women with a prior cesarean delivery. N Engl J Med 2001;345:3–8.

15. Induction of labor. ACOG Practice Bulletin No 107. American College of Obstetricians and Gynecologists. Obstet Gynecol 2009;114:386–97.

16. Boulvain M, Kelly AJ, Irion O. Intracervical prostaglandins for induction of labour. Cochrane Database of Systematic Reviews 2008, Issue 1. Art. No.: CD006971. DOI:10.1002/14651858.CD006971; 10.1002/14651858.CD006971.

Intrapartum Fetal Heart Rate Monitoring

George A. Macones

In 2008, the National Institute of Child Health and Human Development, the American College of Obstetricians and Gynecologists, and the Society for Maternal–Fetal Medicine convened a workshop to standardize and clarify definitions and classification of electronic fetal monitoring tracings (1). A full description of an electronic fetal monitoring tracing requires a qualitative and quantitative description of the following items:

- Uterine contractions
- Baseline fetal heart rate (FHR)
- Baseline FHR variability
- Presence of accelerations
- Periodic or episodic decelerations
- Changes or trends of FHR patterns over time

The features of FHR patterns are categorized as either baseline, periodic, or episodic. Periodic patterns are those associated with uterine contractions, and episodic patterns are those not associated with uterine contractions. The periodic patterns are distinguished on the basis of waveform, currently accepted as either abrupt or gradual onset. Accelerations and decelerations generally are determined in reference to the adjacent baseline FHR. No distinction is made between short-term variability (or beat-to-beat variability or R–R wave period differences in the electrocardiogram) and long-term variability because in actual practice they are visually determined as a unit. There is good evidence that a number of characteristics of FHR patterns are dependent on fetal gestational age and physiologic status as well as and maternal physiologic status. Thus FHR tracings

should be evaluated in the context of many clinical conditions including, gestational age, prior results of fetal assessment, medications, maternal medical conditions, and fetal conditions (eg, growth restriction, known congenital anomalies, fetal anemia, and arrhythmia).

Uterine contractions are quantified as the number of contractions present in a 10-minute window, averaged over 30 minutes. Contraction frequency alone is a partial assessment of uterine activity. Other factors, such as duration, intensity, and relaxation time between contractions are equally important in clinical practice.

The following terminology is used to describe uterine activity:

- Normal—Five or fewer contractions in 10 minutes, averaged over a 30-minute period
- Tachysystole—more than five contractions in 10 minutes, averaged over a 30-minute period
- Characteristics of uterine contractions
  - Tachysystole should always be qualified as to the presence or absence of associated FHR decelerations.
  - The term tachysystole applies to both spontaneous and stimulated labor. The clinical response to tachysystole may differ depending on whether contractions are spontaneous or stimulated.

Fetal heart rate patterns are defined by the characteristics of baseline, variability, accelerations, and decelerations.

The baseline FHR is determined by approximating the mean FHR, rounded to increments of five beats per minute during a 10-minute period, excluding accelerations and decelerations and periods of marked FHR variability (greater than 25 beats per minute). There must be at least 2 minutes of identifiable baseline segments (not necessarily contiguous) in any 10-minute period, or the baseline for that period is indeterminate. In such cases, it may be necessary to refer to the previous 10-minute period for determination of the baseline. Abnormal baseline is termed *bradycardia* when the baseline FHR is fewer than 110 beats per minute; it is termed *tachycardia* when the baseline FHR is greater than 160 beats per minute.

Baseline FHR variability is determined in a 10-minute period, excluding accelerations and decelerations. *Baseline FHR variability* is defined as fluctuations in the baseline FHR that are irregular in amplitude and frequency. The fluctuations are visually quantitated as the amplitude of the peak-to-trough in beats per minute. Variability is classified as follows:

- Absent FHR variability means that the amplitude range is undetectable.
- Minimal FHR variability means that the amplitude range is greater than undetectable and 5 beats per minute or less.
- Moderate FHR variability means that the amplitude range is 6–25 beats per minute.
- Marked FHR variability means that the amplitude range is greater than 25 beats per minute.

An acceleration is a visually apparent abrupt increase in FHR. An *abrupt increase* is defined as an increase in which the time from the onset of acceleration to the peak is less than 30 seconds. To be called an acceleration, the peak must be 15 beats per minute or greater, and the acceleration must last 15 seconds or more from the onset to return. A prolonged acceleration is 2 minutes or longer but less than 10 minutes in duration. An acceleration lasting 10 minutes or longer is defined as a *baseline change*. Before 32 weeks of gestation, accelerations are defined as having a peak of 10 beats per minute or greater and a duration of 10 seconds or longer.

Decelerations are classified as late, early, or variable based on specific characteristics (Box 44). Variable decelerations may be accompanied by other characteristics, the clinical significance of which requires further research investigation. Some examples include a slow return of the FHR after the end of the contraction; biphasic decelerations; tachycardia following variable deceleration(s); accelerations preceding and following decelerations, sometimes called shoulders or overshoots; and fluctuations in the FHR in the trough of the deceleration. Decelerations are defined as *recurrent* if they occur with 50% or more of uterine contractions in any 20-minute period. Decelerations occurring with fewer than 50% of uterine contractions in any 20-minute segment are defined as *intermittent*.

A prolonged deceleration is present when there is a visually apparent decrease in FHR from the baseline that is 15 beats or greater per minute, lasting 2 minutes or

---

Box 44

Characteristics of Fetal Heart Rate Decelerations

Late Deceleration

- Visually apparent usually symmetrical gradual decrease and return of the fetal heart rate associated with a uterine contraction.
- A gradual fetal heart rate decrease is defined as from the onset to the fetal heart rate nadir of 30 seconds or more.
- The decrease in fetal heart rate is calculated from the onset to the nadir of the deceleration.
- The deceleration is delayed in timing, with the nadir of the deceleration occurring after the peak of the contraction.
- In most cases the onset, nadir, and recovery of the deceleration all occur after the beginning, peak, and ending of the contraction, respectively.

Early Deceleration

- Visually apparent usually symmetrical gradual decrease and return of the fetal heart rate associated with a uterine contraction.
- A gradual fetal heart rate decrease is defined as from the onset to the fetal heart rate nadir of 30 seconds or longer.
- The decrease in fetal heart rate is calculated from the onset to the nadir of the deceleration.
- The nadir of the deceleration occurs at the same time as the peak of the contraction.
- In most cases the onset, nadir, and recovery of the deceleration are all coincident with the beginning, peak, and ending of the contraction, respectively.

Variable Deceleration

- Visually apparent abrupt decrease in fetal heart rate.
- An abrupt fetal heart rate decrease is defined as from the onset of the deceleration to the beginning of the fetal heart rate nadir of less than 30 seconds.
- The decrease in fetal heart rate is calculated from the onset to the nadir of the deceleration.
- The decrease in fetal heart rate is 15 beats or greater per minute, lasting 15 seconds or longer and less than 2 minutes in duration.
- When variable decelerations are associated with uterine contractions, their onset, depth, and duration commonly vary with successive uterine contractions.

longer, but less than 10 minutes. A deceleration that lasts greater than or equal to 10 minutes is a *baseline change*.

A *sinusoidal fetal heart rate pattern* is a specific fetal heart rate pattern that is defined as having a visually apparent, smooth, sine wave-like undulating pattern in FHR baseline with a cycle frequency of 3–5 beats per minute that persists for 20 minutes or longer.

The FHR tracing should be interpreted in the context of the overall clinical circumstances, and categorization of a FHR tracing is limited to the time being assessed. The presence of FHR accelerations (either spontaneous or stimulated) reliably predicts the absence of fetal metabolic acidemia. The absence of accelerations does not, however, reliably predict fetal acidemia. Fetal heart rate accelerations can be stimulated with a variety of methods (vibroacoustic technique, transabdominal halogen light, and direct fetal scalp stimulation).

Moderate FHR variability reliably predicts the absence of fetal metabolic acidemia at the time it is observed. Minimal or absent FHR variability alone does not reliably predict the presence of fetal hypoxemia or metabolic acidemia. The significance of marked FHR (previously described as saltatory) variability is unclear.

A three-tier system for the categorization of the interpretation of FHR patterns is recommended (Box 45). Category I FHR tracings are normal. Category I FHR tracings are strongly predictive of normal fetal acid base status at the time of observation. Category I FHR tracings may be followed in a routine manner, and no specific action is required.

Category II FHR tracings are indeterminate. Category II FHR tracings are not predictive of abnormal fetal acid-base status, yet we do not have adequate evidence at present to classify these as Category I or Category III. Category II FHR tracings require evaluation and continued surveillance and reevaluation, taking into account the entire associated clinical circumstances.

Category III FHR tracings are abnormal. Category III tracings are predictive of abnormal fetal acid base status at the time of observation. Category III FHR tracings require prompt evaluation. Depending on the clinical situation, efforts to expeditiously resolve the abnormal FHR pattern may include but are not limited to provision of maternal oxygen, change in maternal position, discontinuation of labor stimulation, and management of maternal hypotension.

Reference

1. Macones GA, Hankins GD, Spong CY, Hauth J, Moore T. The 2008 National Institute of Child Health and Human Development workshop report on electronic fetal monitoring: update on definitions, interpretation, and research guidelines. Obstet Gynecol 2008;112:661–6.

Box 45

Three-Tier Fetal Heart Rate Interpretation System

Category I fetal heart rate tracings include all of the following items:

- Baseline rate—110–160 beats per minute
- Baseline fetal heart rate variability—moderate
- Late or variable decelerations—absent
- Early decelerations—present or absent
- Accelerations—present or absent

Category II fetal heart rate tracings includes all fetal heart rate tracings not categorized as Category I or Category III. Category II tracings may represent an appreciable fraction of those encountered in clinical care. Examples of Category II fetal heart rate tracings include any of the following items:

- Baseline rate
  - Bradycardia not accompanied by absent baseline variability
  - Tachycardia
- Baseline fetal heart rate variability
  - Minimal baseline variability
  - Absent baseline variability with no recurrent decelerations
  - Marked baseline variability
- Accelerations
  - Absence of induced accelerations after fetal stimulation
- Periodic or episodic decelerations
  - Recurrent variable decelerations accompanied by minimal or moderate baseline variability
  - Prolonged deceleration 2 minutes or longer but less than 10 minutes
  - Recurrent late decelerations with moderate baseline variability
  - Variable decelerations with other characteristics such as slow return to baseline, overshoots or "shoulders".

Category III fetal heart rate tracings include either of the following items:

- Absent baseline fetal heart rate variability and any of the following items:
  - Recurrent late decelerations
  - Recurrent variable decelerations
  - Bradycardia
- Sinusoidal pattern

Macones GA, Hankins GD, Spong CY, Hauth J, Moore T. The 2008 National Institute of Child Health and Human Development workshop report on electronic fetal monitoring: update on definitions, interpretation, and research guidelines. Obstet Gynecol 2008;112:661–6.

Cesarean Delivery and Vaginal Birth After Cesarean Delivery

Michael A. Belfort, Clarissa Bonanno, Mary E. D'Alton, and Mark B. Landon

The overwhelming economic burden of cesarean delivery on health care delivery continues to focus efforts on strategies aimed at reducing cesarean delivery rates. Cesarean delivery rates have increased in the United States to 31.1% in 2006 (1). An optimal cesarean delivery rate is difficult to ascertain because an ideal rate must be a function of multiple clinical factors that vary in each population and are influenced by the level of obstetric care provided.

In spite of little consensus regarding the best mode of delivery for many complicated pregnancies, third party payers and institutions continue to rely on expert opinion concerning optimal cesarean delivery rates without the benefit of risk stratification. It follows that institutions involved in tertiary obstetric care, thus managing a large number of preterm deliveries and maternal complications of pregnancy, should have higher cesarean delivery rates than primary care facilities (2).

The American College of Obstetricians and Gynecologists (the College) has developed a simple formula to help institutions and physicians assess their risk-adjusted cesarean delivery rate. Two populations targeted include 1) nulliparous women with a singleton vertex gestation at 37 weeks or greater without other complications and 2) women with one prior low-transverse cesarean delivery, giving birth to a single vertex fetus at 37 weeks of gestation or greater without other complications. For first-time cesarean deliveries, the benchmark rate set by the College for 2010 is 15.5%, which represents the 25th percentile of state rankings (the national rate was 17.9% in 1996). For repeat cesarean delivery, the benchmark rate for vaginal delivery after a prior cesarean delivery is 37%, a figure that represents the 75th percentile of state rankings (the 1996 national vaginal birth after cesarean delivery [VBAC] rate was 30.3%). The use of these simple case-mix adjusted rates should make evaluation of cesarean delivery rates more meaningful.

Vaginal Birth After Cesarean Delivery

At the present time, only 9.2% of women with prior cesarean delivery undergo a trial of labor in the United States (3). It has been established that approximately two thirds of women with a prior cesarean delivery are actually candidates for a trial of labor. Thus, most repeat operations are elective and are often influenced by physician discretion and patient choice. A comparison of trial of labor rates between the United States and several European nations reveals substantial underuse of trial of labor in this country.

Twenty years ago, the College first recommended that each hospital develop its own protocol for the management of VBAC patients and that a woman with one prior low-transverse cesarean delivery should be counseled and encouraged to attempt labor in the absence of a contraindication such as a prior classical incision. This recommendation was supported by the results of several large case series attesting to the safety and effectiveness of trial of labor. With a rise in VBAC use, results from a number of reports appeared in the literature suggesting that risks associated with uterine rupture might be greater than those cited in early reports. Descriptions of uterine rupture with hysterectomy and adverse perinatal outcomes, including death and brain injury, then set the stage for the precipitous decline in VBAC during the last decade.

Acknowledging a statistically small but significant risk of uterine rupture with poor outcomes for both women and their infants exists with trial of labor has lead to a more conservative approach. Nonetheless, most women with one previous cesarean delivery with a low-transverse incision are candidates for VBAC and should be counseled about VBAC and offered a trial of labor. Insufficient data exist to provide counseling for patients presenting with a prior low-vertical incision, multiple gestation, breech presentation, or an estimated fetal weight greater than 4,000 g.

Most women who have had low-transverse uterine incision with prior cesarean delivery and have no contraindications to vaginal birth can be considered candidates for trial of labor (see Box 46). Additionally, research results indicate that it might be reasonable to offer a trial of labor to women in other clinical situations. These would include more than one previous cesarean delivery, macrosomia, gestation beyond 40 weeks, previous low-vertical incision, unknown uterine scar type, and twin gestation. A trial of labor is contraindicated in women at high risk of uterine rupture (Box 47).

Box 46

Selection Criteria for Identifying Candidates for Trial of Labor

- One previous low-transverse cesarean delivery
- Clinically adequate pelvis
- No other uterine scars or previous rupture
- Physicians immediately available throughout active labor capable of monitoring labor and performing an emergency cesarean delivery

The overall success rate for VBAC appears to be in the 70–80% range according to published reports. Predictors of successful trial of labor are well described. The prior indication for cesarean delivery clearly impacts on the likelihood of successful VBAC. A history of prior vaginal birth or a nonrecurring condition, such as breech presentation or nonreassuring fetal well-being, is associated with the highest success rates for VBAC.

Race, age, body mass index, and insurance status have all been demonstrated to impact the success of trial of labor. Obese women are more likely to fail a trial of labor as are women older than 40 years. Success rates for women whose first cesarean delivery was performed for a nonrecurring indication (breech presentation, non-reassuring fetal well-being) are similar to vaginal delivery rates for nulliparous women. Prior cesarean delivery for breech presentation is associated with the highest reported success rate of 89%. In contrast, prior operative delivery for cephalopelvic disproportion or failure to progress is associated with success rates ranging from 50–67%. Prior vaginal delivery, including prior successful VBAC can be considered the greatest predictor for successful trial of labor. Not surprisingly, women who undergo induction of labor are at higher risk for repeat cesarean delivery compared with those who enter spontaneous labor (4).

The principal risk of VBAC is uterine rupture. Results of a review of 10 observational studies providing the best evidence on the occurrence of symptomatic rupture with trial of labor revealed a pooled rupture rate of 3.8 per 1,000 trials of labor (5). A recent large multicenter prospective observational study reported a 0.69% incidence with 124 symptomatic ruptures occurring in 17,898 women undergoing trial of labor (6).

The rate of uterine rupture depends on both the type and location of the previous uterine incision. Uterine rupture rates are highest with previous classical or T-shaped incisions, with a range reported between 4–9%. The risk for rupture with a previous low vertical incision has been difficult to estimate because of imprecision with the diagnosis and the uncommon use of this incision type. Women with unknown scar types do not appear to be at increased risk for uterine rupture. Among 3,206 women with unknown scar types, uterine rupture occurred in 0.5% of the trials of labor (6).

The most serious sequelae of uterine rupture include perinatal death, hypoxic-ischemic encephalopathy, and hysterectomy. Citing six deaths in 74 uterine ruptures among 11 studies, a rate of 0.14 additional perinatal deaths per 1,000 trials of labor was calculated (7). This figure is remarkably similar to the *Eunice Kennedy Shriver* National Institute of Child Health and Human Development Maternal–Fetal Medicine Unit (NICHD MFMU) Network study results in which there were two neonatal deaths among 124 ruptures, for an overall rate of rupture related perinatal death of 0.11 per 1,000 trials of labor (6).

It has been suggested that the risk of uterine rupture is increased in women with multiple prior cesarean deliveries who attempt VBAC. A rate of uterine rupture of 3.7% among such women compared with 0.8% in women with one pervious scar (odds ratio [OR], 4.5; 95% confidence interval [CI], 1.18–11.5) has prompted a recommendation that trial of labor for women with two prior cesarean deliveries be limited to those with a history of prior vaginal delivery (8). In results of a recent report, a uterine rupture rate of 20/1082 (1.8%) in women with two prior cesareans compared with 113/12,535 (0.9%) in women with one prior operation (adjusted OR, 2.3; 95% CI, 1.37–3.85) was documented (9). In contrast, the results of an analysis from the NICHD MFMU Network Cesarean Registry showed no significant difference in rupture rates in women with one prior cesarean delivery, 115/16,916 (0.7%), versus multiple prior cesarean deliveries, 9/982 (0.9%) (3). Thus, it appears that if multiple prior cesarean deliveries are associated with an increased risk for uterine rupture, the magnitude of any additional risk is fairly small. Prior vaginal delivery appears to be protective against uterine rupture following trial of labor. A similar effect of prior vaginal birth has been reported in two large multicenter studies (6, 9).

Induction of labor may be associated with an increased risk of uterine rupture. In results of the prospective NICHD MFMU Network cohort analysis, the risk of uterine rupture was increased nearly threefold (OR, 2.86; 95% CI, 1.75–4.67), with induction in 48 of 4,708 (1%) versus spontaneous labor in 24 of 6,685 (0.4%) (6). It remains unclear whether induction causes uterine rupture or whether an associated risk factor is present. There also are conflicting data concerning whether various induction methods increase the risk for uterine rupture. Results from two large recent series did not indicate an increased risk of rupture associated with the use of prostaglandin agents alone for induction (6, 9). Results of one of these studies did indicate an increased risk for rupture in women undergoing induction only if they received a combination of prostaglandins and oxytocin (9). For this

---

Box 47

Contraindications for Trial of Labor

- Previous classical or T-shaped incision or extensive transfundal uterine surgery
- Previous uterine rupture
- Medical or obstetric complications that precludes vaginal delivery
- Inability to perform emergency cesarean delivery because of unavailable surgeon, anesthesia, sufficient staff, or faculty

reason, it has been recommended that sequential use of prostaglandin E$_2$ and oxytocin be avoided in women with prior cesarean delivery (10). Misoprostol specifically, has been linked to uterine rupture and currently is not recommended for use in women attempting VBAC. Oxytocin use may marginally increase the risk for uterine rupture in women undergoing trial of labor such that judicious use of labor stimulation should be used in this population.

The College recommends that VBAC should be attempted only in institutions equipped to respond to emergencies, with physicians immediately available to provide emergency care. Women attempting VBAC should be encouraged to contact their health care provider promptly when labor or ruptured membranes occurs. Continuous electronic fetal monitoring is prudent, although the need for intrauterine pressure catheter monitoring is controversial. Studies that have examined fetal heart rate patterns before uterine rupture consistently demonstrate that variable decelerations or bradycardia are the most common finding accompanying uterine rupture.

Pregnant women with a previous cesarean delivery are at risk for both maternal and perinatal complications, whether undergoing trial of labor or choosing elective repeat operation. Complications of both procedures should be discussed, and an attempt should be made to include an individualized risk assessment for both uterine rupture and the likelihood of successful VBAC. Future childbearing and the risks of multiple cesarean deliveries, including risks of placenta previa and accreta, should be considered as well. Following complete informed consent detailing the risks and benefits for the individual woman, the delivery plan should be formulated by both the patient and physician. Vaginal birth after cesarean delivery and trial of labor should continue to remain an option for most women with prior cesarean delivery.

Cesarean Delivery on Maternal Request

Cesarean delivery on maternal request is defined as a primary cesarean delivery at the request of the patient, in the absence of any medical or obstetric indication (11). Since 1996, the total cesarean delivery rate has increased yearly, reaching 31.1% in 2006, the highest level ever reported (1). The incidence of cesarean delivery on maternal request and the trend over the past decade are not known because birth certificate and procedural coding data on this entity are lacking. However, increasing demand for cesarean delivery on maternal request may be contributing to the recent increase in the primary cesarean delivery rate (12).

Information on the benefits and risks of cesarean delivery on maternal request is limited. There are no randomized controlled trials comparing cesarean delivery on maternal request with planned vaginal delivery. Most current knowledge is based on observational studies or analogous research on elective cesarean delivery for breech presentation. In March of 2006, a multidisciplinary panel of experts convened at the National Institutes of Health State-of-the-Science Conference on Cesarean Delivery on Maternal Request to review the available literature on this subject (12). The panel concluded that there is insufficient evidence on the benefits and risks of cesarean delivery on maternal request compared with planned vaginal delivery to recommend either mode of delivery.

The consensus statement summarized the best information available on the outcomes of cesarean delivery on maternal request and planned vaginal delivery. Their extensive literature review yielded only three outcome variables supported by moderate-quality evidence:

1. The frequency of postpartum hemorrhage associated with planned cesarean delivery is less than that reported with planned vaginal delivery or unplanned cesarean delivery.
2. Cesarean delivery, planned or unplanned, requires a longer hospital stay than a vaginal delivery.
3. There is a higher rate of neonatal respiratory morbidity with elective cesarean delivery compared with planned vaginal delivery at gestational ages earlier than 39–40 weeks.

All other maternal and neonatal outcomes that supported either planned cesarean delivery or planned vaginal delivery or neither delivery route were based on weak-quality evidence. These results are summarized in Table 30.

Maternal Outcomes

Potential benefits of planned vaginal delivery include a shorter hospital stay, lower rate of infection and anesthetic complications, and a higher breastfeeding initiation rate. Potential benefits of planned cesarean delivery include decreased risk of postpartum hemorrhage and transfusion, lower risk of surgical complications, and a decrease in urinary incontinence during the first year after delivery. Potential risks of cesarean delivery on maternal request include complications in subsequent pregnancies, such as uterine rupture, placenta previa, placenta accreta, and need for hysterectomy. For this reason, the total number of anticipated pregnancies should be discussed and should factor into any decision regarding cesarean delivery on maternal request. Literature on many other maternal outcomes favored neither route of delivery.

Neonatal Outcomes

Potential benefits of planned vaginal delivery include a lower risk of neonatal respiratory problems, lower risk of iatrogenic prematurity, and a shorter hospital stay. Potential benefits of planned cesarean delivery include

Table 30. Potential Outcomes of Planned Cesarean Delivery Based on Weak-Quality Evidence

Potential Benefits	Potential Risks
Maternal	
Decrease in surgical complications	Increase in infection
Decrease in severe vaginal lacerations	Increase in anesthesia complications
Decrease in urinary incontinence	Decrease in breastfeeding initiation
	Increase in subsequent uterine rupture, placenta previa, and hysterectomy
Neonatal	
Decrease in infection	Increase in iatrogenic prematurity
Decrease in birth injury	Increase in length of stay
Decrease in intracranial hemorrhage, neonatal asphyxia, and encephalopathy	
Decrease in fetal mortality	
Outcomes Favoring Neither Vaginal Delivery Nor Cesarean Delivery	
	Anorectal function problems
	Pelvic organ prolapse
	Sexual function problems
	Pelvic pain
	Fistula function problems
	Postpartum depression
	Thromboembolism
	Maternal mortality
	Subsequent stillbirth
	Neonatal mortality
	Long-term neonatal outcomes

decreased rate of infection, and decreased risk of birth injury, intracranial hemorrhage, neonatal asphyxia, and encephalopathy. Epidemiologic models also suggest a potential reduction in fetal mortality because cesarean delivery on maternal request would be performed before 40 weeks of gestation, negating the possibility of stillbirth between 40 weeks of gestation and 42 weeks of gestation. Data on neonatal mortality and other long-term outcomes are limited and favor neither delivery route.

Recommendations

The potential risks and benefits of each mode of delivery should be reviewed with patients who request cesarean delivery. The discussion should be individualized, based on each woman's age, body mass index, accuracy of pregnancy dating, reproductive plans, per-

sonal values, and cultural context (11). The health care provider should inquire about the patient's reason for her request for cesarean delivery so that appropriate information and support can be given to women with anxiety about the birth process because of previous poor obstetric outcomes, personal trauma, or other factors. If the patient's main concern is pain in childbirth, prenatal education, including detailed information on obstetric analgesia and anesthesia, should be offered, and strategies to obtain emotional support in labor should be discussed (13).

Further research on cesarean delivery on maternal request is needed to gather solid evidence for counseling patients about this decision. Until then, a thorough informed consent process is imperative for patients requesting cesarean delivery. Based on the current literature on cesarean delivery on maternal request, the College has provided the following recommendations (11):

- Cesarean delivery on maternal request should not be performed before a gestational age of 39 weeks has been accurately been determined, unless there is documentation of lung maturity
- Cesarean delivery on maternal request should not be motivated by the unavailability of effective pain management.
- Cesarean delivery on maternal request is not recommended for women desiring several children because the risks of placenta previa, placenta accreta, and gravid hysterectomy increase with each cesarean delivery.

Cesarean and Puerperal Hysterectomy

Emergency peripartum hysterectomy refers to the removal of the uterus at the time of a planned or unplanned delivery and complicates 0.3–0.8 per 1,000 births (14, 15). Risk factors include previous cesarean delivery, previous manual removal of placenta, previous myomectomy, and multifetal gestation (16). The most common indications for this procedure are uterine atony unresponsive to medical and less invasive surgical therapy (artery ligation, compression sutures, balloon tamponade), abnormal adherence or invasion of the placenta (accreta or percreta), and rupture or laceration of the uterus.

Planned cesarean hysterectomy is becoming more common as placenta previa with suspected accreta or percreta is increasingly recognized in the antepartum period. In known cases of placenta percreta, appropriate preparations must be made before delivery, such as coordination of multiple disciplines, including blood banks; laboratories; operating rooms; and nursing, surgical, radiologic, and neonatal services (17). Despite adequate preparation, the maternal mortality associated with placenta percreta and cesarean hysterectomy is still high (7%) (18). It is believed that the increase in placenta accreta is related to the rising cesarean delivery rate and the association between prior utrine surgery and placenta previa or accreta in subsequent pregnancies. In a recent series of 186 cesarean hysterectomies, 37% were performed for placenta accreta whereas 35% were performed for atony. Of the 71 accreta cases, 58 (81%) accompanied repeat cesarean delivery (19). Nearly 25% of women with placenta previa and prior cesarean delivery will develop placenta accreta, which in most cases requires hysterectomy to control bleeding. A patient with two or more prior cesarean deliveries and an existing placenta previa has a risk for cesarean hysterectomy that ranges from 30% to 50%. Whereas placenta accreta itself poses a risk for peripartum hysterectomy; its association with prior uterine full thickness incision is responsible for the 50–100-fold increased risk for hysterectomy after cesarean delivery compared with vaginal delivery.

Indications for nonemergent puerperal hysterectomy have changed over time. Although scheduled cesarean hysterectomy is still used in cases of high-grade or early invasive cervical disease, ovarian malignancies, uterine leiomyomas, or abnormal uterine bleeding, peripartum hysterectomy, solely as an elective means of permanent sterilization, is no longer recommended.

Puerperal hysterectomy is associated with increased intraoperative and postoperative maternal morbidity, mainly related to longer operative times, increased blood loss, higher rates of blood transfusion, genitourinary tract and other organ injury, and infection. Given the potential for massive transfusion, care should be taken during surgery to prevent both dilutional coagulopathy and disseminated intravascular coagulation. This includes vigilant monitoring of coagulation function, complete blood count, and arterial blood gases, with early replacement of clotting factors. Recent data from the trauma literature have shown that use of fresh frozen plasma in a 1:1 ratio of fresh frozen plasma to packed red blood cells has been of benefit in terms of earlier correction of coagulopathy, decreased need for packed red blood cells in the intensive care unit, and reduced mortality (20–22). Recombinant activated factor VII (rFVIIa) recently has been reported as being useful for management of massive postpartum hemorrhage. A review of 31 studies reported on 118 cases of massive postpartum hemorrhage treated with rFVIIa (23). A median dose of 71.6 micrograms/kg rFVIIa was reported to be effective in stopping or reducing bleeding in nearly 90% of the reported cases. The authors stated that caution should be exercised in interpreting these results, which were derived from few and uncontrolled studies.

In those cases where there is refractory bleeding after removal of the uterus, placement of a pelvic pressure pack should be considered (24). This temporizing step has been shown to be effective in allowing hemodynamic stabilization of the patient and correction of coagulopathy (24). In cases where there is persistent bleeding, which does not result in hemodynamic collapse but requires continued transfusion, the patient may be transported to the interventional radiology suite for arterial embolization. This procedure is not suitable for the acutely unstable patient (25, 26).

Postoperatively patients who have had prolonged surgery for placenta percreta with massive transfusion may be at risk for a number of problems. These include persistent intraabdominal bleeding, pelvic thromboembolism, renal compromise, bowel ischemia, pulmonary edema, myocardial depression, transfusion-related acute lung injury or acute respiratory distress syndrome or both, and Sheehan syndrome. The postoperative management team should anticipate and be ready for such complications.

References

1. Martin JA, Hamilton BE, Sutton PD, Ventura SJ, Menacker F, Kimeyer S, et al. Births: final data for 2006. Natl Vital Stat Rep 2009;57(7):1–104.

2. Bailit JL, Dooley SL, Peaceman AN. Risk adjustment for interhospital comparison of primary cesarean rates. Obstet Gynecol 1999;93:1025–30.

3. Landon MB, Spong CY, Thom E, Hauth JC, Bloom SL, Varner MW, et al. Risk of uterine rupture with a trial of labor in women with multiple and single prior cesarean delivery. National Institute of Child Health and Human Development Maternal-Fetal Medicine Units Network. Obstet Gynecol 2006;108:12–20.

4. Grinstead J, Grobman WA. Induction of labor after one prior cesarean: predictors of vaginal delivery. Obstet Gynecol 2004;103:534–8.

5. Guise JM, McDonagh MS, Osterweil P, Nygren P, Chan BK, Helfand M. Systematic review of the incidence and consequences of uterine rupture in women with previous caesarean section. BMJ 2004;329:19–25.

6. Landon MB, Hauth JC, Leveno KJ, Spong CY, Leindecker S, Varner MW, et al. Maternal and perinatal outcomes associated with a trial of labor after prior cesarean delivery. National Institute of Child Health and Human Development Maternal-Fetal Medicine Units Network. N Engl J Med 2004;351:2581–9.

7. Chauhan SP, Martin JN Jr, Henrichs CE, Morrison JC, Magann EF. Maternal and perinatal complications with uterine rupture in 142,075 patients who attempted vaginal birth after cesarean delivery: a review of the literature. Am J Obstet Gynecol 2003;189:408–17.

8. Caughey AB, Shipp TD, Repke JT, Zelop CM, Cohen A, Lieberman E. Rate of uterine rupture during a trial of labor in women with one or two prior cesarean deliveries. Am J Obstet Gynecol 1999;181:872–6.

9. Macones GA, Peipert J, Nelson DB, Odibo A, Stevens EJ, Stamilio DM, et al. Maternal complications with vaginal birth after cesarean delivery: a multicenter study. Am J Obstet Gynecol 2005;193:1656–62.

10. Induction of labor for vaginal birth after cesarean delivery. ACOG Committee Opinion No. 342. American College of Obstetricians and Gynecologists. Obstet Gynecol 2006; 108:465–8.

11. Cesarean delivery on maternal request. ACOG Committee Opinion No. 394. American College of Obstetricians and Gynecologists. Obstet Gynecol 2007;110:1501.

12. NIH State-of-the-Science Conference statement on cesarean delivery on maternal request. NIH Consens State Sci Statements 2006;23:1–29.

13. Surgery and patient choice. ACOG Committee Opinion No. 395. American College of Obstetricians and Gynecologists. Obstet Gynecol 2008;111:243–7.

14. Kastner ES, Figueroa R, Garry D, Maulik D. Emergency peripartum hysterectomy: experience at a community teaching hospital. Obstet Gynecol 2002;99:971–5.

15. Kwee A, Bots ML, Visser GH, Bruinse HW. Emergency peripartum hysterectomy: a prospective study in the Netherlands. Eur J Obstet Gynecol Reprod Biol 2006;124: 187–92.

16. Knight M, Kurinczuk JJ, Spark P, Brocklehurst P. Cesarean delivery and peripartum hysterectomy. United Kingdom Obstetric Surveillance System Steering Committee. Obstet Gynecol 2008;111:97–105.

17. Hudon L, Belfort MA, Broome DR. Diagnosis and management of placenta percreta: a review. Obstet Gynecol Surv 1998;53:509–17.

18. O'Brien JM, Barton JR, Donaldson ES. The management of placenta percreta: conservative and operative strategies. Am J Obstet Gynecol 1996;175:1632–8.

19. Shellhaas CS, Gilbert S, Landon MB, Varner MW, Leveno KJ, Hauth JC, et al. The frequency and complication rates of hysterectomy accompanying cesarean delivery. Eunice Kennedy Shriver National Institutes of Health and Human Development Maternal-Fetal Medicine Units Network. Obstet Gynecol 2009;114:224–9.

20. Holcomb JB, Wade CE, Michalek JE, Chisholm GB, Zarzabal LA, Schreiber MA, et al. Increased plasma and platelet to red blood cell ratios improves outcome in 466 massively transfused civilian trauma patients. Ann Surg 2008;248:447–58.

21. Gonzalez EA, Moore FA, Holcomb JB, Miller CC, Kozar RA, Todd SR, et al. Fresh frozen plasma should be given earlier to patients requiring massive transfusion. J Trauma 2007;62:112–9.

22. Gunter OL Jr, Au BK, Isbell JM, Mowery NT, Young PP, Cotton BA. Optimizing outcomes in damage control resuscitation: identifying blood product ratios associated with improved survival. J Trauma 2008;65:527–34.

23. Franchini M, Franchi M, Bergamini V, Salvagno GL, Montagnana M, Lippi G. A critical review on the use of recombinant factor VIIa in life-threatening obstetric postpartum hemorrhage. Semin Thromb Hemost 2008;34: 104–12.

24. Dildy GA, Scott JR, Saffer CS, Belfort MA. An effective pressure pack for severe pelvic hemorrhage. Obstet Gynecol 2006;108:1222–6.

25. Boulleret C, Chahid T, Gallot D, Mofid R, Tran Hai D, Ravel A, et al. Hypogastric arterial selective and superselective embolization for severe postpartum hemorrhage: a retrospective review of 36 cases. Cardiovasc Intervent Radiol 2004;27:344–8.

26. Uchiyama D, Koganemaru M, Abe T, Hori D, Hayabuchi N. Arterial catheterization and embolization for management of emergent or anticipated massive obstetrical hemorrhage. Radiat Med 2008;26:188–97.

Shoulder Dystocia

William A. Grobman

Shoulder dystocia is an infrequent but potentially catastrophic obstetric emergency that has been reported to complicate 0.2–3% of all vaginal deliveries (1). From an anatomical perspective, shoulder dystocia can be defined as the failure of delivery of the fetal shoulder(s) because of a size discrepancy between the shoulders (anterior, posterior, or both) and the pelvic inlet. Shoulder dystocia most often is diagnosed when the typical gentle downward traction on the fetal head that is used to deliver the anterior shoulder is not sufficient to enact this delivery, or when ancillary obstetric maneuvers are required to achieve delivery of the fetal shoulders. In an attempt to establish a more objective definition of this emergency, several investigators have attempted to use a component of time, such as a lapse of more than 60 seconds between delivery of the fetal head and delivery of the body (2). There is no consensus, however, as to the exact time threshold that is optimal to use in order to diagnose a shoulder dystocia.

Although multiple risk factors have been reported to be associated with shoulder dystocia, for many of these factors the associations have not been independent or have been demonstrated inconsistently (3). Moreover, the predictive value of the factors that have been consistently and independently associated with shoulder dystocia is poor (4, 5). For example, it has been established that the frequency of shoulder dystocia increases as birth weight increases. In results of one study, shoulder dystocia occurred in 5.2% of nondiabetic mothers with neonates who weighed 4,000–4,250 g, compared with 21.1% of those mothers whose infants weighed 4,750–5,000 g (6). Nevertheless, approximately 40–60% of cases of shoulder dystocia occur in infants weighing less than 4,000 g (5). One risk factor for shoulder dystocia that deserves attention is history of a shoulder dystocia, because recurrence rates are increased in subsequent pregnancies, particularly when the fetus is of similar or greater size (7). Yet, most parturients will not have this risk factor. Thus, from a prospective point of view, physicians have a poor ability to predict shoulder dystocia for most patients, and there remains no validated predictive model for this obstetric emergency.

Although some experts have advocated ultrasound estimation of fetal weight, performed either during the late third trimester or the intrapartum period, as a tool to estimate the risk and reduce the incidence of shoulder dystocia, estimated weight according to ultrasonography has been shown to display low sensitivity and poor predictive value for birth weight thresholds (greater than 4000 g or greater than 4,500 g) (8). Investigators have found that this technology's accuracy is no better than that provided by clinical palpation (Leopold maneuvers) or that of a parous woman's assessment of her own fetus' weight (9). Furthermore, the strategies that have been theorized, based on estimated fetal weight, to significantly reduce the frequency of shoulder dystocia have not been shown to be effective in practice. Although induction of labor because of suspected or impending fetal macrosomia has been used, there is no good evidence to support this practice. In one prospective clinical trial, nondiabetic patients with ultrasonographic fetal weight estimations of 4,000–4,500 g who were randomized to induction of labor had a frequency of shoulder dystocia that was no different than that of women who were randomized to expectant management (10). The intervention of prophylactic cesarean delivery, likewise, has not consistently been demonstrated by clinical data or decision analysis to be a strategy that can significantly reduce shoulder dystocia without incurring significant increases in cesarean delivery and its associated complications (11, 12). Nevertheless, expert opinion, based on the epidemiologic data that does exist, states that it is reasonable to offer prophylactic cesarean delivery for an estimated fetal weight greater than 5,000 g in women without diabetes mellitus or greater than 4,500 g in women with diabetes mellitus (9).

Once a shoulder dystocia occurs, there is no uniform agreement that a particular alleviating maneuver or sequence of alleviating maneuvers is preferred. In some cases, shoulder dystocia may be heralded by the classic "turtle sign," during which the fetal head, after it has delivered, retracts back tightly against the maternal perineum. Under these circumstances, some clinicians have advocated immediately proceeding to delivery of the fetal shoulders to maintain the forward momentum of the fetus. Alternatively, others support a short delay in delivery of the shoulders, arguing that the endogenous rotational mechanics of the second stage may spontaneously alleviate the obstruction. Regardless, once shoulder dystocia is recognized, either because of a "turtle" sign or the lack of delivery of an anterior shoulder after typical gentle downward traction on the fetal head, alleviating maneuvers should be used. After the patient is asked to temporarily cease expulsive efforts, many providers initially will use the McRoberts maneuver, suprapubic pressure, or both because of ease of implementation, relatively high success rate (approximately 40–60%), and involvement of only maternal manipulation (5). Consisting of exaggerated abduction and hyperflexion of the maternal thighs upon the abdomen, the McRoberts maneuver does not change the actual dimensions of the maternal pelvis. Rather, it relieves shoulder dystocia via marked cephalad rotation of the symphysis pubis and flattening of the sacrum (13). Despite their effectiveness once a shoulder dystocia has occurred, neither the McRoberts maneuver nor suprapubic pressure have been shown to be beneficial as prophylactic measures for patients who are at increased risk of shoulder dystocia (14).

In addition to the previously mentioned maneuvers, techniques that involve fetal manipulation also may be helpful. One such technique is a rotational maneuver, in which the operator rotates the fetus to an oblique, rather than anterior–posterior axis, thereby allowing disimpaction of the anterior shoulder from the symphysis pubis. Many different variations of rotational maneuvers have been described; two that are commonly referred to are the Woods maneuver and Rubin maneuver. In Woods maneuver, the provider places a hand on the anterior aspect of the posterior shoulder and pushes toward the fetal back. In the Rubin maneuver, the practitioner applies pressure to the posterior surface of either the posterior or anterior fetal shoulder and pushes toward the fetal chest, an action that also may assist in the alleviation of the dystocia by causing shoulder adduction (Figure 21). Another type of alleviating action is the delivery of the posterior arm. To perform this maneuver, the provider should attempt to insert their entire hand in the posterior aspect of the vagina and apply pressure at the antecubital fossa to flex the fetal forearm and then sweep the arm across the fetus' chest, with ultimate delivery of the arm over the perineum (Figure 22). After delivery of the arm, there is a 20% reduction in shoulder diameter, thereby allowing the dystocia to be relieved (15).

Although the maneuvers so far described are the ones most commonly performed, others also may be of some help. In the Gaskin maneuver, also known as the "all-fours" technique, the patient is rolled from her existing position onto her hands and knees, a position which has been reported to help with shoulder dystocia resolution. When a shoulder dystocia appears intractable, the operator may need to consider the performance of cephalic replacement (Zavanelli maneuver) and subsequent cesarean delivery. In the originally described Zavanelli maneuver, the head is rotated back to a pre-restitution position, gently flexed, and then pushed back into the vagina with constant firm pressure. Tocolytic agents to relax the uterus may be considered for use in preparation for or during this maneuver. Other reported, but relatively rarely performed, techniques include symphysiotomy, intentional fetal clavicular fracture, and hysterotomy or abdominal rescue. Given that these maneuvers are inherently associated with maternal or fetal trauma, they should be used only in situations when other maneuvers cannot relieve the dystocia. A list

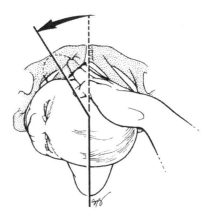

Figure 21. The Rubin maneuver. The more easily accessible fetal shoulder (the anterior is shown here) is pushed toward the anterior chest wall of the fetus. Most often, this results in adduction of both shoulders, reducing the shoulder-to-shoulder diameter and freeing the impacted anterior shoulder. (Cunningham FG, Leveno KJ, Bloom SL, Hauth JC, Gilstrap LC III, Wenstrom KD, editors. Williams obstetrics. 22nd ed. Stamford [CT]: The McGraw-Hill Companies; 2005. Copyright McGraw-Hill Companies, Inc. McGraw-Hill makes no representations or warranties as to the accuracy of any information contained in the McGraw-Hill Material, including any warranties of merchantability or fitness for a particular purpose. In no event shall McGraw-Hill have any liability to any party for special, incidental, tort, or consequential damages arising out of or in connection with the McGraw-Hill Material, even if McGraw-Hill has been advised of the possibility of such damages.)

of the reported techniques that may be used to alleviate a shoulder dystocia is provided in Box 48.

Although episiotomy may be used in the setting of shoulder dystocia, there is not agreement that, in and of itself, it is a maneuver that will alleviate the dystocia. This is because the dystocia is in actuality a "bony dystocia," and, thus, should not be relieved with laceration of only the soft tissue. Nevertheless, the operator may decide, given the individual circumstances, that an episiotomy will allow other maneuvers to be accomplished more easily or effectively, in which case an episiotomy is an acceptable choice. However, one maneuver that should be discouraged is fundal pressure. This action does not alleviate a shoulder dystocia because it simply duplicates the maternal expulsive force that already has failed to deliver the fetal shoulders. In addition, fundal pressure has been associated with both maternal trauma (uterine rupture) and fetal injury (eg, spinal cord injury) (1).

Just as the individual maneuvers that have been described may help the operator to resolve a shoulder dystocia, there is some evidence that experience with simulation of shoulder dystocia also may help a provider (and his or her care team) to manage this event. For example, residents who underwent simulation of a shoulder dystocia, followed by a debriefing period that explored potential areas of improvement, were able

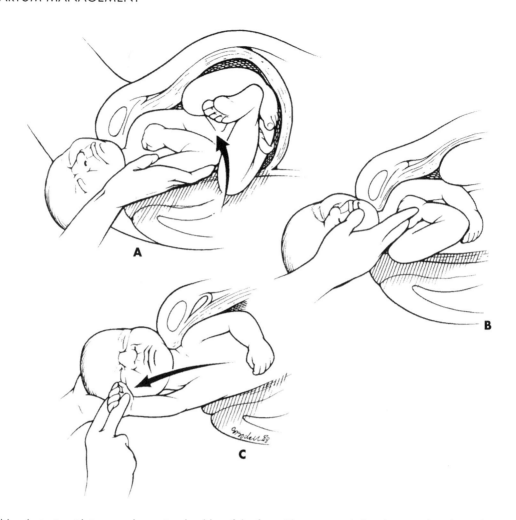

Figure 22. Shoulder dystocia with impacted anterior shoulder of the fetus. The operator's hand is introduced into the vagina along the fetal posterior humerus, which is splinted as the arm is swept across the chest, keeping the arm flexed at the elbow **(A).** The fetal hand is grasped and the arm extended along the side of the face **(B).** The posterior arm is delivered from the vagina **(C).** (Cunningham FG, Leveno KJ, Bloom SL, Hauth JC, Gilstrap LC III, Wenstrom KD, editors. Williams obstetrics. 22nd ed. Stamford [CT]: The McGraw-Hill Companies; 2005. Copyright McGraw-Hill Companies, Inc. McGraw-Hill makes no representations or warranties as to the accuracy of any information contained in the McGraw-Hill Material, including any warranties of merchantability or fitness for a particular purpose. In no event shall McGraw-Hill have any liability to any party for special, incidental, tort, or consequential damages arising out of or in connection with the McGraw-Hill Material, even if McGraw-Hill has been advised of the possibility of such damages.)

to demonstrate better performance during subsequent shoulder dystocia simulations (16, 17). There also is some evidence that simulation is associated not only with performance improvements during subsequent simulations but also with better outcomes during actual clinical shoulder dystocias. In one observational study, investigators found that the introduction of a shoulder dystocia simulation to providers was associated with more maneuvers being used and fewer neonatal injuries occurring in the presence of a shoulder dystocia (18). It should be noted that there is no consensus as to the best form that simulations should take. For example, both low-fidelity simulation (eg, using a simple doll-like mannequin) and high-fidelity simulation (eg, using a mannequin with a high degree of biofidelity) of shoulder dystocia were demonstrated to improve clinician perfor-

mance (19). Furthermore, simulations of shoulder dystocias need not always focus on manual skills relating to specific maneuvers but may instead concentrate on the team communication that is an important component of the successful resolution of a clinical emergency. Drills, which can elucidate systems enhancements that can be made and can allow standardized responses to be practiced and reinforced, may be of benefit (20, 21).

Once a shoulder dystocia occurs, and even if all actions are appropriately taken, there is an increased incidence of both maternal and neonatal trauma. Reported maternal complications related to shoulder dystocia have included third-degree or fourth-degree perineal lacerations, postpartum hemorrhage, vaginal or cervical lacerations, and symphyseal separation with lateral femoral cutaneous neuropathy. Self-limiting neonatal complica-

Box 48

Maneuvers for the Alleviation of Shoulder Dystocia

- Maternal hip hyperflexion and adduction (McRoberts) maneuver
- Suprapubic pressure maneuver
- Rotational maneuvers
  - Woods maneuver
  - Rubin maneuver
- Delivery of the posterior arm
- Gaskin (all fours) maneuver
- Cephalic replacement (Zavanelli) maneuver with cesarean delivery
- Symphysiotomy maneuver
- Intentional fracture of fetal clavicle maneuver
- Abdominal rescue through hysterotomy

tions include clavicular and humeral fracture, which occur in approximately 5–10% of shoulder dystocia cases (5). Additionally, brachial plexus palsies— predominantly Erb–Duchenne paralysis (C-5 through C-6) or Klumpke paralysis (C-8 through T-1)—occur in 10–20% of neonates born after a shoulder dystocia occurs. However, most of these neurologic injuries resolve over time, with an estimated rate of persistence of 1–5% (12). Other long-term neonatal complications that have been reported to occur, albeit infrequently, include permanent central neurologic injury and death (22).

References

1. Shoulder dystocia. ACOG Practice Bulletin No. 40. American College of Obstetricians and Gynecologists. Obstet Gynecol 2002;100:1045–50.

2. Beall MH, Spong C, McKay J, Ross MG. Objective definition of shoulder dystocia: a prospective evaluation. Am J Obstet Gynecol 1998;179:934–7.

3. Dildy GA, Clark SL. Shoulder dystocia: risk identification. Clin Obstet Gynecol 2000;43:265–82.

4. Grobman WA, Stamilio DM. Methods of clinical prediction. Am J Obstet Gynecol 2006;194:888–94.

5. Gherman RB, Ouzounian JG, Goodwin TM. Obstetric maneuvers for shoulder dystocia and associated fetal morbidity. Am J Obstet Gynecol 1998;178:1126–30.

6. Nesbitt TS, Gilbert WM, Herrchen B. Shoulder dystocia and associated risk factors with macrosomic infants born in California. Am J Obstet Gynecol 1998;179:476–80.

7. Lewis DF, Raymond RC, Perkins MB, Brooks GG, Heymann AR. Recurrence rate of shoulder dystocia. Am J Obstet Gynecol 1995;172:1369–71.

8. Chauhan SP, Grobman WA, Gherman RA, Chauhan VB, Chang G, Magann EF, et al. Suspicion and treatment of the macrosomic fetus: a review. Am J Obstet Gynecol 2005; 193:332–46.

9. American College of Obstetricians and Gynecologists. Fetal macrosomia. Practice Bulletin 22. Washington, DC: American College of Obstetricians and Gynecologists; 2000.

10. Gonen O, Rosen DJ, Dolfin Z, Tepper R, Markov S, Fejgin MD. Induction of labor versus expectant management in macrosomia: a randomized study. Obstet Gynecol 1997; 89:913–7.

11. Gonen R, Bader D, Ajami M. Effects of a policy of elective cesarean delivery in cases of suspected fetal macrosomia on the incidence of brachial plexus injury and the rate of cesarean delivery. Am J Obstet Gynecol 2000;183:1296–300.

12. Rouse DJ, Owen J, Goldenberg RL, Cliver SP. The effectiveness and costs of elective cesarean delivery for fetal macrosomia diagnosed by ultrasound. JAMA 1996; 276:1480–6.

13. Gherman RB, Tramont J, Muffley P, Goodwin TM. Analysis of McRoberts' maneuver by x-ray pelvimetry. Obstet Gynecol 2000;95:43–7.

14. Beall MH, Spong CY, Ross MG. A randomized controlled trial of prophylactic maneuvers to reduce head-to-body delivery time in patients at risk for shoulder dystocia. Obstet Gynecol 2003;102:31–5.

15. Poggi SH, Spong CY, Allen RH. Prioritizing posterior arm delivery during severe shoulder dystocia. Obstet Gynecol 2003;101:1068–72.

16. Maslovitz S, Barkai G, Lessing JB, Ziv A, Many A. Recurrent obstetric management mistakes identified by simulation. Obstet Gynecol 2007;109:1295–300.

17. Deering S, Poggi S, Macedonia C, Gherman R, Satin AJ. Improving resident competency in the management of shoulder dystocia with simulation training. Obstet Gynecol 2004;103:1224–8.

18. Draycott TJ, Crofts JF, Ash JP, Wilson LV, Yard E, Sibanda T, et al. Improving neonatal outcome through practical shoulder dystocia training. Obstet Gynecol 2008;112:14–20.

19. Crofts JF, Bartlett C, Ellis D, Hunt LP, Fox R, Draycott TJ. Training for shoulder dystocia: a trial of simulation using low-fidelity and high-fidelity mannequins. Obstet Gynecol 2006;108:1477–85.

20. Thompson S, Neal S, Clark V. Clinical risk management in obstetrics: eclampsia drills. Qual Saf Health Care 2004; 13:127–9.

21. Medical emergency preparedness. ACOG Committee Opinion No. 353. American College of Obstetricians and Gynecologists. Obstet Gynecol 2006;108:1597–9.

22. Gherman RB, Ouzounian JG, Goodwin TM. Obstetric maneuvers for shoulder dystocia and associated fetal morbidity. Am J Obstet Gynecol 1998;178:1126–30.

Episiotomy and Pelvic Floor Disorders

Tristi W. Muir

The use of episiotomy has decreased substantially over the past two decades. In 2004, 24.5% of women who had a vaginal delivery had an episiotomy (1) compared with 65% of women giving birth vaginally in 1979 (2). The health care provider's decision to perform an episiotomy remains a clinical judgment. To understand the effects of this surgical procedure on subsequent pelvic floor disorders has been the subject of numerous studies and debates.

There is no evidence to support the routine use of episiotomy for maternal or neonatal benefit. The use of the episiotomy should be restricted to select cases and remains a clinical judgment by the health care provider. The purported benefits of the episiotomy compared with a laceration, such as a more efficient and efficacious repair of a surgical incision rather than a laceration, have not been substantiated (3).

Complications

Current data and clinical opinion suggest that there are insufficient objective evidence-based criteria to recommend episiotomy, especially routine use of episiotomy, and that clinical judgment remains the best guide for use of this procedure (4, 5). Complications associated with episiotomy may occur at the time of the delivery or in the postpartum period and may have life-long consequences. As with any incision, there is the risk of subsequent hemorrhage or hematoma formation, this is especially true given the increased vascular supply in pregnancy. Episiotomy is a risk factor for postpartum hemorrhage (more than 500 cc of blood loss, based on the World Health Organization definition) (6). In results of a recent prospective cohort study including over 11,000 vaginal deliveries, postpartum hemorrhage occurred in 19.4% of women who had an episiotomy as compared with 7.7% of women without an episiotomy (bivariate analysis confirmed the significance of episiotomy as a risk factor for postpartum hemorrhage-adjusted odds ratio [OR], 1.70; 95% confidence interval [CI], 1.15–2.5) (6).

Infection

Infections at the episiotomy sites are relatively uncommon because of the increased vascularity in pregnancy. When infection does occur, especially in connection with a third-degree or fourth-degree laceration, it may be associated with substantial morbidity. Diagnosis generally is based on purulent discharge in association with redness and induration. Treatment consists of opening the episiotomy. The episiotomy should be irrigated with copious fluid, followed by debridement of the wound. The infected area should be inspected for any dead tissue suggesting necrotizing fasciitis. Proper care requires that the wound subsequently be cleaned at least twice daily; irrigation with a sitz bath or a handheld shower device should be used liberally. Broad-spectrum antibiotics also should be prescribed.

When an anal sphincter laceration is involved, the risk of infection at the time of injury may be decreased with the use of a broad-spectrum antibiotic and copious irrigation at the time of repair. A prospective, randomized trial evaluated the use of antibiotics at the time of an anal sphincter laceration. Women who received antibiotics had a significantly lower rate of perineal wound complications when compared with women who received placebo (8.2% versus 24.1%, $P=.037$) (7). Infection of a third-degree or fourth-degree laceration may result in fecal incontinence, rectovaginal fistula, pain, and a gaping introitus (or cloaca). This may affect defecatory and sexual function. A change in body image also may occur.

Episiotomy Dehiscence

The repaired episiotomy may break down because of multiple etiologies inclusive of hematoma formation, infection, surgeon error, or (rarely) excessive strain. Infection is the most common etiology of episiotomy breakdown (8, 9). The open wound may then be addressed through treatment of any underlying infection, evacuation of a hematoma and control of persistent bleeding and treatment of constipation. Expectant management with healing by secondary intent may be appropriate for superficial wound breakdown or to avoid further infection. Early or late closure of the episiotomy wound may be needed in the case of more extensive episiotomies (particularly with third-degree or fourth-degree episiotomies). Results from case series indicate that with appropriate preoperative care, primarily wound debridement and antibiotics, early closure of the dehiscence is safe and effective (8–10)

Pain and Sexual Function

Results from a systematic review of the literature on episiotomies over the past 50 years indicated that the initial perineal pain associated with routine (liberal) use of episiotomy is greater than in women in whom episiotomy was restricted to a maternal or fetal indication. This pain typically resolves with time and is equivalent between the two groups by 6 weeks and 6 months. Women with an episiotomy are slower to resume having intercourse and initially have more dyspareunia. Mediolateral episiotomy is associated with more initial pain than median episiotomy (4).

The method of episiotomy repair may affect immediate postpartum pain. Subcutaneous closure of the epithelium of the incision is associated with less immediate postpartum pain than the interrupted suture technique (26.5% versus 44%, respectively) (11). This difference dissipated by 3 months postpartum.

Pelvic Floor Function

Pelvic organ prolapse occurs more frequently in women with vaginal deliveries than those who undergo a cesarean delivery or are nulliparous (12). The contribution of an episiotomy to the development of prolapse is not clearly elucidated. Episiotomy is associated with levator ani muscle injury (OR, 3.1; 95% CI, 1.4–7.2) (13). Damage to these pelvic floor muscles may contribute to the subsequent development of pelvic organ prolapse. Additionally, the injury to the support over the rectum and to the perineal body leaves scar tissue that is not as strong as the native tissue. This weaker tissue may give way with time to the development of pelvic organ prolapse in the posterior compartment. The supportive tissue may not be repaired correctly at the time of delivery, leaving a defect that may grow over the years, particularly with the persistence or development of obesity, constipation, or injury to the pelvic floor muscles.

Urinary Incontinence

Urinary incontinence has been found to be equally prevalent after delivery regardless of the performance of an episiotomy (Table 31) (14). A systematic review of the literature on episiotomy revealed no difference in the postpartum occurrence of urinary incontinence between restricted and routine use of episiotomy (4). A Danish Registry provided long-term data on the prevalence of urinary incontinence twelve years following delivery. There was no significant difference between women who had an episiotomy and those who did not have an episiotomy (46% versus 38.5%, $P=.24$) (15). Risk factors for postpartum urinary incontinence include antenatal urinary incontinence, absence of a college education, and higher predelivery body mass index (16). In this analysis, cesarean delivery was found to be protective (OR, 0.5; 95% CI, 0.3–0.9).

Anal Incontinence

Anal incontinence is defined as the leakage of gas, mucus, liquid stool, or solid stool by accident. Anal continence is a complex interaction between the intact, innervated pelvic floor and anal sphincter muscles as well as compliance and sensation of the rectum. In addition to the outlet mechanism of continence (anal sphincters and pelvic floor muscles) the consistency of the stool and the speed in which it arrives may influence continence. Disorders of transit, such as diarrhea-

Table 31. Prevalence of Urinary and Bowel Symptoms 6 Weeks Postpartum and 6 Months Postpartum in Primiparous Women

	Sphincter Tear (n = 365)	Vaginal Delivery Without Sphincter Tear (n = 356)	Elective Cesarean Delivery (n = 116)	P Value (Sphincter Tear versus Vaginal Control)	P Value (Vaginal Delivery versus Cesarean Delivery)
Urinary Incontinence					
6 weeks postpartum	34.8%	35.4%	25.0%	.76	.32
6 months postpartum	33.7%	31.3%	22.9%	.66	.44
Fecal Incontinence					
6 weeks postpartum	26.6%	11.2%	10.3%	Less than .001	.82
6 months postpartum	17.0%	8.2%	7.6%	.01	.98
Fecal Urgency					
6 weeks postpartum	37.5%	27.8%	34.5%	.02	.13
6 months postpartum	31.6%	23.2%	28.6%	.04	.02

Data from Borello-France D, Burgio KL, Richter HE, Zyczynski H, Fitzgerald MP, Whitehead W, et al. Fecal and urinary incontinence in primiparous women. Pelvic Floor Disorders Network. Obstet Gynecol 2006;108:863–72.

predominant irritable bowel syndrome or inflammatory bowel disease, may send women rushing to the toilet. Women may lose continence on their way to the toilet if it is too far away or if mobility issues are present.

Episiotomy and operative vaginal delivery are risk factors strongly associated with anal sphincter laceration in both primiparous and multiparous women. Decreasing the use of both may be associated with preservation of anal continence. A retrospective study analyzed over 16,000 vaginal deliveries occurring between 1996 and 2004. During the study period the use of episiotomy decreased from 9% to 8% (operative vaginal delivery decreased from 5% to 3%), and the anal sphincter laceration rate decreased from 11.2% to 7.9% (17). Women who had an episiotomy were 36% more likely to have an anal sphincter laceration as compared with those without an episiotomy.

Anal sphincter laceration occurs in 2–19% of vaginal deliveries in the United States (18). In primiparous women, the risk of an anal sphincter laceration varies with size of the fetus, fetal position at birth, length of second stage of labor, and the associated obstetric interventions, including episiotomy. Many of these risk factors persist in the multiparous woman, with the important caveat that once a woman has had an anal sphincter laceration, that scar is more prone to tear again with a subsequent vaginal delivery (Table 32). The identified risk factors often occur simultaneously. For example, a practitioner caring for a woman with a prolonged second stage of labor is more likely to hasten delivery by performing an episiotomy and an instrumental delivery. When an episiotomy is performed during a forceps delivery of an infant in the occiput posterior position, the risk of anal sphincter laceration increases dramatically (OR, 33.8; 95% CI, 4.8–239.5) (18). Episiotomy is an independent risk factor for subsequent fecal incontinence, independent of maternal and fetal factors

and other intrapartum interventions such as instrumental delivery.

Incontinence of flatus or stool occurs in up to one half of women after delivery. Women who have midline episiotomies at the time of delivery are more likely than women without an episiotomy to have an anal sphincter laceration (8.3% versus 3.8%, respectively) (2). Fecal incontinence occurs in 0.7–6% of women during the year after having a vaginal delivery (19). The Childbirth and Pelvic Symptoms cohort study of primiparous women evaluated fecal incontinence symptoms after delivery. Fecal incontinence symptoms were significantly more common in women after a vaginal delivery with an anal sphincter tear than women who delivered vaginally without a recognized anal sphincter laceration or who underwent a cesarean delivery before labor (17%, 8%, and 8%, respectively) (14).

After the repair of a recognized anal sphincter defect, 40–86% of women continue to have an external anal sphincter defect detectable by endoanal ultrasonography (19). Episiotomy has been identified as a risk factor for persistent sphincter defects (20). The other continence mechanisms, such as functioning pelvic floor muscles, may compensate for the injured anal sphincter to maintain continence. This compensation may deteriorate with subsequent delivery and with aging effects on the connective tissue, innervation and muscular strength of the pelvic floor, as well as the internal and external anal sphincters. Consequently, fecal incontinence may present itself later in life.

The risk of an anal sphincter laceration during the subsequent vaginal delivery is greater among women who have had a prior anal sphincter laceration than women who have not (adjusted OR, 4.3; 95% CI, 3.8–4.8) (21). A recurrent laceration is related to a number of factors, including infant birth weight and operative delivery procedures (episiotomy and forceps delivery). As

Table 32. Risk Factors for Anal Sphincter Laceration in Nulliparous and Multiparous Women

Risk Factors	Nulliparous Women	Multiparous Women
Fetal	Increased birthweight Larger head circumference	Birthweight greater than 4,000 g
Maternal	Nulliparity	Prior anal sphincter laceration
Delivery	Occiput posterior position Prolonged second stage of labor Epidural anesthesia	
Physician	Episiotomy Operative vaginal delivery	Episiotomy Forceps delivery

Data from Fitzgerald MP, Weber AM, Howden N, Cundiff GW, Brown MB. Risk factors for anal sphincter tear during vaginal delivery. Pelvic Floor Dysfunction Network. Obstet Gynecol 2007;109:29–34 *and* DiPiazza D, Richter HE, Chapman V, Cliver SP, Neely C, Chen CC, et al. Risk factors for anal sphincter tear in multiparas. Obstet Gynecol 2006;107:1233–7.

fetal weight increases, the risk of recurrence increases. The risk of a recurrent anal sphincter laceration increases from 1.3% for infant birth weight less than 3,000 g to 23.3% for birth weight greater than 5,000 g (21). Performing an episiotomy during the subsequent delivery in a woman with a prior anal sphincter laceration more than doubles her risk of another anal sphincter laceration (OR, 2.6; 95% CI, 2.25–3.04) (22).

References

1. Frankman EA, Wang L, Bunker CH, Lowder JL. Episiotomy in the United States: has anything changed? Am J Obstet Gynecol 2009;200:573.e1–7.

2. Weber AM, Meyn L. Episiotomy use in the United States, 1979-1997. Obstet Gynecol 2002;100:1177–82.

3. Alperin M, Krohn MA, Parviainen K. Episiotomy and increase in the risk of obstetric laceration in a subsequent vaginal delivery. Obstet Gynecol 2008;111:1274–8.

4. Hartmann K, Viswanathan M, Palmieri R, Gartlehner G, Thorp J Jr, Lohr KN. Outcomes of routine episiotomy: a systematic review. JAMA 2005;293:2141–8.

5. Episiotomy. ACOG Practice Bulletin No. 71. American College of Obstetricians and Gynecologists. Obstet Gynecol 2006;107: 957–62.

6. Sosa CG, Althabe F, Belizan JM, Buekens P. Risk factors for postpartum hemorrhage in vaginal deliveries in a Latin-American population. Obstet Gynecol 2009;113:1313–9.

7. Duggal N, Mercado C, Daniels K, Bujor A, Caughey AB, El-Sayed YY. Antibiotic prophylaxis for prevention of postpartum perineal wound complications: a randomized controlled trial. Obstet Gynecol 2008;111:1268–73.

8. Ramin SM, Ramus RM, Little BB, Gilstrap LC 3rd. Early repair of episiotomy dehiscence associated with infection. Am J Obstet Gynecol 1992;167:1104–7.

9. Uygur D, Yesildaglar N, Kis S, Sipahi T. Early repair of episiotomy dehiscence. Aust N Z J Obstet Gynaecol 2004;44:244–6.

10. Hankins GD, Hauth JC, Gilstrap LC 3rd, Hammond TL, Yeomans ER, Snyder RR. Early repair of episiotomy dehiscence. Obstet Gynecol 1990;75:48–51.

11. Kettle C, Hills RK, Jones P, Darby L, Gray R, Johanson R. Continuous versus interrupted perineal repair with standard or rapidly absorbed sutures after spontaneous vaginal birth: a randomised controlled trial. Lancet 2002;359:2217–23.

12. Lukacz ES, Lawrence JM, Contreras R, Nager CW, Luber KM. Parity, mode of delivery, and pelvic floor disorders. Obstet Gynecol 2006;107:1253–60.

13. Kearney R, Miller JM, Ashton-Miller JA, DeLancey JO. Obstetric factors associated with levator ani muscle injury after vaginal birth. Obstet Gynecol 2006;107:144–9.

14. Borello-France D, Burgio KL, Richter HE, Zyczynski H, Fitzgerald MP, Whitehead W, et al. Fecal and urinary incontinence in primiparous women. Pelvic Floor Disorders Network. Obstet Gynecol 2006;108:863–72.

15. Viktrup L, Rortveit G, Lose G. Risk of stress urinary incontinence twelve years after the first pregnancy and delivery. Obstet Gynecol 2006;108:248–54.

16. Burgio KL, Borello-France D, Richter HE, Fitzgerald MP, Whitehead W, Handa VL, et al. Risk factors for fecal and urinary incontinence after childbirth: the childbirth and pelvic symptoms study. The Pelvic Floor Disorders Network. Am J Gastroenterol 2007;102:1998–2004.

17. Minaglia SM, Ozel B, Gatto NM, Korst L, Mishell DR Jr, Miller DA. Decreased rate of obstetrical anal sphincter laceration is associated with change in obstetric practice. Int Urogynecol J Pelvic Floor Dysfunct 2007;18:1399–404.

18. Fitzgerald MP, Weber AM, Howden N, Cundiff GW, Brown MB. Risk factors for anal sphincter tear during vaginal delivery. Pelvic Floor Disorders Network. Obstet Gynecol 2007;109:29–34.

19. Wang A, Guess M, Connell K, Powers K, Lazarou G, Mikhail M. Fecal incontinence: a review of prevalence and obstetric risk factors. Int Urogynecol J Pelvic Floor Dysfunct 2006;17:253–60.

20. Bradley CS, Richter HE, Gutman RE, Brown MB, Whitehead WE, Fine PM, et al. Risk factors for sonographic internal anal sphincter gaps 6-12 months after delivery complicated by anal sphincter tear. Pelvic Floor Disorders Network. Am J Obstet Gynecol 2007;197:310.e1–310.e5.

21. Spydslaug A, Trogstad LI, Skrondal A, Eskild A. Recurrent risk of anal sphincter laceration among women with vaginal deliveries. Obstet Gynecol 2005;105:307–13.

22. Dandolu V, Gaughan JP, Chatwani AJ, Harmanli O, Mabine B, Hernandez E. Risk of recurrence of anal sphincter lacerations. Obstet Gynecol 2005;105:831–5.

Fetal Death

Catherine Y. Spong

In the United States, a fetal death refers to any pregnancy lost after 20 weeks of gestation. Although most states use a lower limit of 20 weeks of gestation only to report fetal death, some also include fetal weight limits (1). In the United States, the incidence of fetal death has decreased for all races from 18.4 fetal deaths per 1,000 births in 1950 to 6.2 per 1,000 births in 2005 (2). Although this number represents a substantial decrease in fetal mortality, significant differences exist among maternal races (from 4.79 for non-Hispanic white women to 11.3 for non-Hispanic Black women) (2). Black women have a 2.3-fold increased risk of fetal death compared with white women.

Expert groups have been working to establish criteria, including biologic plausibility, epidemiologic data, and dose response to determine the cause of death (3). Among the many possible causes of fetal loss, the most common are genetic abnormalities, infection, maternal–fetal hemorrhage, and maternal medical conditions (Box 49).

Various risk factors associated with an increased risk of fetal death. Women of advance maternal age are at higher risk of stillbirth throughout gestation, with a peak risk at 37–41 weeks of gestation, whereas the risk of stillbirth for women aged 35–39 years with pregnancies at this gestational age was 1 in 382 ongoing pregnancies (relative risk, 1.32; 95% confidence interval, 1.22–1.43). This risk increases to 1 in 267 ongoing pregnancies for women aged 40 years and older (4). Cigarette smoking is the most common preventable cause of stillbirth (5). Research on maternal smoking during pregnancy shows that fetal mortality is increased by 35%, from 7.2 cases per 1,000 births in fetuses of women who do not smoke to 9.7 cases per 1,000 births in fetuses of women who do smoke. Increasing the number of cigarettes smoked per day is likewise associated with increasing fetal mortality. Women who stop smoking in the first trimester of pregnancy have stillbirth rates equal to those who never smoked (6). Alcohol use during pregnancy was associated with a fetal mortality of 13.3 cases per 1,000 births, whereas fetal mortality was 7.5 cases per 1,000 births among women who did not drink during pregnancy. Fetal mortality was four times higher among women who consumed five or more drinks per week than among those who consumed one drink per week during pregnancy (7).

The latency period (the interval between fetal death and delivery) is inversely proportional to gestational age at fetal loss. Spontaneous labor generally occurs within 2 weeks in 80–90% of cases of fetal death. A dead fetus poses little medical risk for the mother unless coagulopathy occurs (usually more than 3 weeks after fetal death). Weekly measurement of plasma fibrinogen levels may alert the clinician to clinically significant coagulopathy.

The method and timing of delivery after a fetal death depends on the gestational age at which the death occurred, the history of a previous uterine scar, and maternal preference. In the second trimester, dilation and evacuation can be offered if an experienced provider is available, although these modalities may limit efficacy of autopsy for the detection of macroscopic fetal abnormalities. Before 28 weeks of gestation, the use of vaginal misoprostol appears to be the most efficient method of

---

Box 49

Possible Causes of Fetal Loss

- Infection
- Maternal medical conditions
  - Hypertensive disorders
  - Diabetes mellitus
  - Thyroid disease
  - Renal disease
  - Liver disease
  - Connective tissue disease (systemic lupus erythematosus)
  - Cholestasis
- Antiphospholipid antibody syndrome
- Inheritable thrombophilias
- Red cell alloimmunization
- Platelet alloimmunization (also known as alloimmune thrombocytopenia)
- Congenital anomaly and malformations
- Chromosomal abnormalities, including confined placental mosaicism
- Maternal–fetal hemorrhage
- Placental abnormalities including vasa previa and placental abruption
- Umbilical cord pathology, including velamentous insertion, prolapse, occlusion, and entanglement
- Multifetal gestation, including twin–twin transfusion syndrome and twin reversed arterial perfusion
- Amniotic band sequence
- Uterine complications, including rupture and septate uterus
- Intrapartum stillbirth
- Trauma

induction (8–10), although high-dose oxytocin infusion also is acceptable. Misoprostol can be given vaginally or orally. Typical vaginal dosing strategies for misoprostol use are adjusted to gestational age: between 13–17 weeks, 200 micrograms, every 6 hours; between 18–26 weeks, 100 micrograms, every 6 hours; and more than 27 weeks, 25–50 micrograms, every 4 hours (11). Oral misoprostol can be given at 100–400-microgram doses, every 2–6 hours. The use of vaginal misoprostol has been shown to be as effective as the use of oral misoprostol at achieving delivery in cases of fetal death within 48 hours, but less effective within 24 hours, with fewer side effects than with the use of oral misoprostol (12).

Before induction of labor, cervical ripening should be considered. Effective methods for cervical ripening include the use of mechanical cervical dilators and administration of synthetic prostaglandin E$_1$ and prostaglandin E$_2$ (13–16). Mechanical dilation methods are effective in ripening the cervix and include hygroscopic dilators, osmotic dilators (*Laminaria japonicum*), Foley catheters (14–26 French) with inflation volume of 30–80 mL, double balloon devices (Atad Ripener Device), and extraamniotic saline infusion, using infusion rates of 30–40 mL/h (17–25).

Every effort should be undertaken to determine the cause of fetal death. Accurate identification of an etiologic agent or process can be used to start the emotional healing process for the couple and to counsel them accurately about the risk of recurrence and the need for preconception or antenatal management in a subsequent pregnancy. Using a formal algorithm for evaluation, such as those provided in Figure 23 and Appendix C will ensure that the search for the cause of death occurs in an orderly and systematic fashion, which will facilitate identification of causality. Research is under way to identify the optimal evaluation plan. At this time, testing for the most common causes of stillbirth and those that predispose to recurrent stillbirth are of highest priority.

Careful review of the prenatal laboratory evaluation and record may be informative. A carefully performed autopsy and placental examination (gross and microscopic) have been shown to significantly increase the probability of finding a cause for fetal death. Laboratory evaluation should include complete blood count with platelet count, maternal antibody screen, rapid plasma reagent or VDRL test, Kleihauer–Betke test or other test for maternal–fetal hemorrhage, and urine toxicology sample. Selected patients may benefit from thyroid function tests, lupus anticoagulant and anticardiolipin antibody screening, glucose screening, or other specialized testing. Chromosomal analysis is valuable and should be offered to all women with a fetal death at greater than 20 weeks of gestation. An abnormal karyotype can be found in approximately 8–13% of stillbirths (26–28). The rate of karyotypic abnormalities exceeds 20% in fetuses with anatomic abnormalities or in those with growth restriction, but the rate of chromosomal anomalies found in normally formed fetuses was found to be 4.6% in the results of one large series (28). If an abnormal karyotype is found in association with stillbirth, the most common abnormalities are monosomy X (23%), trisomy 21 (23%), trisomy 18 (21%), and trisomy 13 (8%). Confined placental mosaicism also has been associated with an increased risk of stillbirth but currently is not part of standard testing (29). Karyotypic analysis underestimates the contribution of genetic abnormalities to stillbirth because in up to 50% of karyotype attempts, cell culture is unsuccessful (27). One strategy to increase the yield of cell culture is to perform an amniocentesis before the delivery. This typically is performed after the woman has had an opportunity to process the death of her baby and after an epidural is placed. In the results of a large Dutch study, invasive testing had a much greater tis-

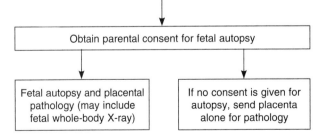

Figure 23. Flowchart for fetal and placental evaluation. (Management of stillbirth. ACOG Practice Bulletin No. 102. American College of Obstetricians and Gynecologists. Obstet Gynecol 2009;113:748–61.)

sue culture rate (85%) than fetal tissue sampling after birth (28%) (28). In addition, routine assessments for single-gene defects and microdeletions currently are not recommended because of uncertainty of the role of these genetic anomalies. However, it is likely that no single-gene defect is likely to be responsible for a substantial proportion of stillbirths. Genetic evaluation for specific abnormalities should be guided by the clinical history and detected fetal abnormalities. Approximately 20% of stillborn fetuses have dysmorphic features or skeletal abnormalities and 15–20% have a major malformation (26, 30). In addition, chromosomal analysis may be particularly informative in cases of recurrent pregnancy losses, family or personal history of a fetal anomaly, malformations, growth restriction, or ultrasound or morphologic stigmata of aneuploidy (Box 50).

After careful evaluation, 25–50% of all fetal deaths remain unexplained. Couples with unexplained fetal deaths are likely to be more apprehensive during a subsequent pregnancy and require special support. Maternal assessment of fetal movement should begin at approximately 28 weeks of gestation. Antepartum fetal testing (a weekly nonstress tests and amniotic fluid index or biophysical profile) may be initiated at 32 weeks of gestation or 1–2 weeks before the gestational age of the previous stillbirth (3). The timing of delivery depends on a combination of maternal anxiety, cervical ripeness, and the cause of the previous loss. Most authorities would recommend elective delivery at 37–38 weeks after confirmation of fetal lung maturity.

References

1. Martin JA, Hoyert DL. The national fetal death file. Semin Perinatol 2002;26:3–11.

2. MacDorman MF, Kirmeyer S. Fetal and perinatal mortality, United States, 2005. Natl Vital Stat Rep 2009;57:1–19.

3. Reddy UM. Prediction and prevention of recurrent stillbirth. Obstet Gynecol 2007; 110:1151–64.

4. Reddy UM, Ko CW, Willinger M. Maternal age and the risk of stillbirth throughout pregnancy in the United States. Am J Obstet Gynecol 2006;195:764–70.

5. Dodd JM, Robinson JS, Crowther CA, Chan A. Stillbirth and neonatal outcomes in South Australia 1991-2000. Am J Obstet Gynecol 2003;189:1731–6.

6. Wisborg K, Kesmodel U, Henriksen TB, Olsen SF, Secher NJ. Exposure to tobacco smoke in utero and the risk of stillbirth and death in the first year of life. Am J Epidemiol 2001;154:322–7.

7. Hoyert DL. Medical and life-style risk factors affecting fetal mortality, 1989–90. Vital Health Stat 20 1996;(31):1–32.

8. Dodd J, Crowther C. Induction of labour for women with a previous Caesarean birth: a systematic review of the literature. Aust N Z J Obstet Gynaecol 2004;44:392–5.

9. Dickinson JE, Evans SF. The optimization of intravaginal misoprostol dosing schedules in second-trimester pregnancy termination [published erratum appears in Am J Obstet Gynecol 2005;193:597]. Am J Obstet Gynecol 2002;186:470–4.

10. Tang OS, Lau WN, Chan CC, Ho PC. A prospective randomised comparison of sublingual and vaginal misoprostol in second trimester termination of pregnancy. BJOG 2004;111:1001–5.

11. Gomez Ponce de Leon R, Wing D, Fiala C. Misoprostol for intrauterine fetal death. Int J Gynaecol Obstet 2007;99 (suppl 2):S190–3.

12. Gomez Ponce de Leon R, Wing DA. Misoprostol for termination of pregnancy with intrauterine fetal demise in the second and third trimester of pregnancy - a systematic review. Contraception 2009;79:259–71.

Box 50

Evaluation of Stillbirth

Generally Accepted Tests

- Fetal autopsy
- Placental evaluation
- Karyotype evaluation
- Indirect Coombs test
- Serologic test for syphilis
- Screen for maternal–fetal hemorrhage (Kleihauer–Betke test)
- Drug screen
- Fasting glucose test (to exclude diabetes mellitus)

Useful in Some Cases

- Lupus anticoagulant screen
- Anticardiolipin antibodies test
- *Factor V Leiden* mutation test
- *Factor II–prothrombin G20210A* mutation test
- Screen for protein C, protein S, and antithrombin III deficiency

Uncertain Utility

- Thyroid-stimulating hormone test
- Glycohemoglobin test
- Toxoplasmosis, other agents, rubella, cytomegalovirus, and herpes simplex titers
- Parvovirus serology
- Placental cultures
- Testing for other thrombophilias

Developing Technology

- Comparative genomic hybridization
- Testing for single-gene mutations
- Testing for confined placental mosaicism
- Nucleic acid based testing for infection

Silver RM, Varner MW, Reddy U, Goldenberg R, Pinar H, Conway D, et al. Work-up of stillbirth: a review of the evidence. Am J Obstet Gynecol 2007;196:433–44.

13. Krammer J, Williams MC, Sawai SK, O'Brien WF. Pre-induction cervical ripening: a randomized comparison of two methods. Obstet Gynecol 1995;85:614–8.

14. Fletcher HM, Mitchell S, Simeon D, Frederick J, Brown D. Intravaginal misoprostol as a cervical ripening agent. Br J Obstet Gynaecol 1993;100:641–4.

15. Porto M. The unfavorable cervix: methods of cervical priming. Clin Obstet Gynecol 1989;32:262–8.

16. Wing DA, Jones MM, Rahall A, Goodwin TM, Paul RH. A comparison of misoprostol and prostaglandin E2 gel for preinduction cervical ripening and labor induction. Am J Obstet Gynecol 1995;172:1804–10.

17. Atad J, Hallak M, Ben-David Y, Auslender R, Abramovici H. Ripening and dilatation of the unfavourable cervix for induction of labour by a double balloon device: experience with 250 cases. Br J Obstet Gynaecol 1997;104:29–32.

18. Blumenthal PD, Ramanauskas R. Randomized trial of Dilapan and Laminaria as cervical ripening agents before induction of labor. Obstet Gynecol 1990;75:365–8.

19. Chua S, Arulkumaran S, Vanaja K, Ratnam SS. Preinduction cervical ripening: prostaglandin E2 gel vs hygroscopic mechanical dilator. J Obstet Gynaecol Res 1997;23:171–7.

20. Gilson GJ, Russell DJ, Izquierdo LA, Qualls CR, Curet LB. A prospective randomized evaluation of a hygroscopic cervical dilator, Dilapan, in the preinduction ripening of patients undergoing induction of labor. Am J Obstet Gynecol 1996;175:145–9.

21. Lin A, Kupferminc M, Dooley SL. A randomized trial of extra-amniotic saline infusion versus laminaria for cervical ripening. Obstet Gynecol 1995;86:545–9.

22. Lyndrup J, Nickelsen C, Weber T, Molnitz E, Guldbaek E. Induction of labour by balloon catheter with extra-amniotic saline infusion (BCEAS): a randomised comparison with PGE2 vaginal pessaries. Eur J Obstet Gynecol Reprod Biol 1994;53:189–97.

23. Mullin PM, House M, Paul RH, Wing DA. A comparison of vaginally administered misoprostol with extra-amniotic saline solution infusion for cervical ripening and labor induction. Am J Obstet Gynecol 2002;187:847–52.

24. Boulvain M, Kelly AJ, Lohse C, Stan CM, Irion O. Mechanical methods for induction of labour. Cochrane Database of Systematic Reviews 2001, Issue 4. Art. No.: CD001233. DOI: 10.1002/14651858.CD001233; 10.1002/14651858.CD01233.

25. Guinn DA, Davies JK, Jones RO, Sullivan L, Wolf D. Labor induction in women with an unfavorable Bishop score: randomized controlled trial of intrauterine Foley catheter with concurrent oxytocin infusion versus Foley catheter with extra-amniotic saline infusion with concurrent oxytocin infusion. Am J Obstet Gynecol 2004;191:225–9.

26. Pauli RM, Reiser CA, Lebovitz RM, Kirkpatrick SJ. Wisconsin Stillbirth Service Program: I. Establishment and assessment of a community-based program for etiologic investigation of intrauterine deaths. Am J Med Genet 1994;50:116–34.

27. Laury A, Sanchez-Lara PA, Pepkowitz S, Graham JM Jr. A study of 534 fetal pathology cases from prenatal diagnosis referrals analyzed from 1989 through 2000. Am J Med Genet A 2007;143A:3107–20.

28. Korteweg FJ, Bouman K, Erwich JJ, Timmer A, Veeger NJ, Ravise JM, et al. Cytogenetic analysis after evaluation of 750 fetal deaths: proposal for diagnostic workup. Obstet Gynecol 2008;111:865–74.

29. Kalousek DK, Barrett I. Confined placental mosaicism and stillbirth. Pediatr Pathol 1994;14:151–9.

30. Pauli RM, Reiser CA. Wisconsin Stillbirth Service Program: II. Analysis of diagnoses and diagnostic categories in the first 1,000 referrals. Am J Med Genet 1994;50:135–53.

POSTPARTUM MANAGEMENT

Neonatal Resuscitation

Jay P. Goldsmith, George A. Little, and Gilbert I. Martin

Derived from the Latin verb *resuscitare* (to arouse again), resuscitation in the delivery room is a process to assist the newly born infant during the transition from dependent fetal to independent neonatal life. A cascade of physiologic events occurs at birth during which the placenta is replaced by the lungs as the primary organ of gas exchange. Ensuring a smooth transition during the first moments of life and optimizing outcomes requires excellent communication and collaborative care before, during, and after birth by obstetric and pediatric care providers, especially in complicated pregnancies.

Anticipation

Ongoing risk assessment during prenatal, antepartum, and intrapartum care can identify many of the infants who will require special attention, including resuscitation during the neonatal period. Such identification allows neonatal care providers to be fully prepared and parents counseled and involved in decision-making regarding their baby.

At least one person capable of initiating neonatal resuscitation and responsible for the newborn must be present for every birth (1). That person or someone immediately available should have the skills to perform a complete resuscitation, including ventilation with bag and mask, endotracheal intubation, chest compressions, and administration of medications (1). Standards of the Joint Commission on Accreditation of Healthcare Organizations state that resuscitative services must be available throughout an organization and that qualifications must be consistent with responsibilities (2). Each hospital with perinatal services should have a program in place that ensures the competency of the resuscitation personnel through periodic credentialing (1). Thus, providers of obstetric care, including physicians, nurse–midwives, and nurses, should be able to initiate neonatal resuscitation and stabilization from the moment of birth as unexpected depression and complications occur. When problems are anticipated, communication and consultation with other providers who are skilled in neonatal care is advised. The birth of an extremely preterm infant should occur whenever possible in a center capable of providing a team of trained caregivers to begin intensive care from the moment of birth (3). Communication to the potential resuscitation team should include all pertinent information and the

acronym "HANDS" may be helpful in this regard: H for **h**emorrhage, A for **a**mniotic fluid (meconium stained), N for **n**umber of neonates expected, D for **d**ates (gestational age), and S for fetal monitoring **s**trip (category 1, 2 or 3). If clinical circumstances allow, certain conditions might warrant maternal–fetal transfer to another institution in a regional system where subspecialty services, such as neonatology, pediatric surgery, neurology, and cardiology, are available.

Resuscitation

Approximately 10% of neonates require some help with breathing at birth, and 1% require advanced intervention. Full resuscitation, including chest compressions and drug administration, is a rare event, occurring in 1–2 per 1,000 live births. The Neonatal Resuscitation Program is a standardized clinical provider course jointly created and sponsored by the American Heart Association and the American Academy of Pediatrics. Derived from the Consensus on Science and Treatment Recommendations as developed by the International Liaison Committee on Resuscitation, the Neonatal Resuscitation Program is the foundation of practically all current instruction in resuscitation in the United States and a growing portion of international teaching (4, 5).

Immediately after birth, specific steps should be taken, including drying, suctioning, and tactile stimulation. Subsequently, continuous evaluation and judgment are used according to specific guidelines resulting in intervention along specific pathways. Intervention is less if the clinician notes spontaneous respirations and a heart rate of more than 100 beats per minute. Conversely, a low heart rate (less than 60 beats per minute) with inadequate respiration or response to positive-pressure ventilation leads to additional interventions, including chest compressions and, possibly, the use of medications. Effective gas exchange can be accomplished with a bag and mask in most situations. Intubation should be performed if clinically indicated and a skilled provider is available. Laryngeal mask airway is an alternative therapy able to provide positive airway pressure where a skilled intubator is not present or the intubation process is difficult. The use of supplemental oxygen should be reserved for those infants who do not respond to the initial steps with an increase in heart rate. Results from recent studies have shown it may take 5–10 minutes in normal healthy term infants to reach an oxygen saturation of 90% and that use of oxygen to treat cyanosis alone may be harmful (6). The premature infant, less than 28 weeks of gestation, is at particular risk of cold stress, and special steps should be taken to maintain body temperature, including warming the delivery room and placing the neonate from the neck down in a food-grade reclosable one-gallon polyethylene bag (2).

The Apgar score is a traditional and useful tool to assess neonatal status in the minutes immediately after birth. It should be recorded by an independent observer at 1 minute and 5 minutes after delivery and every 5 minutes thereafter until a score of 7 is achieved. Assessment and initiation of resuscitation when necessary must begin immediately at birth and should not depend on the 1-minute Apgar score. The score depicts the physiologic state of the moment; alone, it is not evidence of appropriateness of care or a predictor of neurologic sequelae. Apgar scores of infants who undergo resuscitation ("assisted scores") should be appropriately noted in the medical record in an expanded Apgar score form (4, 7).

Stabilization

Resuscitation progresses into ongoing stabilization and care based on need. Many neonates that require resuscitation efforts improve rapidly, are observed for a period of time, and are transitioned to routine care, including being with their mothers and breastfeeding. The resuscitation algorithm in the *Textbook of Neonatal Resuscitation* indicates that neonates given positive pressure ventilation should be observed in postresuscitation care, which includes temperature control, close monitoring of vital signs (including blood pressure), and anticipation of complications (4). The likelihood of developing postresuscitation complications depends on the conditions that required the interventions and increases with the length and extent of the resuscitation performed. Problems such as prematurity and respiratory distress may need ongoing support. Problems identified before labor or delivery (congenital anomalies) may require additional assessment (genetic consultation and studies). Initiation of antibiotic therapy for suspected perinatally acquired infections should take place immediately. Concerns regarding group B streptococci infection should be addressed before and after birth according to national prevention guidelines (8).

Special Concerns

Meconium

Resuscitation and stabilization in the presence of meconium has been a controversial subject for years. Meconium-stained amniotic fluid is present in 10–20%

of term and late-preterm deliveries, and most neonates with meconium staining do not develop problems. Meconium aspiration syndrome is thought to occur in 1 in 120 liveborn neonates, or approximately 6–8% of all neonates with meconium staining. Severe cases have high mortality and morbidity, including pneumonitis, pneumothorax, and pulmonary artery hypertension.

Care of such an infant does not depend on the viscosity of the meconium-stained fluid. Current evidence does not support the routine intrapartum suctioning of the oropharynx and nasopharynx on the perineum after delivery of the head because this procedure does not prevent or alter the course of meconium aspiration syndrome (9). If the infant is not vigorous at birth and meconium is present, the Neonatal Resuscitation Program recommends intubation and suctioning to remove material below the glottis before positive-pressure ventilation is begun. If the infant is active, suctioning and intubation are therapeutic options that are part of ongoing stabilization and care (1).

Resuscitation at the Threshold of Viability

The survival rate for neonates born at the threshold of viability increases and the incidence of neurodevelopmental disability decreases with each additional week of gestation. Resuscitation is not indicated in cases in which gestation, birth weight, or both are associated with almost certain death and unacceptably high morbidity in the rare survivors. In situations in which prognosis is uncertain, parents should be counseled regarding potential outcomes, and their decisions whether to institute resuscitation and intensive care should be honored. The decision to perform a cesarean delivery indicated for a fetus with an abnormal heart rate at the threshold of viability should include counseling the mother as to the short-term and long-term risks of the procedure as well as the neonatal outcomes. Local outcomes and available national data, which include gestational age, birth weight, sex, number of infants, and whether steroids have been administered, all significantly impact prediction of outcome and should be part of the parental counseling (10). A calculator available through the National Institutes of Child Health and Human Development web site (see Appendix A) should be used to provide additional perspective on outcomes to health care providers and parents (10).

Some parents will decide that resuscitation should not be initiated. Many elect to provide individualized care that involves ongoing decisions concerning the extent and duration of resuscitation based on the clinical course and further discussions. Parents may be present while perinatal care is being provided to neonates, including procedures, resuscitation, and stabilization. Parents should be informed about and involved in the care of their children within the principles of family-centered care (11).

Neonatal Encephalopathy and Cerebral Palsy

Factors often used to define perinatal asphyxia, such as the need for resuscitation, Apgar score, and presence of meconium, as well as category III fetal heart rate patterns, are not specific to the pathophysiologic process involved with neurologic damage. False-positive rates are significant. Approximately 70% or more of cases of neonatal encephalopathy apparently have causality that began before the onset of labor (12). This knowledge reinforces the need for anticipation and risk assessment well before delivery and promotes caution when discussing prognosis and outcomes after neonatal resuscitation has been necessary. Criteria that help with the definition of the relationship between acute intrapartum events and neurologic outcomes, such as cerebral palsy, are available (12). The use of head or body cooling after a significant asphyxial episode has been shown to improve neurodevelopmental outcome and should be considered in those infants who meet criteria for treatment (13).

Oxygen

Long-standing recommendations for the use of supplemental oxygen during the initial acute phase of resuscitation have been revised. Most term and late-preterm infants can be successfully resuscitated with positive-pressure ventilation with air or low levels of oxygen. Recent research and evolving knowledge about the immediate effectiveness and the possibility of long-term sequelae of oxygen administration raise significant concerns especially in the preterm infant. The Neonatal Resuscitation Program now recommends that blended oxygen and a pulse oximeter be available in the delivery room of hospitals that routinely care for premature infants less than 32 weeks of gestation (4). In the unusual circumstance when supplemental oxygen is not available, positive-pressure resuscitation with air (21% oxygen) should be used.

References

1. American Academy of Pediatrics, American College of Obstetricians and Gynecologists. Guidelines for perinatal care. 6th ed. Elk Grove Village (IL): AAP; Washington, DC: American College of Obstetricians and Gynecologists; 2007.

2. The Joint Commission. Comprehensive accreditation manual for hospitals: CAMH. Oakbrook Terrace (IL): The Commission; 2009.

3. Vento M, Aguar M, Leone TA, Finer NN, Gimeno A, Rich W, et al. Using intensive care technology in the delivery room: a new concept for the resuscitation of extremely preterm neonates. Pediatrics 2008;122:1113–6.

4. Kattwinkel J, Bloom RS, editors. Textbook of Neonatal Resuscitation. 5th ed. Dallas (TX): American Heart Association; Elk Grove Village (IL): American Academy of Pediatrics; 2006.

5. Niermeyer S, Kattwinkel J, Van Reempts P, Nadkarni V, Phillips B, Zideman D, et al. International Guidelines for Neonatal Resuscitation: An excerpt from the Guidelines 2000 for Cardiopulmonary Resuscitation and Emergency Cardiovascular Care: International Consensus on Science. Contributors and Reviewers for the Neonatal Resuscitation Guidelines. Pediatrics 2000;106:E29.

6. Richmond S, Goldsmith JP. Refining the role of oxygen administration during delivery room resuscitation: what are the future goals? Semin Fetal Neonatal Med 2008;13: 368–74.

7. The Apgar score. ACOG Committee Opinion No. 333. American College of Obstetricians and Gynecologists. Obstet Gynecol 2006;107:1209–12.

8. Schrag S, Gorwitz R, Fultz-Butts K, Schuchat A. Prevention of perinatal group B streptococcal disease. Revised guidelines from CDC. MMWR Recomm Rep 2002;51(RR-11): 1–22.

9. Vain NE, Szyld EG, Prudent LM, Wiswell TE, Aguilar AM, Vivas NI. Oropharyngeal and nasopharyngeal suctioning of meconium-stained neonates before delivery of their shoulders: multicentre, randomised controlled trial. Lancet 2004;364:597–602.

10. Tyson JE, Parikh NA, Langer J, Green C, Higgins RD, National Institute of Child Health and Human Development Neonatal Research Network. Intensive care for extreme prematurity--moving beyond gestational age. N Engl J Med 2008;358:1672–81.

11. Harrison H. The principles for family-centered neonatal care. Pediatrics 1993;92:643–50.

12. American Academy of Pediatrics, American College of Obstetricians and Gynecologists. Neonatal encephalopathy and cerebral palsy: defining the pathogenesis and pathophysiology. Elk Grove Village (IL): AAP; Washington, DC: American College of Obstetricians and Gynecologists; 2003.

13. Jacobs SE, Hunt R, Tarnow-Mordi WO, Inder TE, Davis PG. Cooling for newborns with hypoxic ischaemic encephalopathy. Cochrane Database of Systematic Reviews 2007, Issue 4. Art. No.: CD003311. DOI: 10.1002/14651858. CD003311.pub2; 10.1002/14651858.CD003311.pub2.

Breastfeeding

Wendy F. Hansen

The American Academy of Pediatrics recommends exclusive breastfeeding of infants for the first 6 months of life, with continuation for at least 12 months or longer if mutually desired by the mother and child. Healthy People 2010 published national health objectives, including those regarding breastfeeding, that call for 75% of women to initiate breastfeeding, 50% of women to be breastfeeding at 6 months (25% exclusive), and 25% of women to be breastfeeding for 1 year (1).

Epidemiology

In October 2008, the Centers for Disease Control and Prevention (CDC), using data from the National Immunization Survey, published statistics describing breastfeeding practices in the United States (2). Of mothers of children born in 2005, 74% initiated breastfeeding, whereas 43% were breastfeeding at 6 months (32% exclusively), and 21% at 12 months (12% exclusively). In another report, based on data from the Pediatric Nutrition Surveillance System, the CDC published their 2007 statistics on breastfeeding practices of nearly 8 million low-income mothers (3). This report is not as optimistic as the 2005 data, showing that 59.8 % of mothers ever breast fed, 25.4 % of mothers breastfed for at least 6 months, and 17.6 % of mothers breastfed for at least 12 months. Nevertheless, although short of the Healthy People 2010 goal, both reports show substantial increases for all indicators of breastfeeding over the past decade. Several factors influence a woman's choice to breastfeed. It is clear that maternal age (older is better) and formal education along with strong family support are powerful influences on a woman's choice to breastfeed and her ability to be successful regardless of her ethnic heritage or her geographic location.

Benefits

There is widespread consensus that breastfeeding is optimal in undeveloped countries. Conversely, for many years, formula was thought to be an equal substitute for breastfeeding, especially in the United States.

Nevertheless, the evidence of the benefits of breastfeeding in the United States became clear with considerable advances in scientific knowledge. The Agency for Health Care Research and Quality reviewed over 400 individual studies and over 9,000 abstracts from developed countries through 2006 in an attempt to better define the evidence for benefits of breastfeeding for both mother and infant (4). These studies found that infants who were breastfed for at least 3–4 months had protection from common childhood diseases, such as nonspecific gastrointestinal problems, otitis media, and lower respiratory tract infections, for far longer than the actual duration of breastfeeding; they were protected for up to 1 year. There also was an association between increased duration and exclusivity of breastfeeding for some infant outcomes, modeling a dose response effect. Partial benefits also could be seen with the presence of breast milk even when supplementation is required.

The authors also concluded that in infants and children, breastfeeding also decreased the incidence of atopic dermatitis, asthma (young children), obesity, type 1 diabetes mellitus and type 2 diabetes mellitus, childhood leukemia, sudden infant death syndrome, and necrotizing enterocolitis. There was no relationship between breastfeeding in term infants and cognitive performance.

For maternal outcomes, a history of breastfeeding was associated with a reduced risk of type 2 diabetes mellitus and breast cancer and ovarian cancer. There was no relationship between a history of breastfeeding and the risk of osteoporosis. The effect of breastfeeding in mothers on return to prepregnancy weight was negligible, and the effect of breastfeeding on postpartum weight loss was unclear.

This benefit to infants and children is thought largely to be from the composition of human milk. Breast milk is a complex fluid that is species specific. The exact composition of breast milk varies between stage of lactation, breastfeeding pattern, individuals, season, and parity. Foremilk, the milk released at the beginning of a feed, is watery, low in fat, and high in carbohydrates, relative to the creamier hind milk that is released as the feed progresses. Human milk contains 0.8–0.9% of protein, 3–5% of fat, 6.9–7.2% of carbohydrates, and 0.2% of ash (minerals). The principal protein of human milk is β-casein, the principal carbohydrate is lactose, and the principal fat is triglycerides. Human milk also contains several bioactive substances that have important nonnutritional functions and include procytokines and antiinflammatory substances, hormones, growth modulators, and digestive enzymes that are specific to the immature gastrointestinal tract of the infant.

Contraindications

It is estimated that most women are able to establish and maintain breastfeeding for an extended period if they are motivated and have the support from their families, employer, community, and the medical system. Despite motivation and support, however, women with certain conditions should not breastfeed and, in rare situations, certain infants should not be breastfed (5). Although contraindications to breastfeeding are few, they are important to recognize (6). They include the following factors:

- The infant with galactosemia, a rare genetic metabolic disorder
- The infant whose mother:
  - Has been infected with the human immunodeficiency virus (HIV)
  - Is taking antiretroviral medications
  - Has untreated, active tuberculosis
  - Is infected with human T-cell lymphotropic virus type I or type II
  - Is using or is dependent on an illicit drug
  - Is taking prescribed cancer chemotherapy agents, such as antimetabolites, which interfere with DNA replication and cell division
  - Is undergoing radiation therapies; however, many nuclear medicine therapies require only at temporary interruption in breastfeeding

Formula Feeding

In cases in which breastfeeding is not an option, physicians should reassure women that formulas available today provide the infants with sufficient amounts of the right nutrients. There are three major types of infant formula currently on the market in the United States:

1. Cow's milk-based formulas—appropriate for full-term and preterm infants with no special nutritional requirements
2. Soy-based formulas—appropriate for term infants with galactosemia and hereditary lactase deficiency and in situations in which a vegetarian diet is preferred. Infants with documented cow milk protein-induced enteropathy or enterocolitis frequently are as sensitive to soy protein and should not be given isolate soy protein-based formula (7)
3. Hydrolyzed protein formulas—appropriate for infants with documented cow milk and soy protein allergies (7)

Women should be encouraged to discuss their options with their infants' health care providers.

Physiology

The first hormonal changes of pregnancy bring changes to the breast tissue. For many women this is the first sign of pregnancy. Progesterone, prolactin, and placental lactogen play essential roles in the development and differentiation of glandular tissue, especially the alveoli. Estrogen is thought to stimulate ductal growth while inhibiting milk synthesis. In the first half of pregnancy, there is intense alveolar and lobular proliferation, along with ductile sprouting and branching. By midpregnancy there is some secretory development with colostrum present in the alveoli and milk ducts. The breasts are capable of full lactation from 16 weeks of gestation onwards.

Common Problems

Mastitis

Mastitis is an acute inflammation of the connective tissue of the mammary gland: a mammary cellulitis. The incidence of mastitis is highest in the first few weeks postpartum and gradually decreases thereafter (8). Results from two studies within the United States suggest an incidence range of 9.3–9.5% (9, 10). Risk factors include a history of mastitis with a previous child, blocked duct, cracked nipples, use of creams, and the use of a manual breast pump. Traditional teaching holds that nipple trauma allows the portal of entry for microorganisms and that inadequate emptying causes milk stasis allowing a medium for bacterial growth. The diagnosis of mastitis is a clinical one. It most commonly presents with unilateral breast tenderness or pain, redness in an area that often demarcates the underlying lobe involved, fever (often greater than 38.9 °C [102 °F]), and flulike symptoms. Although mastitis is a connective tissue infection, cultured breast milk has been used in identifying the pathogenic microorganism. *Staphylococcus aureus* accounts for most identified pathogens (35–50% of isolates) along with coagulase-negative staphylococci, followed by group A hemolytic streptococci and B hemolytic streptococci, *Escherichia coli, Haemophilus influenzae, Klebsiella* species, and *Bacteroides* species. Recent experience has shown an emergence of community acquired methicillin-resistant *Staphylococcus aureus* (MRSA) in postpartum mastitis infections. In results from a single-center case–control study from 1998–2005, an increase in MRSA with 81% of MRSA cases occurring in 2005 was found (11). In results of a second study from a single center from 1997–2005, it was found that community-acquired MRSA was most commonly associated with breast abscess (10) and no increase over time was noticed. Interestingly, women with breast abscesses and culture results positive for MRSA improved clinically with drainage and the use of antibiotics not directed against MRSA (before culture results were known), suggesting that drainage of the abscess and emptying of the breast are essential to complete resolution. Until recently, culture of breast milk has not been routinely performed. The practitioner needs to be aware of the emergence of MRSA and have a low threshold for culture.

First-line clinical treatment includes the use of antibiotics and continued emptying of the breast. There is widespread belief that emptying the breast is essential in preventing complication of mastitis, mainly breast abscess and prolonged infection. Penicillinase-resistant penicillins and cephalosporins, such as dicloxacillin or cephalexin, are commonly used. Resolution of symptoms should occur within 2 days of antibiotic treatment and breast emptying in most women (8). Symptoms can be treated with nonsteroidal antiinflammatory drugs, fluids, and rest. Mastitic milk is associated with increased concentrations of immune components and inflammatory molecules, which resolve within 1 week of treatment. Adverse effects on infants have not been reported, and mastitic milk poses no threat to an infant. When mastitis goes untreated or does not respond to initial treatment, 5–11% of patients will go on to develop a breast abscess. If signs and symptoms do not improve in 48 hours, the women should be reexamined, a culture of the milk should be done, and strong consideration should be given to the administration of an antibiotic for MRSA. If results of the physical examination are suggestive of an abscess, ultrasonography of the breast can be performed for confirmation. Traditionally, incision and drainage has been the standard treatment. More recently, ultrasound-guided percutaneous drainage has been described.

Lactational Atrophic Vaginitis

Lactational atrophic vaginitis is a common consequence of the hypoestrogenic state resulting from breastfeeding. Decreased estrogen levels can cause urogenital atrophy, including epithelial thinning, decreased elasticity, and diminished vaginal blood flow. Consequent symptoms include vaginal dryness, itching, burning, irritation, and pain with intercourse. Topical estrogen cream applied to the vulvovaginal area can improve symptoms without affecting milk supply.

Breast Pain

Pain associated with breastfeeding is the second most commonly cited reason for cessation of breastfeeding. Breast pain may result from engorgement, mastitis, pain from erythematous, fissured nipples and fissured areola. Breast pain with initiation of breastfeeding is common and most often transient with proper instruction on feeding techniques. However, persistent breast pain after 2 weeks postpartum that radiates through the breast during and after feeding requires evaluation. Evaluation of breast pain is based on clinical symptoms. In the absence of clinical mastitis, there is little evidence to guide either diagnosis or treatment. Despite the lack of evidence, there is widespread empiric use of antifungals for presumed infection of the breast by *Candida* species. A recent prospective comparative study exploring the relationship between the presence of *Candida* species in women with and without breast pain produced results that indicated an association with the presence of *Candida* species, but it remains unclear whether this is causative because most women with pain had no *Candida* species identified (12).

Delayed Lactation

Delayed lactation has been described in women with a history of type 1 diabetes mellitus and gestational diabetes mellitus, obesity, and cesarean delivery (13). The causes are not well understood. Flat or inverted nipples can cause problems with suckling, thereby causing a delay. Ineffective or infrequent milk removal also will cause a delay, especially in women who are very ill or who have infants who are very premature or ill.

Insufficient Milk Supply

Insufficient milk supply is the most cited reason given by women worldwide for cessation of breastfeeding. This reason may be real or perceived. Real anatomical and physiological reasons include the following conditions:

- Breast surgery, most commonly breast reduction, which often severs ducts and removes glandular tissue.
- Congenital tubular hypoplastic breasts, which have an inadequate glandular development.
- Insufficient feeding or pumping best defined as infrequent feeding or pumping or ineffective pumping as in the case of a premature infant (13).

Perceived insufficient milk is thought to be secondary to lack of education, lack of support, and ambivalence about breastfeeding. Once a real anatomic reason is excluded, management should be centered on support of the woman along with safety, nutritional, and hydration issues for the infant.

Breast Reduction Mammoplasty

As mentioned previously, women who have undergone breast reduction surgery often encounter problems with insufficient milk supply. Their ability to breastfeed will depend on how much glandular tissue remains, how well the ductal attachments to the nipple have been preserved, and their residual sensation or nerve status. Many women can partially breastfeed.

Breast Implants

Breast milk in women with silicone and saline implants is safe and poses no threat to an infant (6). Many women with breast implants can breastfeed successfully, whereas others cannot. An Institute of Medicine Study in 2000 reported that 28–64% of such women reported lactational insufficiency. The periareolar approach (incision around the nipple) was the factor highly suggestive of lactational insufficiency, most likely secondary to damage of the nerve and underlying tissue (14).

Medications

Questions regarding safe use of medications while breastfeeding are perhaps the most common questions a physician encounters. Information regarding the effect of infant exposure to many medications is inadequate. Given the rapidly changing information, it is important to have resources that you are familiar with and readily available, such as those listed in Box 51.

Contraception and Breastfeeding

The lactational amenorrhea method is a method of avoiding pregnancy that is based on the natural postpartum infertility that occurs when a woman is amenorrheic and fully breastfeeding (15). The lactational amenorrhea method is more than 98% effective during the first 6 months postpartum under the following conditions:

- Breastfeeding must be the infant's only source of nutrition. Feeding formula or other liquids, including water, pumping instead of breastfeeding, and feeding solids all reduce the effectiveness of this method.

- The infant must be breastfed at least every 4 hours during the day and at least every 6 hours at night

- The infant must be younger than 6 months

- The woman must not have had a menstrual period after 56 days postpartum (when determining fertility, bleeding before 56 days postpartum can be ignored) (5).

References

1. U.S. Department of Health and Human Services. Maternal, infant, and child health: increase the proportion of mothers who breastfeed their babies. Healthy people 2010: with understanding and improving health and objectives for improving health. 2nd ed. Washington, DC: U.S. Government Printing Office; 2000. p. 16–46.

2. Breastfeeding among U.S. children born 1999-2006. Centers for Disease Control and Prevention National Immunization Survey. Atlanta (GA): CDC; 2009. Available at: http://www.cdc.gov/breastfeeding/data/NIS_data/index.htm. Retrieved September 15, 2009.

3. Polhamus B, Dalenius K, Borland E, Mackintosh H, Smith B, Grummer-Strawn L. Pediatric Nutrition Surveillance 2007 Report. Atlanta (GA): U.S. Department of Health and Human Services, Centers for Disease Control and Prevention; 2009. Available at: http://www.cdc.gov/PEDNSS/pdfs/PedNSS_2007.pdf. Retrieved September 15, 2009.

4. Breastfeeding and maternal and infant health outcomes in developed countries. Evidence Report/Technology Assessment No. 153. Rockville (MD): Agency for Health-

---

Box 51

Web Resources on Safe Use of Medications During Lactation

- Motherisk

  http://www.motherisk.org/women/index.jsp

  This resource of the Hospital for Sick Children in Toronto, Ontario, Canada, is a clinical, research and teaching program dedicated to antenatal drug, chemical, and disease risk counseling. It is affiliated with the University of Toronto. Created in 1985, Motherisk provides evidence-based information and guidance about the safety or risk to the developing fetus or infant, of maternal exposure to drugs, chemicals, diseases, radiation, and environmental agents.

- Organization of Teratology Information Specialists

  http://www.otispregnancy.org/

  This resource of the Organization of Teratology Information Specialists provides accurate evidence-based, clinical information to patients and health care professionals about exposures during pregnancy and lactation.

- *The Transfer of Drugs and Other Chemicals Into Human Milk*

  http://aappolicy.aappublications.org/cgi/reprint/pediatrics;108/3/776.pdf

  This resource is published by the American Academy of Pediatrics, Committee on Drugs.

- Medication Use During Pregnancy and Breastfeeding

  http://www.cdc.gov/ncbddd/meds/

  This resource is provided by the Centers for Disease Control and Prevention.

- Drugs and Lactation Database (LactMed)

  http://toxnet.nlm.nih.gov/cgi-bin/sis/htmlgen?LACT

  The National Library of Medicine sponsors this peer-reviewed and fully referenced database of drugs to which breastfeeding mothers may be exposed.

---

care Research and Quality; 2007. Available at: http://www.ahrq.gov/downloads/pub/evidence/pdf/brfout/brfout.pdf. Retrieved September 15, 2009.

5. American Academy of Pediatrics, American College of Obstetricians and Gynecologists. Breastfeeding handbook for physicians. Elk Grove Village (IL): AAP; Washington, DC: American College of Obstetricians and Gynecologists; 2006.

6. Transfer of drugs and other chemicals into human milk. American Academy of Pediatrics Committee on Drugs. Pediatrics 2001;108:776–89.

7. Bhatia J, Greer F. Use of soy protein-based formulas in infant feeding. American Academy of Pediatrics Committee on Nutrition. Pediatrics 2008;121:1062–8.

8. Barbosa-Cesnik C, Schwartz K, Foxman B. Lactation mastitis. JAMA 2003;289:1609–12.

9. Foxman B, D'Arcy H, Gillespie B, Bobo JK, Schwartz K. Lactation mastitis: occurrence and medical management among 946 breastfeeding women in the United States. Am J Epidemiol 2002;155:103–14.

10. Stafford I, Hernandez J, Laibl V, Sheffield J, Roberts S, Wendel G Jr. Community-acquired methicillin-resistant Staphylococcus aureus among patients with puerperal mastitis requiring hospitalization. Obstet Gynecol 2008; 112:533–7.

11. Reddy P, Qi C, Zembower T, Noskin GA, Bolon M. Postpartum mastitis and community-acquired methicillin-resistant Staphylococcus aureus. Emerg Infect Dis 2007; 13:298–301.

12. Andrews JI, Fleener DK, Messer SA, Hansen WF, Pfaller MA, Diekema DJ. The yeast connection: is Candida linked to breastfeeding associated pain? Am J Obstet Gynecol 2007; 197:424.e1–424.e4.

13. Eglash A, Montgomery A, Wood J. Breastfeeding. Dis Mon 2008;54:343–411.

14. Bondurant S, Ernster VL, Herdman R, editors. Safety of silicone breast implants. Washington, DC: National Academy Press; 2000.

15. FFPRHC Guidance (July 2004): contraceptive choices for breastfeeding women. Faculty of Family Planning & Reproductive Health Care. J Fam Plann Reprod Health Care 2004;30:181–9; quiz 189.

Postpartum Contraception

Anne E. Burke

Whereas discussion of contraception ideally begins during the antepartum period, contraceptive options should be reviewed postpartum. Ovulation can occur as early as 27 days after delivery (1). Recommendations for contraceptive use may differ depending on whether or not a woman is breastfeeding. The highest risk for thromboembolic complications is immediately postpartum. Thus, nonlactating women can safely initiate the use of combined hormonal contraceptives (pill, patch, or ring) 3–4 weeks after delivery, unless contraindicated (2). However, the estrogen component in these medications has been associated with a reduction in milk supply (3). For fully lactating women who decline other options, estrogen-containing contraceptives should be deferred for 3 months postpartum, or until lactation is well established (1). Many experts recommend a longer delay, or complete avoidance of estrogen-containing methods while breastfeeding. The World Health Organization, for example, advises against use of combined methods until at least 6 months after delivery (2).

A more favorable alternative in the breastfeeding population may be the use of a progestin-only contraceptive that does not appear to impair lactation. Such alternatives include the daily progesterone-only pill, depot medroxyprogesterone acetate injections, and the etonogestrel implant. Many experts have recommended that initiation of progestin methods, especially high-dose formulations, such as depot medroxyprogesterone acetate injections, be delayed until 6 weeks after delivery in women who breastfeed (4). This delay is based on theoretical concerns for neonatal hormone exposure or early interference with lactogenesis. However, study results indicate that lactation is not impaired (5, 6), and for many women, the proven contraceptive benefit of immediate postpartum initiation may outweigh theoretical risks. Thus, women who are not breastfeeding can initiate progestin-only contraception any time after delivery.

The postpartum period is an appropriate time to initiate long-term contraception if the woman desires. Options include intrauterine contraception and implantable contraception. An intrauterine device can safely be placed at least 4–6 weeks after delivery. Placement of the levonorgestrel intrauterine system should be delayed until 6 weeks after delivery in lactating women (4, 7). A copper intrauterine device also can be placed within 48 hours of placental delivery if a woman is not breastfeeding, although the risk of expulsion is higher (8). This is considered an off-label use for the two types of intrauterine contraception currently available in the United States. Placement between 48 hours and 4 weeks postpartum is not recommended because of increased risk of perforation (2, 9).

The single-rod etonogestrel contraceptive implant is labeled for insertion at least 4 weeks postpartum (10). However, this implant can be inserted immediately postpartum, even in breastfeeding women. There do not appear to be any adverse effects on lactation or infant health (11).

Barrier methods are safe to initiate immediately after childbirth. Diaphragm or cervical cap refitting is best delayed for at least 6 weeks, or until uterine involution is complete. The lactational amenorrhea method of contraception may be used in motivated patients. To be most effective (approximately 98%) in the first 6 months, this technique requires amenorrhea, breastfeeding at least every 4 hours during the day (every 6 hours at night), and essentially no supplemental feeding (4).

Some women may opt for postpartum sterilization. This decision should ideally be made in the antepartum period. Proper preoperative counseling is essential regardless of when the decision is made. Immediate postpartum tubal ligation is reasonable if the woman and newborn are stable and if other aspects of patient care will not be compromised (12, 13). Alternatively, postpartum tubal ligation can be performed before hospital discharge, or performed via laparoscopic approach 6 weeks after delivery. Hysteroscopic sterilization should be deferred until 6 weeks postpartum (14).

References

1. Speroff L, Mishell DR Jr. The postpartum visit: it's time for a change in order to optimally initiate contraception. Contraception 2008;78:90–8.

2. World Health Organization. Medical eligibility criteria for contraceptive use. 3rd ed. Geneva: WHO; 2004.

3. Tankeyoon M, Dusitsin N, Chalapati S, Koetsawang S, Saibiang S, Sas M, et al. Effects of hormonal contraceptives on milk volume and infant growth. WHO Special Programme of Research, Development and Research Training in Human Reproduction Task force on oral contraceptives. Contraception 1984;30:505–22.

4. Kennedy KI, Trussell J. Postpartum contraception and lactation. In: Hatcher RA, Trussell J, Cates WCJ, Stewart F, Kowal D, editors. Contraceptive technology. 19th revised ed. New York (NY): Ardent Media; 2007. p. 403–31.

5. Shaamash AH, Sayed GH, Hussien MM, Shaaban MM. A comparative study of the levonorgestrel-releasing intra-uterine system Mirena versus the Copper T380A intrauterine device during lactation: breast-feeding performance, infant growth and infant development. Contraception 2005;72:346–51.

6. Halderman LD, Nelson AL. Impact of early postpartum administration of progestin-only hormonal contraceptives compared with nonhormonal contraceptives on short-term breast-feeding patterns. Am J Obstet Gynecol 2002;186:1250–6; discussion 1256–8.

7. Mirena: package insert. Wayne (NJ): Bayer Healthcare; 2008. Available at: http://berlex.bayerhealthcare.com/html/products/pi/Mirena_PI.pdf. Retrieved September 15, 2009.

8. Grimes DA, Schulz KF, Van Vliet Huib HA, Stanwood NL, Lopez LM. Immediate post-partum insertion of intrauterine devices. Cochrane Database of Systematic Reviews 2001, Issue 2. Art. No.: CD003036. DOI: 10.1002/14651858. CD003036; 10.1002/14651858.CD003036.

9. Van Houdenhoven K, van Kaam KJ, van Grootheest AC, Salemans TH, Dunselman GA. Uterine perforation in women using a levonorgestrel-releasing intrauterine system. Contraception 2006;73:257–60.

10. Implanon: package insert. Kenilworth (NJ): Schering-Plough; 2009. Available at: http://www.spfiles.com/piimplanon.pd.pdf. Retrieved September 15, 2009.

11. Isley MM, Edelman A. Contraceptive implants: an overview and update. Obstet Gynecol Clin North Am 2007;34:73–90, ix.

12. Bucklin BA. Postpartum tubal ligation: timing and other anesthetic considerations. Clin Obstet Gynecol 2003;46:657–66.

13. American Academy of Pediatrics, American College of Obstetricians and Gynecologists. Guidelines for perinatal care. 6th ed. Elk Grove Village (IL): AAP; Washington, DC: American College of Obstetricians and Gynecologists; 2007.

14. Simon H. Grand rounds: an update on hysteroscopic tubal sterilization. Contemp Ob Gyn 2006;51(8):43,44,47–8.

Appendix A
Information Resources

Patient Safety

Agency for Healthcare Research and Quality
www.ahrq.gov

The Joint Commision
www.jointcommission.org

National Center for Patient Safety
www.patientsafety.gov

National Patient Safety Foundation
www.npsf.org

Preconception Care and Routine Care

American Dietetic Association
www.eatright.org

HealthierUS.gov
www.healthierus.gov

March of Dimes
www.marchofdimes.com

Maternal Child Health Bureau of HRSA
www.mchb.hrsa.gov

MEDLINEplus
www.medlineplus.gov

National Birth Defection Prevention Network
www.nbdpn.org

National Center on Birth Defects and
Developmental Disabilities
www.cdc.gov/ncbddd

Centers for Disease Control and Prevention
Pregnancy-Planning Education Program
www.cdc.gov/ncbddd/pregnancy

National Council on Folic Acid
www.folicacidinfo.org

National Guideline Clearinghouse
www.guideline.gov

National Women's Health Information Center
www.4woman.gov

Nutrition.gov
www.nutrition.gov

Reprotox
An Information System on Environmental Hazards to
Human Reproduction and Development
www.reprotox.org

Smallstep.gov
www.smallstep.gov

U.S. Department of Agriculture, National Agriculture
Library, Food, and Nutrition Information Center
www.nal.usda.gov/fnic

Selected Patient Education Resources

American College of Obstetricians and Gynecologists
Patient Page
http://www.acog.org/publications/patient_education/
patientPage.cfm

American Academy of Pediatrics Parenting Corner
http://www.aap.org/parents.html

March of Dimes: Pregnancy and Newborn
http://www.marchofdimes.com/pnhec/pnhec.asp

UpToDate for Patients
http://www.uptodate.com/patients/about/toc.
do?full_url_key = true&tocKey = table_of_contents/
patient_information/pregnancy

Substance Abuse

American Cancer Society: Tobacco and Cancer
www.cancer.org/docroot/PED/PED_10.asp

Substance Abuse and Mental Health Services
Administration (SAMHSA)
www.samhsa.gov

National Institute on Drug Abuse
www.nida.nih.gov

Teratogenic Exposures

American Society of Health-System Pharmacists
www.ashp.org

American Pharmaceutical Association
www.pharmacist.com

National Toxicology Program: Center for the
Evaluation of Risks to Human Reproduction
cerhr.niehs.nih.gov

Clinical Teratology Web
depts.washington.edu/terisweb

U.S. Food and Drug Administration
www.fda.gov

MEDLINEplus Drug Information
www.nlm.nih.gov/medlineplus/druginformation.html

Motherisk
www.motherisk.org/prof/index.jsp
or
www.motherisk.org/women/index.jsp

National Center on Birth Defects and Developmental Disabilities
www.cdc.gov/ncbddd

National Center for Complementary and Alternative Medicine: Herbs at a Glance
nccam.nih.gov/health/herbsataglance.htm

National Institute on Drug Abuse
www.nida.gov

National Institute for Occupational Safety and Health
www.cdc.gov/niosh

Occupational Safety & Health Administration
www.osha.gov

Organization for Teratology Information Services
www.otispregnancy.org

Reprotox
www.reprotox.org

U.S. Pharmacopoeia
www.usp.org

Ultrasonography

American College of Obstetricians and Gynecologists
www.acog.org

American Institute of Ultrasound in Medicine
www.aium.org

ClinicalTrials.gov
http://ClinicalTrials.gov

National Institute of Child Health and Human Development
www.nichd.nih.gov

Society of Diagnostic Medical Sonography
www.sdms.org

Society for Maternal–Fetal Medicine
www.smfm.org

Prenatal Diagnosis of Genetic Disorders

American College of Medical Genetics
www.acmg.net

Genetics Home Reference
www.ghr.nlm.nih.gov

The Human Genome Resources
www.ncbi.nlm.nih.gov/projects/genome/guide/human

March of Dimes
www.marchofdimes.com

National Center on Birth Defects and Developmental Disabilities
www.cdc.gov/ncbddd

National Human Genome Research Institute
www.genome.gov

National Institute of Child Health and Human Development
www.nichd.nih.gov

National Newborn Screening & Genetics Resource Center
genes-r-us.uthscsa.edu

NINDS Cerebral Palsy Information
www.ninds.nih.gov/disorders/cerebral_palsy/cerebral_palsy.htm

Fetal Therapy

American Academy of Pediatrics
www.aap.org

North American Fetal Therapy Network (NAFTNet)
www.naftnet.org

Complications of Pregnancy*

American Academy of Pediatrics
www.aap.org

American Heart Association
www.americanheart.org

American Society of Hypertension
www.ash-us.org

MEDLINEplus
Medlineplus.gov

March of Dimes
www.marchofdimes.com

National Heart, Lung, and Blood Institute
www.nhlbi.nih.gov

National Institute of Child Health and Human Development
www.nichd.nih.gov

National Organization of Mothers of Twins Clubs
www.nomotc.org

National Women's Health Information Center
www.4woman.gov

Society for Maternal Fetal Medicine
www.smfm.org

Cardiac Disease and Chronic Hypertension

American Heart Association
www.americanheart.org

National Heart, Lung, and Blood Institute
www.nhlbi.nih.gov

*These resources may enhance information provided in the sections on "Preeclampsia and Gestational Hypertension," "Pregnancy-Related Hemorrage," "Multiple Gestation," "Intrauterine Growth Restriction," "Preterm Labor and Delivery," "Premature Rupture of Membranes," and "Postterm Gestation."

Obesity

Centers for Disease Control and Prevention—
  Overweight and Obesity
www.cdc.gov/NCCDPHP/DNPA/obesity

KidsHealth.org
kidshealth.org/teen/food_fitness/dieting/obesity.html

MEDLINEplus
Medlineplus.gov

The Obesity Society
www.obesity.org

Obesity in America (from the Endocrine Society)
www.obesityinamerica.org

Deep Vein Thrombosis and Pulmonary Embolism

American Heart Association
www.americanheart.org

American Lung Association
www.lungusa.org

MEDLINEplus
Medlineplus.gov

National Heart, Lung, and Blood Institute
www.nhlbi.nih.gov

Pulmonary Disorders

American Academy of Allergy Asthma and
  Immunology
www.aaaai.org

American Lung Association
www.lungusa.org

Asthma and Allergy Foundation of America
www.aafa.org

CDC's Division of Tuberculosis Elimination
www.cdc.gov/tb

CDC's Seasonal Influenza (Flu) Homepage
www.cdc.gov/flu

CDC's National Asthma Control Program
www.cdc.gov/ASTHMA

Cystic Fibrosis Foundation
www.cff.org

MEDLINEplus
Medlineplus.gov

National Heart, Lung, and Blood Institute
www.nhlbi.nih.gov

Liver and Alimentary Tract Diseases

American Association for the Study of Liver Diseases
www.aasld.org

Healthfinder
www.healthfinder.gov

March of Dimes
www.marchofdimes.com

MEDLINEplus
Medlineplus.gov

National Institute of Diabetes and Digestive and
  Kidney Disease
www.niddk.nih.gov

National Women's Health Information Center
www.4woman.gov

Neurologic Diseases

Epilepsy Foundation
www.epilepsyfoundation.org

Massachusetts General Hospital Center for Women's
  Mental Health
www.womensmentalhealth.org

National Institute of Neurological Disorders
  and Stroke
www.ninds.nih.gov

Diabetes Mellitus

American Diabetes Association
www.diabetes.org/home.jsp

National Diabetes Education Program
www.ndep.nih.gov

National Institute of Child Health and Human
  Development
www.nichd.nih.gov

National Institute of Diabetes and Digestive
  and Kidney Diseases
www2.niddk.nih.gov

Thyroid Diseases

American Thyroid Association
www.thyroid.org/index.html

Hormone Foundation
www.hormone.org

March of Dimes
www.marchofdimes.com

National Institute of Diabetes and Digestive and
  Kidney Diseases
www2.niddk.nih.gov

Hematologic Disorders

American Society of Hematology
www.bloodthevitalconnection.org/default.aspx

Centers for Disease Control and Prevention—
  Division of Blood Disorders
www.cdc.gov/ncbddd/hbd/default.htm

March of Dimes
www.marchofdimes.com

National Heart, Lung, and Blood Institute
www.nhlbi.gov

Renal Disease

National Institute of Diabetes and Digestive and
  Kidney Diseases
www.niddk.nih.gov

National Kidney Foundation
www.kidney.org

Society for Maternal–Fetal Medicine
www.smfm.org

Immunologic Disorders

American Autoimmune Related Diseases Association
www.aarda.org

Lupus Foundation of America
www.lupus.org/webmodules/webarticlesnet/
  templates/new_index.aspx

National Institute of Arthritis and Musculoskeletal
  and Skin Diseases
www.niams.nih.gov

Organization of Teratology Information Specialists
  (OTIS)—Autoimmune Diseases in Pregnancy Project
autoimmunediseasesandpregnancy.org

Infection

Centers for Disease Control and Prevention
www.cdc.gov

March of Dimes
www.marchofdimes.com

National Center for Infectious Diseases
www.cdc.gov/ncidod

National Institute of Allergy and Infectious Diseases
www.niaid.nih.gov

U.S. Department of Health and Human Services:
  AIDSInfo
AIDSinfo.nih.gov

Chronic Pain and Headache

American Council for Headache Education
www.achenet.org

American Pain Foundation
www.painfoundation.org

National Institute of Neurological Disorders
  and Stroke
www.ninds.nih.gov

NIH Pain Consortium
painconsortium.nih.gov

Surgical Complications

American Association of Gynecologic Laparoscopists
www.aagl.org

Depression

MGH Center for Women's Mental Health
www.womensmentalhealth.org

National Institute of Mental Health
www.nimh.nih.gov

Postpartum Support International
www.postpartum.net

Labor Stimulation

American College of Nurse-Midwives
www.acnm.org

Association of Women's Health, Obstetric and
  Neonatal Nurses
www.awhonn.org

March of Dimes
www.marchofdimes.com

Intrapartum Fetal Heart Rate Monitoring

Association of Women's Health, Obstetric and
  Neonatal Nurses
www.awhonn.org

Cesarean Delivery and Vaginal Birth After Cesarean Delivery

March of Dimes
www.marchofdimes.com

Shoulder Dystocia

March of Dimes
www.marchofdimes.com

Epsiotomy and Pelvic Floor Disorders

American College of Nurse-Midwives
www.acnm.org

American Urogynecologic Society
www.augs.org

Society of Pelvic Reconstructive Surgeons
www.sprs.org

Fetal Death

Association of Women's Health, Obstetric and
  Neonatal Nurses
www.awhonn.org

March of Dimes
www.marchofdimes.com

National Fetal and Infant Mortality Review Program
www.acog.org/departments/dept_web.cfm?recno = 10

Neonatal Resuscitation

American Academy of Pediatrics
www.aap.org

Association of Women's Health, Obstetric and
  Neonatal Nurses
www.awhonn.org

Eunice Kennedy Shriver National Institute of Child
  Health and Human Development
  Neonatal Research Network: Extremely Preterm
  Birth Data
http://www.nichd.nih.gov/about/org/cdbpm/pp/
  prog_epbo/epbo_case.cfm

Breastfeeding

La Leche League International
www.llli.org

Drugs and Lactation Database (LactMed)
toxnet.nlm.nih.gov/cgi-bin/sis/htmlgen?LACT

National Institute of Child Health and
  Human Development
www.nichd.nih.gov

United States Breastfeeding Committee
www.usbreastfeeding.org

Postpartum Contraception

Association of Reproductive Health Professionals
www.arhp.org

National Institute of Child Health and Human
  Development
www.nichd.nih.gov

Appendix B

Antepartum Record

DATE _____

NAME _____

      LAST   FIRST   MIDDLE

ID # _____ HOSPITAL OF DELIVERY _____

NEWBORN'S PHYSICIAN _____ REFERRED BY _____

PRIMARY PROVIDER/GROUP _____

FINAL EDD _____	ADDRESS _____

BIRTH DATE AGE RACE MARITAL STATUS MONTH DAY YEAR S M W D SEP	ADDRESS
OCCUPATION EDUCATION (LAST GRADE COMPLETED)	ZIP PHONE (H) (O)
LANGUAGE ETHNICITY	INSURANCE CARRIER/MEDICAID #
HUSBAND/DOMESTIC PARTNER PHONE	POLICY #
FATHER OF BABY PHONE	EMERGENCY CONTACT PHONE

TOTAL PREG	FULL TERM	PREMATURE	AB, INDUCED	AB, SPONTANEOUS	ECTOPICS	MULTIPLE BIRTHS	LIVING

MENSTRUAL HISTORY

LMP ☐ DEFINITE ☐ APPROXIMATE (MONTH KNOWN)   MENSES MONTHLY ☐ YES ☐ NO   FREQUENCY: Q _____ DAYS   MENARCHE _____ (AGE ONSET)

     ☐ UNKNOWN ☐ NORMAL AMOUNT/DURATION   PRIOR MENSES _____ DATE   ON BCP AT CONCEPT ☐ YES ☐ NO   hCG + ___/___/___

     ☐ FINAL _____

PAST PREGNANCIES (LAST SIX)

DATE MONTH/ YEAR	GA WEEKS	LENGTH OF LABOR	BIRTH WEIGHT	SEX M/F	TYPE DELIVERY	ANES.	PLACE OF DELIVERY	PRETERM LABOR YES/NO	COMMENTS/ COMPLICATIONS

MEDICAL HISTORY

	○ Neg. + Pos.	DETAIL POSITIVE REMARKS INCLUDE DATE & TREATMENT		○ Neg. + Pos.	DETAIL POSITIVE REMARKS INCLUDE DATE & TREATMENT
1. DIABETES			17. D (Rh) SENSITIZED		
2. HYPERTENSION			18. PULMONARY (TB, ASTHMA)		
3. HEART DISEASE			19. SEASONAL ALLERGIES		
4. AUTOIMMUNE DISORDER			20. DRUG/LATEX ALLERGIES/ REACTIONS		
5. KIDNEY DISEASE/UTI					
6. NEUROLOGIC/EPILEPSY			21. BREAST		
7. PSYCHIATRIC			22. GYN SURGERY		
8. DEPRESSION/POSTPARTUM DEPRESSION			23. OPERATIONS/ HOSPITALIZATIONS (YEAR & REASON)		
9. HEPATITIS/LIVER DISEASE					
10. VARICOSITIES/PHLEBITIS					
11. THYROID DYSFUNCTION			24. ANESTHETIC COMPLICATIONS		
12. TRAUMA/VIOLENCE			25. HISTORY OF ABNORMAL PAP		
13. HISTORY OF BLOOD TRANSFUS.			26. UTERINE ANOMALY/DES		

	AMT/DAY PREPREG	AMT/DAY PREG	# YEARS USE			
				27. INFERTILITY		
14. TOBACCO				28. ART TREATMENT		
15. ALCOHOL				29. RELEVANT FAMILY HISTORY		
16. ILLICIT/RECREATIONAL DRUGS				30. OTHER		

COMMENTS _____

Version 6. Copyright © 2007 The American College of Obstetricians and Gynecologists, 409 12th Street, SW, PO Box 96920, Washington, DC 20090-6920   AA128   1 2 3 4 5 / 1 0 9 8 7

ACOG ANTEPARTUM RECORD (FORM A)

Patient Addressograph

SYMPTOMS SINCE LMP

GENETIC SCREENING/TERATOLOGY COUNSELING
INCLUDES PATIENT, BABY'S FATHER, OR ANYONE IN EITHER FAMILY WITH:

	YES	NO		YES	NO
1. PATIENT'S AGE 35 YEARS OR OLDER AS OF ESTIMATED DATE OF DELIVERY			13. HUNTINGTON'S CHOREA		
2. THALASSEMIA (ITALIAN, GREEK, MEDITERRANEAN, OR ASIAN BACKGROUND): MCV LESS THAN 80			14. MENTAL RETARDATION/AUTISM		
			IF YES, WAS PERSON TESTED FOR FRAGILE X?		
3. NEURAL TUBE DEFECT (MENINGOMYELOCELE, SPINA BIFIDA, OR ANENCEPHALY)			15. OTHER INHERITED GENETIC OR CHROMOSOMAL DISORDER		
4. CONGENITAL HEART DEFECT			16. MATERNAL METABOLIC DISORDER (EG, TYPE 1 DIABETES, PKU)		
5. DOWN SYNDROME			17. PATIENT OR BABY'S FATHER HAD A CHILD WITH BIRTH DEFECTS NOT LISTED ABOVE		
6. TAY–SACHS (ASHKENAZI JEWISH, CAJUN, FRENCH CANADIAN)			18. RECURRENT PREGNANCY LOSS, OR A STILLBIRTH		
7. CANAVAN DISEASE (ASHKENAZI JEWISH)			19. MEDICATIONS (INCLUDING SUPPLEMENTS, VITAMINS, HERBS OR OTC DRUGS)/ILLICIT/RECREATIONAL DRUGS/ALCOHOL SINCE LAST MENSTRUAL PERIOD		
8. FAMILIAL DYSAUTONOMIA (ASHKENAZI JEWISH)			IF YES, AGENT(S) AND STRENGTH/DOSAGE		
9. SICKLE CELL DISEASE OR TRAIT (AFRICAN)					
10. HEMOPHILIA OR OTHER BLOOD DISORDERS			20. ANY OTHER		
11. MUSCULAR DYSTROPHY					
12. CYSTIC FIBROSIS					

COMMENTS/COUNSELING _____

INFECTION HISTORY	YES	NO		
1. LIVE WITH SOMEONE WITH TB OR EXPOSED TO TB			4. HEPATITIS B, C	YES ☐ NO ☐
2. PATIENT OR PARTNER HAS HISTORY OF GENITAL HERPES			5. HISTORY OF STD, GONORRHEA, CHLAMYDIA, HPV, HIV, SYPHILIS (CIRCLE ALL THAT APPLY)	
3. RASH OR VIRAL ILLNESS SINCE LAST MENSTRUAL PERIOD			6. OTHER (SEE COMMENTS)	

COMMENTS _____

INTERVIEWER'S SIGNATURE _____

INITIAL PHYSICAL EXAMINATION

DATE _____ / _____ / _____   WEIGHT _____   HEIGHT _____   BMI _____   BP_____

1. HEENT	☐ NORMAL	☐ ABNORMAL	12. VULVA	☐ NORMAL	☐ CONDYLOMA	☐ LESIONS
2. FUNDI	☐ NORMAL	☐ ABNORMAL	13. VAGINA	☐ NORMAL	☐ INFLAMMATION	☐ DISCHARGE
3. TEETH	☐ NORMAL	☐ ABNORMAL	14. CERVIX	☐ NORMAL	☐ INFLAMMATION	☐ LESIONS
4. THYROID	☐ NORMAL	☐ ABNORMAL	15. UTERUS SIZE	_____ WEEKS		☐ FIBROIDS
5. BREASTS	☐ NORMAL	☐ ABNORMAL	16. ADNEXA	☐ NORMAL	☐ MASS	
6. LUNGS	☐ NORMAL	☐ ABNORMAL	17. RECTUM	☐ NORMAL	☐ ABNORMAL	
7. HEART	☐ NORMAL	☐ ABNORMAL	18. DIAGONAL CONJUGATE	☐ REACHED	☐ NO	_____ CM
8. ABDOMEN	☐ NORMAL	☐ ABNORMAL	19. SPINES	☐ AVERAGE	☐ PROMINENT	☐ BLUNT
9. EXTREMITIES	☐ NORMAL	☐ ABNORMAL	20. SACRUM	☐ CONCAVE	☐ STRAIGHT	☐ ANTERIOR
10. SKIN	☐ NORMAL	☐ ABNORMAL	21. SUBPUBIC ARCH	☐ NORMAL	☐ WIDE	☐ NARROW
11. LYMPH NODES	☐ NORMAL	☐ ABNORMAL	22. GYNECOID PELVIC TYPE	☐ YES	☐ NO	

COMMENTS (Number and explain abnormals) _____

EXAM BY _____

ACOG ANTEPARTUM RECORD (FORM B)

NAME _____
　　　　　LAST　　　　　　　　　　　FIRST　　　　　　　　　MIDDLE

| DRUG ALLERGY_____ | LATEX ALLERGY ☐ YES ☐ NO |

| IS BLOOD TRANSFUSION ACCEPTABLE?　☐ YES　☐ NO | ANTEPARTUM ANESTHESIA CONSULT PLANNED　☐ YES　☐ NO |

PROBLEMS/PLANS

1. _____
2. _____
3. _____
4. _____
5. _____
6. _____

MEDICATION LIST
(Include Dosage)　　　Start date　　　Stop date

1. _____　___/___/___　___/___/___
2. _____　___/___/___　___/___/___
3. _____　___/___/___　___/___/___
4. _____　___/___/___　___/___/___
5. _____　___/___/___　___/___/___
6. _____　___/___/___　___/___/___

EDD CONFIRMATION

INITIAL EDD

LMP　　　　___/___/___　=　EDD ___/___/___

INITIAL EXAM　___/___/___ = ___ WKS = EDD ___/___/___

ULTRASOUND　___/___/___ = ___ WKS = EDD ___/___/___

INITIAL EDD　___/___/___　INITIALED BY _____

18–20-WEEK EDD UPDATE

QUICKENING　___/___/___　+22 WKS = ___/___/___

FUNDAL HT. AT UMBIL.　___/___/___　+20 WKS = ___/___/___

ULTRASOUND　___/___/___ = ___ WKS = ___/___/___

FINAL EDD　___/___/___　INITIALED BY _____

PREPREGNANCY WEIGHT
_____

Column headers (diagonal):
WEEKS GEST. (BEST EST.) / FUNDAL HEIGHT (CM) / PRESENTATION / FHR / FETAL MOVEMENT / PRETERM LABOR SIGNS/SYMPTOMS; +=PRESENT 0=ABSENT / CERVIX EXAM (DIL./EFF./STA.) ULTRASOUND LENGTH / BLOOD PRESSURE / WEIGHT / URINE (ALBUMIN/GLUCOSE) / EDEMA / PAIN SCALE* (0-10) / NEXT APPOINTMENT / PROVIDER (INITIALS)

COMMENTS

_____
_____
_____
_____
_____
_____
_____
_____
_____
_____
_____
_____
_____
_____
_____
_____
_____

PROBLEMS _____

COMMENTS _____

*Describe the intensity of discomfort ranging from 0 (no pain) to 10 (worst possible pain).

ACOG ANTEPARTUM RECORD (FORM C)

LABORATORY AND EDUCATION

INITIAL LABS	DATE	RESULT	REVIEWED
BLOOD TYPE	/ /	A B AB O	
D (Rh) TYPE	/ /		
ANTIBODY SCREEN	/ /		
HCT/HGB/MCV	/ /	_____ % _____ g/dL	
PAP TEST	/ /	NORMAL/ABNORMAL/_____	
VARICELLA	/ /		
RUBELLA	/ /		
VDRL	/ /		
URINE CULTURE/SCREEN	/ /		
HBsAg	/ /		
HIV COUNSELING/TESTING*	/ /	POS. NEG. DECLINED	

OPTIONAL LABS	DATE	RESULT	
HEMOGLOBIN ELECTROPHORESIS	/ /	AA AS SS AC SC AF ↑A$_2$ POS. NEG. DECLINED	
PPD	/ /		
CHLAMYDIA	/ /		
GONORRHEA	/ /		
CYSTIC FIBROSIS	/ /	POS. NEG. DECLINED	
TAY-SACHS	/ /	POS. NEG. DECLINED	
FAMILIAL DYSAUTONOMIA	/ /	POS. NEG. DECLINED	
HEMOGLOBIN			
GENETIC SCREENING TESTS (SEE FORM B)	/ /		
OTHER			

8–20-WEEK LABS (WHEN INDICATED/ELECTED)	DATE	RESULT	
ULTRASOUND	/ /		
1ST TRIMESTER ANEUPLOIDY RISK ASSESSMENT	/ /	POS. NEG. DECLINED	
MSAFP/MULTIPLE MARKERS	/ /	POS. NEG. DECLINED	
2ND TRIMESTER SERUM SCREENING	/ /	POS. NEG. DECLINED	
AMNIO/CVS	/ /		
KARYOTYPE	/ /	46,XX OR 46,XY/OTHER_____	
AMNIOTIC FLUID (AFP)	/ /	NORMAL_____ ABNORMAL_____	
ANTI-D IMMUNE GLOBULIN (RHIG)	/ /		

COMMENTS/ADDITIONAL LABS

*Check state requirements before recording results.   *(CONTINUED)*

PROVIDER SIGNATURE (AS REQUIRED) _____

ACOG ANTEPARTUM RECORD (FORM D)

LABORATORY AND EDUCATION *(continued)*

24–28-WEEK LABS (WHEN INDICATED)	DATE	RESULT		COMMENTS/ADDITIONAL LABS
HCT/HGB/MCV	/ /	_____ % _____ g/dL		
DIABETES SCREEN	/ /	1 HOUR_____		
GTT (IF SCREEN ABNORMAL)	/ /	_____FBS _____1 HOUR _____2 HOUR _____3 HOUR		
D (Rh) ANTIBODY SCREEN	/ /			
ANTI-D IMMUNE GLOBULIN (RhIG) GIVEN (28 WKS OR GREATER)	/ /	SIGNATURE _____		

32–36-WEEK LABS	DATE	RESULT		
HCT/HGB	/ /	_____ % _____ g/dL		
ULTRASOUND (WHEN INDICATED)	/ /			
HIV (WHEN INDICATED)*				
VDRL (WHEN INDICATED)	/ /			
GONORRHEA (WHEN INDICATED)	/ /			
CHLAMYDIA (WHEN INDICATED)	/ /			
GROUP B STREP	/ /			

*Check state requirements before recording results.

COMMENTS
_____
_____
_____
_____
_____
_____

ACOG ANTEPARTUM RECORD (FORM D, *continued*)

PROVIDER SIGNATURE (AS REQUIRED)_____

Patient Addressograph

NAME _____
          LAST   FIRST   MIDDLE

PLANS/EDUCATION
(COUNSELED ☐)—BY TRIMESTER. INITIAL AND DATE WHEN DISCUSSED.

	COMPLETED	NEED FOR FURTHER DISCUSSION
FIRST TRIMESTER		☐ FOLLOW-UP IN 3RD TRIMESTER, IF NEEDED
☐ HIV AND OTHER ROUTINE PRENATAL TESTS		
☐ RISK FACTORS IDENTIFIED BY PRENATAL HISTORY		
☐ ANTICIPATED COURSE OF PRENATAL CARE		
☐ NUTRITION AND WEIGHT GAIN COUNSELING; SPECIAL DIET		
☐ TOXOPLASMOSIS PRECAUTIONS (CATS/RAW MEAT)		
☐ SEXUAL ACTIVITY		
☐ EXERCISE		
☐ INFLUENZA VACCINE		
☐ SMOKING COUNSELING		
☐ ENVIRONMENTAL/WORK HAZARDS		
☐ TRAVEL		
☐ TOBACCO (ASK, ADVISE, ASSESS, ASSIST, AND ARRANGE)		
☐ ALCOHOL		
☐ ILLICIT/RECREATIONAL DRUGS		
☐ USE OF ANY MEDICATIONS (INCLUDING SUPPLEMENTS, VITAMINS, HERBS, OR OTC DRUGS)		
☐ INDICATIONS FOR ULTRASOUND		
☐ DOMESTIC VIOLENCE		
☐ SEAT BELT USE		
☐ CHILDBIRTH CLASSES/HOSPITAL FACILITIES		
SECOND TRIMESTER		
☐ SIGNS AND SYMPTOMS OF PRETERM LABOR		
☐ ABNORMAL LAB VALUES		
☐ INFLUENZA VACCINE		
☐ SELECTING A NEWBORN CARE PROVIDER		
☐ SMOKING COUNSELING		
☐ DOMESTIC VIOLENCE		
☐ POSTPARTUM FAMILY PLANNING/TUBAL STERILIZATION		

(CONTINUED)

COMMENTS
_____
_____
_____
_____
_____
_____

ACOG ANTEPARTUM RECORD (FORM E)

PLANS/EDUCATION *(continued)*
(COUNSELED ☐)—BY TRIMESTER. INITIAL AND DATE WHEN DISCUSSED.

THIRD TRIMESTER	COMPLETED	NEED FOR FURTHER DISCUSSION
☐ ANESTHESIA/ANALGESIA PLANS		
☐ FETAL MOVEMENT MONITORING		
☐ LABOR SIGNS		
☐ VBAC COUNSELING		
☐ SIGNS AND SYMPTOMS OF PREGNANCY-INDUCED HYPERTENSION		
☐ POSTTERM COUNSELING		
☐ CIRCUMCISION		
☐ BREAST OR BOTTLE FEEDING		
☐ POSTPARTUM DEPRESSION		
☐ INFLUENZA VACCINE		
☐ SMOKING COUNSELING		
☐ DOMESTIC VIOLENCE		
☐ NEWBORN EDUCATION (NEWBORN SCREENING, JAUNDICE, SIDS, CAR SEAT)		
☐ FAMILY MEDICAL LEAVE OR DISABILITY FORMS		

REQUESTS

TUBAL STERILIZATION CONSENT SIGNED   DATE   INITIALS

___/___/___   _____

HISTORY AND PHYSICAL HAVE BEEN SENT TO HOSPITAL, IF APPLICABLE.   DATE   INITIALS

___/___/___   _____

COMMENTS

ACOG ANTEPARTUM RECORD (FORM E, *continued*)

Plans/Education Notes

_____

_____

_____

_____

_____

_____

_____

_____

_____

_____

_____

_____

_____

_____

_____

_____

_____

_____

_____

_____

_____

_____

_____

_____

ACOG ANTEPARTUM RECORD (FORM E, _continued_)

Appendix C

Assessment of Fetal Death

Physician Responsibilities	**Nursing Responsibilities** Page i

Physician Responsibilities

_____ Review of prenatal records and laboratory results

_____ Maternal testing

    All patients
- ☐ Random glucose
- ☐ CBC with platelet count
- ☐ Antibody screen
- ☐ VDRL
- ☐ Kleihauer-Betke
- ☐ Urine toxicology screen

    Selected patients
- ☐ Thyroid function testing
- ☐ CMV titer (IgM, acute and convalescent IgG)
- ☐ Lupus anticoagulant/anticardiolipin antibody

_____ Genetic w/u indicated _____/ contacted_____

_____ Confirm completion of stillbirth/fetal examination (page ii) and placement on mother's chart

Consents obtained:

_____ Autopsy

_____ Others (eg, photographs)

_____

_____

_____ Placenta sent to pathology

_____ Fetal death/stillborn autopsy form (page iii) completed

Additional studies:

_____ Photographs

_____ Viral cultures

_____ X-rays

_____ Bacterial cultures

_____ Others _____

_____

Nursing Responsibilities   Page i

Saw baby: ☐ Mother   ☐ Father   ☐ Other

Held baby: ☐ Mother   ☐ Father   ☐ Other

Baby's name _____

_____ Keepsakes given to family by hospital:
- ☐ Commemorative card
- ☐ Footprints
- ☐ Photo
- ☐ Blanket
- ☐ Bracelet
- ☐ Tape measure
- ☐ Baptismal card/blessing card
- ☐ Referral to support organization
- ☐ Lock of hair
- ☐ Booklets (specify) _____

_____

_____

_____

Unit chosen:
    ☐ Ob   ☐ Gyn

Resources:
    ☐ Social services   ☐ Chaplain
    ☐ Community support   ☐ Mental health groups

☐ Burial options explained
    Option chosen _____

☐ Grief process explained to:
    ☐ Mother   ☐ Father   ☐ Other

☐ Address/telephone number on in-patient admission record verified for follow-up call

Comments _____

_____

_____

_____

_____

(Continued)

Fetal Death/Stillborn Examination   Page ii

Key: +, present; –, absent; ?, unsure

Date _____

Weight _____   Head circumference _____   Crown–heel length (stretched) _____

General _____   Macerated _____   Intact _____

Other (describe) _____

Head
___ Normal
___ Hydrocephalic
___ Scalp defects
___ Anencephalic
___ Abnormal skull shape
___ Collapsed
___ Other (describe) _____
_____

Eyes
___ Normal
___ Close together
___ Far apart
___ Straight
___ Up slanting
___ Down slanting
___ Abnormally small
___ Abnormally large
___ Epicanthus
___ Other (describe) _____
_____

Nose
___ Normal
___ Other (describe) _____

Mouth
___ Normal
___ Cleft palate
___ Cleft lip
___ Large tongue
___ Small chin
___ Other (describe) _____
_____

Ears
___ Normal
___ Lowset (top below eyes)
___ Tags
___ Pits
___ Symmetric
___ Other (describe) _____
_____

Neck
___ Normal
___ Excess skin

Neck *(continued)*
___ Cystic mass
___ Other (describe) _____
_____

Chest
___ Normal
___ Asymmetric
___ Small
___ Other (describe) _____
_____

Abdomen
___ Normal
___ Distension
___ Omphalocele
___ Gastroschisis
___ Hernia
___ 3-vessel cord
___ Other (describe) _____
_____

Back
___ Normal
___ Spina bifida (defect level____)
___ Scoliosis
___ Kyphosis
___ Other (describe) _____
_____

Limbs
Length: nl, short, long
Form: nl, symmetric missing parts
Position: nl, abnl

Arms	*Length*	*Form*	*Position*
Right	_____	_____	_____
Left	_____	_____	_____

Legs	*Length*	*Form*	*Position*
Right	_____	_____	_____
Left	_____	_____	_____

Hands
Right
___ Fingers (#)
___ Webbing/syndactyly
___ Transverse crease
___ Other (describe) _____
_____

Hands *(continued)*
Left
___ Fingers (#)
___ Webbing/syndactyly
___ Transverse crease
___ Other (describe) _____
_____

Feet
Right
___ Toes (#)
___ Webbing
___ Wide space between toes 1-2
___ Other (describe) _____

Left
___ Toes (#)
___ Webbing
___ Wide space between toes 1-2
___ Other (describe) _____
_____

Nails
___ Normal
___ Small (which ones?_____)
___ Other (describe) _____
_____

Genitalia
___ Normal
___ Imperforate anus
___ Ambiguous genitalia (describe)
_____

Male
___ Hypospadias
___ Chordee
___ Undescended testes
___ Other (describe) _____
_____

Female
___ Normal urethral opening
___ Clitoromegaly
___ Other (describe) _____
_____

(Continued)

Fetal Death/Stillborn Autopsy

Page iii

To accompany body to morgue: Fill in as completely as possible

Date_____

Medical record #_____

Mother _____

Fetus _____

Name_____

LMP _____

Estimated gestational age_____Weeks

Gravida_____ Para_____ A_____ Living children_____

Ultrasound dx _____

_____

_____

Placenta examination _____

_____

_____

Cord examination _____

_____

_____

Cytogenetics obtained:

   Blood: ☐ Yes   ☐ No

   Skin: ☐ Yes   ☐ No

Alpha-fetoprotein _____

Prenatal assessment _____

Labor:

   Spontaneous _____

   Induced _____

Delivery:

   Date _____   Time _____

   Vaginal _____

   Cesarean _____

Pregnancy complications _____

_____

_____

_____

_____

Delivery complications _____

_____

_____

_____

_____

Indication(s) for pathologic examination _____

_____

_____

_____

_____

_____

Special requests for gross and microscopic evaluation

_____

_____

_____

_____

Attending clinician _____

Phone number _____

Courtesy of the Virginia Commonwealth University Medical Center.

Index

Note: Page numbers followed by *b*, *f*, and *t* denote boxes, figures, and tables, respectively.

A

Abdomen, acute. *See* Acute abdomen
Abdominal palpation, small fetus and, 81
Abortifacients, herbal, 30
Abruptio placentae. *See* Placental abruption
Acamprosate, 23
Acetaminophen
  for headache, use in pregnancy, 172*t*
  for rheumatoid arthritis, 153
  use in pregnancy, 168
Acute abdomen, 176–178, 176*b*
Acute chest syndrome, in sickle cell disease, 145
Acute fatty liver of pregnancy, 124–125, 125*b*
Acyclovir, for herpes simplex virus infection, 162
Adnexal masses
  in pregnancy, 178
  ultrasound characteristics, 178, 178*b*
Adverse Outcome Index, 3–4
Air travel, during pregnancy, 15
Albuterol, for asthma, 117–119, 118*t*
Alcohol
  detection in urine and blood, limits of, by time from last use, 23*t*
  teratogenicity, 21, 26
  abuse
    interventions for, 22–23
    laboratory diagnosis, 21
    maternal–fetal effects, 20–21
    preconception management, 13–14
    prevalence, 17
    screening for, 17–18, 18*b*
    and stillbirth, 208
  withdrawal
    severity, assessment, 21
    signs and symptoms, 21
    treatment, 21
Alcoholics Anonymous, 23
Alimentary tract disease, 124–129, 223
Alloimmune thrombocytopenia, 54–55, 146
Alpha-adrenergic drugs, for chronic hypertension, 103*t*
Alpha-fetoprotein, maternal serum (MSAFP)
  in Down syndrome screening, 44–45
  in neural tube defect screening, 46
  in twin pregnancy, 74
Alpha-methyldopa, for hypertension, in renal disease, 148–149

Alternative and complementary medicine, preconception management, 12
Amantadine, 119
Amitriptyline, for headache prevention, use in pregnancy, 173*t*
Amniocentesis
  for detection of aneuploidy, 48
  for diagnosis of genetic disorders, 48
  in multifetal pregnancy, 74
  safety, 48
Amnioreduction
  for twin reversed arterial perfusion syndrome, 73
  for twin–twin transfusion syndrome, 56, 72
Amniotic fluid volume, monitoring, for postterm pregnancy, 97
Amniotomy, for labor induction, 188
Amphetamines, detection in urine and blood, limits of, by time from last use, 23*t*
Anal incontinence, postpartum, 205–207, 205*t*
Anal sphincter lacerations, 206–207, 206*t*
Anemia. *See also* Iron-deficiency anemia
  in chronic disease, 144
  fetal
    detection, 37
    management, 52–55
  macrocytic, 145
  microangiopathic hemolytic, 146
  in pregnant women
    definition, 143
    diagnostic assessment, 143, 143*f*
  in renal disease, 150
  sickle-cell. *See* Sickle cell disease
Anesthesia
  for delivery, maternal substance abuse and, 22
  myasthenia gravis and, 130
  obesity and, 105, 107–108
Aneuploidy
  disorders associated with, 44, 46, 47*t*
  fetal, detection, 48–49
  risk
    in dichorionic twin gestation, 74
    in multifetal pregnancy, 74
Angiotensin-converting enzyme inhibitors
  contraindications to, 102–103
  fetal effects, 11
  teratogenicity, 27
Angiotensin-receptor antagonists
  contraindications to, 102–103
  fetal effects, 11
  teratogenicity, 27
Ankylosing spondylitis, 159
Antepartum Record, 14, 226–233

Antibiotics
  for acute pyelonephritis, 163–164
  for bacterial pneumonia, 121
  for group B streptococci, 164
  in management of premature rupture of membranes (PROM), 94
  prophylactic
    with cesarean delivery, in obese patient, 108
    for group B streptococci, 164
  teratogenic, 27–28
Anticardiolipin antibodies, testing for, 156, 157*b*
Anticholinesterase drugs, 130–131
Anticoagulants
  for deep vein thrombosis, 112–114
  for patient with mechanical heart valve, 115
  preconception management, 11
  prophylactic administration
    postpartum, 112
    in pregnancy, 112
  for pulmonary embolism, 112–114
  teratogenicity, 28
Anticonvulsants
  for chronic pain, use in pregnancy, 169*t*, 170
  for eclamptic seizures, 60
  preconception management, 12, 13
  teratogenicity, 12, 28, 129–130
Antidepressants
  adverse effects on fetus or newborn, 12, 183
  for chronic pain, use in pregnancy, 168
  for depression, 183
  preconception management, 12
  teratogenicity, 26–27
Anti-D immune globulin, 52–53
Antiepileptic medication. *See* Anticonvulsants
Antihypertensive agents
  for chronic hypertension, 102–103, 103*t*
  for preeclampsia or eclampsia, 60
  teratogenicity, 27
Antiphospholipid antibodies
  and preeclampsia, 59–60, 61
  and stroke risk, 132
  in systemic lupus erythematosus (SLE), 155, 156
  testing for, 156
Antiphospholipid antibody syndrome, 155–158
  catastrophic, 157, 158
  clinical manifestations, 156
  diagnostic criteria for, 156*b*
  fetal risks in, 157
  maternal risks in, 157